Delmar's
PEDIATRIC

NURSING
CARE PLANS

3rd Edition

Delmar's
PEDIATRIC

NURSING
CARE PLANS

3rd Edition

KARLA L. LUXNER, RNC, ND

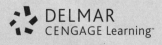
DELMAR
CENGAGE Learning™

Australia • Brazil • Japan • Korea • Mexico • Singapore • Spain • United Kingdom • United States

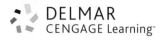

**Delmar's Pediatric Nursing Care Plans,
Third Edition**
Karla L. Luxner

Vice President, Health Care Business Unit:
William Brottmiller

Editorial Director: Cathy L. Esperti

Acquisitions Editors: Matthew Filimonov,
Melissa Martin

Senior Developmental Editor:
Elisabeth F. Williams

Marketing Director: Jennifer McAvey

Marketing Coordinator: Kip Summerlin

Editorial Assistant: Patricia Osborn

Technology Director: Laurie K. Davis

Art and Design Coordinators:
Connie Lundberg-Watkins, Alex Vasilakos

Production Coordinator: Bridget Lulay

Project Editor: Jennifer Luck

For product information and technology assistance, contact us at
Cengage Learning Customer & Sales Support, 1-800-354-9706

For permission to use material from this text or product,
submit all requests online at **www.cengage.com/permissions**
Further permissions questions can be emailed to
permissionrequest@cengage.com

Library of Congress Control Number: 2003048936

ISBN-13: 978-0-7668-5994-4

ISBN-10: 0-7668-5994-0

Delmar
Executive Woods
5 Maxwell Drive
Clifton Park, NY 12065
USA

Cengage Learning is a leading provider of customized learning solutions with office locations around the globe, including Singapore, the United Kingdom, Australia, Mexico, Brazil, and Japan. Locate your local office at
www.cengage.com/global

Cengage Learning products are represented in Canada by Nelson Education, Ltd.

To learn more about Delmar, visit **www.cengage.com/delmar**

Purchase any of our products at your local bookstore or at our preferred online store **www.ichapters.com**

Notice to the Reader

Publisher does not warrant or guarantee any of the products described herein or perform any independent analysis in connection with any of the product information contained herein. Publisher does not assume, and expressly disclaims, any obligation to obtain and include information other than that provided to it by the manufacturer. The reader is expressly warned to consider and adopt all safety precautions that might be indicated by the activities described herein and to avoid all potential hazards. By following the instructions contained herein, the reader willingly assumes all risks in connection with such instructions. The publisher makes no representations or warranties of any kind, including but not limited to, the warranties of fitness for particular purpose or merchantability, nor are any such representations implied with respect to the material set forth herein, and the publisher takes no responsibility with respect to such material. The publisher shall not be liable for any special, consequential, or exemplary damages resulting, in whole or part, from the readers' use of, or reliance upon, this material.

Printed in the United States of America
4 5 6 7 11 10 09

CONTENTS

PREFACE

Health promotion, restoration, and disease prevention in children require the care and attention of parents and family as well as health care providers. Children are not simply small adults, but have their own unique physiologic, psychological, and cognitive processes at each stage of development. Pediatric nurses work with parents and families in the community as well as acute care settings to protect and enhance the well-being of infants and children so they may reach their full potential. Awareness and respect for cultural variation is essential to modern nursing as is sound scientific knowledge providing the framework for evidence-based practice.

CONCEPTUAL APPROACH

The nursing process serves as a learning tool for readers and as a practice and documentation format for clinicians. Based on a thorough assessment, the nurse formulates a specific care plan for each individual client. The care plans in this book are provided to facilitate that process for readers and practitioners. To that end, each care plan solicits specific client data and prompts the nurse to individualize the interventions, consider cultural relevance, and evaluate the client's individual response. The book provides basic nursing care plans for common diagnoses related to each body system followed by care plans and flow charts for specific illnesses commonly encountered in the pediatric population.

ORGANIZATION

Delmar's Pediatric Nursing Care Plans, 3rd edition, includes care plans that have been developed to reflect comprehensive pediatric nursing care based on the most common psychosocial and physiologic alterations. Because care is based on solid application of principles of growth and development, and respect and appreciation of the parents and family as partners in the care of their children, the book opens with an overview of growth and development of children. Subsequent chapters offer an overview of each body system, covering basic and diseasespecific care plans. The diagnoses are cross-referenced, and the practitioner is encouraged to add, subtract, delete, and otherwise adapt the diagnoses to provide individualized care for a specific client.

Nursing care begins with a comprehensive review and assessment of each individual client. The data are then analyzed and a specific plan of care developed. Interventions for each diagnosis must again be individualized for each client. The format for each nursing care plan in this book is summarized below.

- Nursing diagnoses as approved by the North American Nursing Diagnosis Association (NANDA) taxonomy (2003–2004); the complete NANDA listing is found in Appendix A (new to this edition).

- Related factors (etiology) for each diagnosis are suggested and the user is prompted to choose the most appropriate for the specific client.

- Defining characteristics for each actual diagnosis are listed with prompts to the user to include specific client data from the nursing assessment.

- Goals are related to the nursing diagnosis and include a time frame for evaluation to be specified by the user.

- Appropriate outcome criteria specific for the client are suggested. In keeping with current practice, this edition includes a Nursing Outcome Classification (NOC) label for each nursing diagnosis. Appendix B offers a complete listing of NOC labels.

- Nursing interventions and rationales are comprehensive. They include pertinent continuous assessments and observations. Common therapeutic actions originating from nursing and those resulting from collaboration with the primary caregiver are suggested with prompts for creativity and individualization. Client and family teaching and psychosocial support are provided with respect for cultural variation and individual needs. Consultation and referral to other caregivers is suggested when indicated.

- Nursing Intervention Classification (NIC) labels are provided in this new edition for each nursing diagnosis. These are inserted after the interventions and rationales to assist the user in becoming familiar with this classification process for nursing interventions. Appendix C provides the complete listing of NIC labels.

- Evaluation of the client's goal and presentation of data related to the outcome criteria is followed by consideration of the next step for the client.

A new, descriptive introductory chapter outlines how to customize care plans for an individual client based on the standardized care plans found in this book.

A CD is included in the back of this book that contains electronic files for all the care plans in the book. Readers can create new care plans, customize care plans, add and delete nursing diagnoses and interventions, and print the plans of care for use in the clinical setting.

ACKNOWLEDGMENTS

I am grateful to editors for their encouragement and support, and to my students, nurse colleagues, and the many infants, children, and parents who have enriched my understanding of pediatrics. This book is dedicated to my own children: Sam, Julie, John, Mary, and Rebecca, who provided me with first-hand experience and many excellent stories about infants and children.

Karla L. Luxner

REVIEWERS

Kathy Pearson, RN, BSN, MSN, CS
Instructor of Nursing
Temple College
Temple, Texas

Annette Gibson, BSN, MEd, MSN
Instructor of Nursing
Miami Dade Community College
Miami, Florida

Vera V. Cull, RN, DSN
Assistant Professor
University of Alabama at Birmingham
   School of Nursing
Birmingham, Alabama

AN INTRODUCTION TO THE USE OF THE NURSING CARE PLANS

INTRODUCTION

Excellent nursing practice reflects proficient use of the nursing process demonstrated by skillful assessment, diagnosis, planning, outcome identification, intervention, and evaluation. The nursing process provides the framework that directs nursing practice. Nursing care planning is the application of the nursing process to a specific client situation. Written nursing care plans are a means of communication among health care providers, clients, and families. They ensure that care is coordinated to achieve desired health care outcomes.

A thorough assessment is the foundation of the nursing process. The assessment data are then reviewed and organized according to client needs. Nursing diagnoses, derived from the assessment, provide the basis for selection of interventions to achieve outcomes for which the nurse is accountable (NANDA, 2003). "Now, as never before, today's nurse must make more complex professional decisions, determine what things to do and what things not to do for which clients. Priorities are critical: often the nurse must make hard choices between what is essential and what is merely beneficial" (Barnum, 1999). The primary purpose of the nursing diagnostic processes applied by nurses is to design a plan of care for and in conjunction with the client that results in the prevention, reduction, or resolution of the client's health problem (Harkreader, 2004).

In the current multidisciplinary health care environment, nurses are positioned for a high level of accountability. The nurse is required to make many independent decisions and to coordinate the various disciplines working together and sharing responsibility for client outcome achievement. This environment affords nursing an opportunity to define its boundaries and to use the nursing process to coordinate care across disciplines. Nurses need to develop strong assessment skills, organize the data obtained to prioritize client needs, predict achievable, measurable client outcomes, and tailor interventions for

the individual client. This text is designed to assist the user in that process.

NURSING CARE PLANS AND INDIVIDUAL CLIENT CARE NEEDS

This book is intended to facilitate the care planning process for nurses working with pediatric clients based on recognized nursing standards. Each of the nursing diagnoses is from NANDA's Taxonomy II (NANDA, 2003). The outcome criteria include the appropriate Nursing Outcome Classification (NOC) as well as prompts to assist the user in developing individualized outcomes. This text also contains suggested Nursing Intervention Classifications (NIC) for each nursing diagnosis in addition to suggested comprehensive and individualized interventions for each diagnosis.

Each section begins with essential introductory information about the condition and the current medical management when appropriate. A thorough assessment of the client is essential to developing a plan of care. The user is prompted to insert specific client data into the care plan at strategic points in each diagnosis. The user is offered a variety of common and additional nursing diagnoses for each condition including:

1. The etiology (related to) for each diagnosis using specific client data obtained in the assessment.

2. Possible defining characteristics, with prompts for individualization, which support the diagnosis.

3. A client goal related to the nursing diagnosis with a prompt to identify an appropriate time frame for evaluation of the outcomes.

4. Measurable outcome criteria requiring the use of specific client data and individualized parameters.

5. Comprehensive and detailed nursing interventions with guidance to individualize care for the specific client.

6. Rationales for the nursing interventions to demonstrate evidence-based practice.

7. Evaluation based on individual client information. The user is prompted to evaluate goal achievement and present the specific client data called for in the outcome criteria.

The nursing care plans provided in this text are intended to serve as a framework on which to design individualized client care reflecting current nursing standards of care. The user must first obtain comprehensive, reliable, and detailed assessment information for the particular client using all available sources. The initial assessment data should then be interpreted and organized into categories reflecting prioritized client needs. Frequently, after reflecting on the initial assessment, the nurse will find that additional focused assessment data must be obtained before care can be planned. Appropriate nursing diagnoses are then selected and prioritized. Individual client data are the defining characteristics that support the choice of nursing diagnosis. A specific goal and the necessary outcome criteria that will be used to identify when the goal has been met should be based on the defining characteristics. Outcome criteria reflect the individual client's capabilities and expectations. The nurse then selects a comprehensive array of interventions to provide current evidence-based client care directed toward the outcomes and resolution of the problem. Interventions should also be prioritized and may include additional ongoing assessments, therapeutic nursing activities, collaborative interventions, client and family teaching, and referrals. Current standards of care for pediatric nursing practice have been incorporated throughout the text. Every effort has been made to prompt the user to insert individual client data and to specify the parameters of care as the care plan is developed. Thoughtful use of this text will guide the user to develop comprehensive individualized care plans based on current scientific knowledge and evidence for best practices.

The process for planning individualized care involves the same steps as the nursing process.

1. Collect assessment data from all available sources including the client, the family, other providers, and the chart. Chart data may include: nurse's notes or flow sheets; laboratory, diagnostic, or surgical reports; progress notes from dietary, rehab, or physical therapy; the physician's history and physical, and progress notes. Assess the client's current status through the interview, observation, and physical examination. After studying the health record and obtaining assessment data, organize the information into prioritized problem or client need categories.

2. Identify viable nursing diagnoses and potential client risks suggested by the categories of assessment data. Review the appropriate chapter in this text and review the nursing diagnoses provided for the condition. Choose the diagnoses that fit the specific client. The diagnostic process is individualized by identifying "related to" factors and "defining characteristics" that flow from the comprehensive client assessment. For example, "Acute pain related to surgical incision" is supported by the client data, "verbalizes pain at a 9 on a scale of 0–10." The client's own words and pain rating support the diagnosis and guide the nurse to choose an outcome criteria of "verbalizes pain as less than 9 on a scale of 1–10" and interventions that must include assessment of pain using a scale of 1–10.

3. Plan to identify and meet client goals using specific outcomes as evidence. The goal pertains to the diagnosis and moves the client toward resolution of the problem within a reasonable time frame. The outcome criteria included in the text indicate options to measure goal attainment and encourage specific qualifiers such as when, how much, and individual client variables to be added to individualize the plan. "Client will experience decreased pain within 24 hours" is a clear goal with an achievable target time. "Verbalizes pain as 5 or less on a scale of 1–10" would be a measurable outcome that, if based on the particular client situation and capabilities, individualizes the plan and indicates goal attainment.

4. Design interventions to meet the goal and resolve the nursing diagnosis. Choose interventions pertinent to the client that are consistent with the medical orders. Ongoing assessment of the client's pain perception,

positioning, teaching the client to ask for medication before pain becomes severe, and the administration of pain medications, specifying the drug, dose, route, and times as ordered, are examples of both independent and collaborative nursing interventions, which would achieve the outcome, attain the goal, and resolve the "Acute Pain" diagnosis.

5. Evaluate the effectiveness of the plan. By setting a client goal and specific observable outcomes, the plan communicates the need for ongoing evaluation and updating. Evaluation of the outcome criteria at the specified time will either indicate resolution of the problem or the need to continue or revise the care plan.

CRITICAL THINKING, THE NURSING PROCESS, AND CARE PLAN DEVELOPMENT

Critical thinking and decision-making skills are used to identify nursing diagnoses. Critical thinking entails purposeful, goal-directed thinking and analysis of information. The nurse uses critical thinking to make clinical judgments based on evidence. The nurse synthesizes the information collected in the assessment and then makes judgments about how to put the information together to form nursing diagnoses. The format of this book encourages the nurse to review the client history and obtain thorough assessment data that are significant for a particular condition. The nurse is then prompted to insert relevant assessment findings as appropriate to formulate an individualized nursing care plan.

The following case study illustrates how to apply individual client data to a care plan in this book.

PEDIATRIC ASTHMA CASE STUDY

A 14-year-old African-American female is brought to the pediatrician's office by her mother. She has just started running on her high school track team, but has been complaining to her mother that her running "feels different this year." When she ran in middle school she could race longer distances without becoming winded. She now says her "chest burns" and she is running fewer miles before she has to stop to catch her breath. Her girlfriend told her she could

hear her wheezing and she should go to the nurse. The school nurse confirmed her wheezing and notified her mother to come pick her up from school. There is no history of asthma in the family but her parents both smoke cigarettes. The school nurse advised that cigarettes could be contributing to the child's respiratory complaints. At the pediatrician's office her peak flow is 380 L/min, which is within 5% of her predicted value for her height and weight. She does complain of coughing at night. Her lung sounds are now clear with no wheezing noted. Her ECG and heart sounds appear normal. She has no significant past medical history except for occasional ear infections. Immunizations are up-to-date, she is allergic to penicillin, and she denies smoking or drug use.

The family nurse practitioner (FNP) discusses the possibility of exercise-induced asthma with the client and her mother. She directs the client to measure her peak flow before running and if she experiences symptoms to stop running and again measure her peak flow. She is to repeat these measurements five times, five minutes apart, and return to the office with her records. The FNP writes a note to the track coach and school nurse outlining the procedure. On one week follow-up peak flow pattern shows recovery after 30 minutes but her peak flow diminishes to 70%–85% of her estimated level. The FNP prescribes Albuterol, 2 puffs MDI, 15 minutes before exercise. The FNP reviews the peak flow guidelines with the mother and client and directs her to keep a daily record for two weeks and to return for reassessment.

Three months later the client awoke in the middle of the night coughing and experiencing shortness of breath. She was suffering from a cold and her parents had a holiday party that evening with the house filled with cigarette smoke. She checked her peak flow and found she was in the yellow zone. She used her Albuterol inhaler and woke her mother. Her peak flow was repeated for her mother and was now in the red zone. She self-administered more Albuterol and her mother took her to the emergency room where she was given a nebulizer treatment, oxygen, and steroids. Her peak flow remained at 200 L/min and she was admitted to the pediatric unit with acute asthma. Her vital signs were: temperature 99°F, heart rate 124, respiratory rate 34 breaths per minute and shallow with expiratory wheezing. Her O_2 saturation was 88%. She was placed on O_2 at 4L/min.

Upon admission the client's mother indicated awareness of the need for change by stating, "We have to do something to prevent this."

NURSING DIAGNOSIS #1

Ineffective Airway Clearance

Related to: Bronchospasm and increased pulmonary secretions.

Defining Characteristics: Shallow respirations with expiratory wheeze, respiratory rate 34, SaO_2 88%, peak flow 200L/min after medications.

Goal: Client will maintain a clear airway throughout admission.

Outcome Criteria:

✔ Respiratory rate less than 24, lungs clear to auscultation, SaO_2 greater than 95%.

NOC: *Respiratory Status: Ventilation*

INTERVENTIONS

Assess respirations for rate (count one full minute), pattern depth, and ease, auscultate lung sounds, and note use of accessory muscles and retractions q 4 h. Assess for cough, characteristics of cough and sputum q 4 h. Administer humidified oxygen at 4 L/min via nasal canula per physician's order. Monitor O_2 saturation continuously reporting saturation that remains less than 93% to the physician.

Assess skin for pallor or cyanosis every 4 hours, note distribution or duration of cyanosis (nail beds, skin, mucous membranes, circumoral).

Position with head elevated at least 30° or seated upright with head on pillows; position on side if more comfortable; avoid tight clothing or bedding; use pillows and/or padding as needed to maintain positioning.

Demonstrate and instruct to parents and child possible positions for comfort and ventilation during activities and sleep.

Teach parents and child correct disposal of tissues; appropriate covering of mouth and nose when coughing to avoid respiratory infections.

Pace activities and exercises and allow for rest periods and energy conservation. Instruct child in relaxation exercises, quiet play, and controlled breathing.

Teach and demonstrate use of oxygen saturation monitor to parents (application, settings, alarm, electric source).

NIC: *Airway Management*

NURSING DIAGNOSIS #2

Health Seeking Behaviors: Prevention of Asthma Attack

Related to: Expressed desire for information about preventive measures for child's asthma.

Defining Characteristics: Mother states, "we have to do something to prevent this".

Goal: Client and family will obtain information about asthma prevention during hospitalization.

Outcome Criteria:

✔ Parents and child verbalize understanding of triggering agents and prevention measures for asthma attacks.

NOC: *Health-Promoting Behavior*

INTERVENTIONS

Assess for knowledge of factors related to attacks, past history of respiratory infections, and measures taken to maintain health of child.

Assess health history of allergies in family members, what does or does not precipitate attack, and what behaviors result from the attack.

Teach parents and child handwashing technique; allow for demonstration.

Teach child to avoid contact with those who have respiratory infections, how to cover mouth and nose when coughing or sneezing, and to dispose of tissues properly.

Discuss with parents/child about physiology and signs and symptoms of the disease and possible precipitating factors influencing an attack.

Discuss with parents and child the signs and symptoms indicating the onset of an attack (change in respirations, wheezing, dyspnea).

Teach parents of the effect of cigarette smoke and allergens, and how to avoid exposure to offending environmental factors (cold air, humidity, air pollution, sprays, plants).

Assist parents to identify ways to change the home environment to reduce smoke, dust, exposure to pets, and indoor plants, changing of filters, avoidance of foods (yellow dye), and drugs (aspirin).

Teach the child breathing exercises and controlled breathing and relaxation techniques.

INTERVENTIONS

Teach parent and child about medication administration as ordered at discharge (specify drug, dose route, and times to be given) and how to manage method of administration. Advise to avoid over-the-counter drugs without physician advice.

Refer to community health department for additional information and adolescent asthma support group.

NIC: *Health Education*

CLINICAL PATHWAYS: A METHOD OF ACHIEVING OUTCOMES ACROSS THE CONTINUUM OF CARE

Health care consumers expect affordable care and optimal outcomes. Third-party providers scrutinize client outcomes to validate the need for expensive health care services. Health care organizations report outcomes to state, federal, and independent agencies to verify practice standards and attract consumers and providers. The demand for the most effective and cost-efficient manner of restoring clients to health has led to collaborative responsibility for client care demonstrated by the clinical pathway. Clinical pathways, also known as "care maps," are care management tools that outline the expected clinical course and outcomes for a specific client type (Kelly-Heidenthal, 2003). The manner in which a pathway is constructed is usually agency-specific but typically it follows the client's length of stay on a day-by-day basis for the specific disease process or surgical intervention. Clinical pathways are a clinical tool that organizes, directs, and times the major care activities and interventions of the entire multidisciplinary team for a particular diagnosis or procedure. Their design is intended to minimize delays, maximize appropriate resource utilization, and promote high-quality care. "The clinical pathway describes a blended plan of care constructed by all providers, considering the subject together" (Barnum, 1999).

Clinical pathways identify standard client outcomes against which the efficiency of care may be measured. The pathway guides the care team along a sequence of interdisciplinary interventions that incorporate standardized aspects such as client and family teaching, nutrition, medications, activities, diagnostic studies, and treatments. The tool is developed collaboratively by all health team members and includes predictable and established time frames, usually by delineating each hospital day as an event requiring new intervention along a continuum. A care map provides consistency of client care activities. Clinical pathways also, because of their standardization of practice, allow for measuring performance improvement within an agency and between similar agencies over time.

Clinical pathways can only guide rather than dictate the course of care for an individual. They do not take into account additional client problems that may affect the client's recovery. Therefore, the process of incorporating clinical pathways is the same as in individualizing care plans. The nurse must include the individualized client needs in conjunction with the standard clinical pathway. When the client's needs vary from the expected outcome time frame, the nurse must reassess, report, and manage the variance to meet the client's needs. The manner of reporting variances is agency-specific. Not all clients' care can be organized into a clinical pathway model. For more complex client care situations an individualized care plan applying the various nursing diagnoses in this text, is more appropriate.

Well-designed nursing care plans and/or care maps move the client from one level of care on the health continuum to another. These tools help the nurse to monitor and guide the progress of the client through a particular health condition including preventive and restorative phases and end-of-life care. Care planning organizes and coordinates client care according to relevant standards, promotes consistency and communication between caregivers, and incorporates the problem-solving process which integrates responsiveness to client needs and cost-efficiency.

UNIT 1

GROWTH AND DEVELOPMENT OF CHILDREN

CHAPTER 1.0

GROWTH AND DEVELOPMENT

A solid understanding of growth and development is essential for planning and providing nursing care for infants and children. The child's ability to cope with stress, illness, hospitalization, or terminal illness is related to physical, cognitive, and psychosocial growth and development. Nursing care is designed to foster the individual child's growth and support his or her developmental needs.

DEVELOPMENTAL THEORIES

PSYCHOSOCIAL DEVELOPMENT (ERICKSON)

- **Trust Versus Mistrust, Infant (birth to 1 year):** Characterized by taking in through all the senses; loving care of a mothering person is essential to develop trust; must have basic needs met; attachment to primary caretaker.

  The favorable outcome is faith and optimism.

- **Autonomy Versus Shame and Doubt, Toddler (1 to 3 years):** Characterized by increasing ability to control bodies, themselves, and their environment; seek independence, negativism, threatened by changes in routine, curious explorer.

  The favorable outcome is self-control and will power.

- **Initiative Versus Guilt, Preschool (3 to 6 years):** Characterized by enterprise and a strong imagination; develop conscience; feelings of being punished; egocentric, inquisitive, rich fantasy life, and magical thinking.

  The favorable outcome is direction and purpose.

- **Industry Versus Inferiority, School-Age (6 to 12 years):** Active learners, well-developed language skills and concept of time, concerns about body image, understands concept of death. Enjoy sorting and ordering, making collections, and super heroes. Exhibit cognitive conceit. Can assist with own care and appreciates rewards. Physically graceful and skilled; sports and clubs of same-sex peers are important.

  The favorable outcome is competence.

- **Identity Versus Role Confusion, Adolescent (13 to 18 years):** Characterized by ability to deal with reality and abstractions, mood swings, changing body image; preoccupied with the way they appear in the eyes of others as compared to their own self-concept. Peers of both same and opposite-sex are very important to identity formation.

  The favorable outcome is devotion and fidelity to others and to values and ideologists.

PSYCHOSEXUAL DEVELOPMENT (FREUD)

- **Oral Stage (birth to 1 year):** Characterized by infant-seeking pleasure via oral activities such as biting, sucking, chewing, and vocalizing.

- **Anal Stage (1 to 3 years):** Characterized by interest in the anal region and sphincter muscles (child is able to withhold or expel feces); toilet training is a major milestone (method of parent discipline, may have lasting effects on child's personality development).

- **Phallic State (3 to 6 years):** Characterized by interest and recognition in differences between the sexes and becomes very curious about these differences; often described as interest by females as penis envy and by males as castration anxiety.

- **Latency period (6 to 12 years):** Characterized by gaining increased skill on newly acquired traits and skills; interested in acquiring knowledge and vigorous play. Sexuality lies dormant while energy is focused elsewhere.

- **Genital stage (12 years and over):** Characterized by maturation of the reproductive system and production of sex hormones; genital organs become a source of tension and pleasure; interested in forming friendships and preparation for marriage as an adult.

INTERPERSONAL DEVELOPMENT (SULLIVAN)

■ **Infant (0 to 1 year):** Receive gratification and comfort from loving, tender care; develops trust and ability to count on others.

■ **Childhood (2 to 5 years):** Engage in peer, family, neighborhood activities; need adult participation; learn to delay gratification and accept interference with wishes: gradually seek attention and approval from peers.

■ **Juvenile (5 to 12 years):** Engage in socialization, competition, cooperation, and compromise; develop shared interests and genuine friendships with peers of same sex, and later with opposite sex; give more allegiance to peers than to family; promote personal identity

COGNITIVE DEVELOPMENT (PIAGET)

■ **Sensorimotor (birth to 2 years):** Characterized by progression from reflex activity through simple repetitive behaviors to imitative behaviors; information is gained through the senses and developing motor abilities; develop a sense of "cause and effect"; problem-solving is by trial and error; high level of curiosity, experimentation, and enjoyment in novelty; begin to separate self from others; develop sense of "object permanence"; begin language development.

■ **Preoperational (2 to 7 years):** Characterized by egocentrism (inability to put oneself in the place of others); interpret objects and events in terms of their relationships or use of them; cannot see another's point of view; thinking is concrete, tangible; inability to make deductions or generalizations; display high level of imagination and questioning; reasoning is intuitive.

■ **Concrete Operations (7 to 11 years):** Characterized by thoughts; become increasingly logical and coherent; able to classify, sort, organize facts, and begin to problem-solve; develop conservation (realize volume, weight, and number remain the same even though outward appearances are changed); solve problems in a concrete, systematic fashion, based on visual perceptions.

■ **Formal Operations (11 to 13 years):** Characterized by thoughts which are adaptable and flexible; possess abstract thinking; able to make logical conclusions; able to make hypotheses and test them; can consider abstract, theoretical, philosophical issues.

MORAL DEVELOPMENT (KOHLBERG)

Based on cognitive development theory and consists of 3 major levels.

■ **Preconventional Level (2 to 7 years):** Parallels Piaget's preoperational level of cognitive development and intuitive thinking. Characterized by development of: cultural values; sense of right and wrong; integrate things in terms of physical or pleasurable consequences of their actions. Initially, determines goodness or badness in terms of its consequences (attempt to avoid punishment). Later, determines right behavior consists of what satisfies own needs (and sometimes those of others).

■ **Conventional Level (7 to 11 years):** Parallels Piaget's stage of concrete operations of cognitive development. Characterized by a concern with conformity and loyalty; value a specific group (i.e., the family, group, or national expectations); behavior that conforms to specific group considered good and earns approval. Values such as fairness, give and take, and sharing interpreted in a practical manner without loyalty, gratitude, or justice.

■ **Postconventional, Autonomous, or Principled Level (11 to 15 years):** Parallels Piaget's stage of formal operations. Characterized by tendency/desire to display correct behavior in terms of individual rights and standards; begins to question possibility of changing existing laws/ rules in terms of societal needs.

SPIRITUAL DEVELOPMENT (FOWLER)

Five stages of development of faith; four are closely associated with parallel cognitive (Piaget) and psychosocial (Erickson) development in childhood.

■ **Stage 0, (Undifferentiated):** Characterized by infant period of development, in which the infant is unable to determine concept of right or wrong. Development of basic trust lays the foundation for beginning faith.

■ **Stage 1, (Intuitive-projectile):** Characterized by toddler period of development, in which the primary behavior is referred to as imitating religious gestures and behaviors of others. Unable to comprehend meaning or significance of religious practices; begin to assimilate religious values and beliefs held by parents; do not attempt to understand basic concepts of religion.

- **Stage 2, (Mythical-literal):** Characterized by school-age period of development, in which the child's spiritual development parallels cognitive development. Belief that spiritual development is associated with previous experiences and societal interactions. Newly-acquired conscience influences actions (good vs. bad; bad actions create guilt); petitions to an omnipotent being important; able to articulate their faith.

- **Stage 3, (Synthetic-convention):** Characterized by early phase of adolescent period of development, in which become aware of spiritual disappointments (i.e., prayers are not always answered); may begin to abandon or modify previous religious practices and those established by their parents.

- **Stage 4, (Individuating-reflexive):** Characterized by middle phase of adolescent period of development, in which the adolescent may become skeptical and begin to compare religious standards of their parents and significant others. The adolescent will begin to compare religious beliefs with scientific facts, described as a period of searching for answers; and to be uncertain about their religious ideas.

SELECTED MILESTONES

GROSS MOTOR

- **0 to 4 months:** Lifts head if in prone position with head erect or bobbing and back rounded; raises chest with support of arms flexed limbs; 0 to 1 month, startle and rooting reflex are very strong, Moro reflex begins to fade at 2 months; 2 to 4 months, decrease in head lag when pulled up to sitting position.

- **4 to 8 months:** Holds head up and erect without support; lifts head and shoulders to 90 degree angle and rolls from back to side; turns over both ways; supports weight on legs and may pull self into sitting position; beginning at 4 months, able to sit with support; head lag disappears; by 7 months, able to sit alone without support; likes to bounce on legs when held in standing position; Moro reflex has disappeared.

- **8 to 12 months:** Sits alone, creeps, crawls, cruises, sits from standing position without assistance, prefers being up instead of lying down; at 9 months, stands while holding onto furniture and able to pull self to standing position; at 11 months walks while holding onto furniture or with both hands held; at 12 months may be able to walk with one hand held.

- **12 to 15 months:** Walks alone with side-based gait, creeps up stairs, throws things.

- **15 to 24 months:** Walks alone with improvement, runs, pulls toys when walking, walks on toes, walks backwards, climbs up steps, climbs on furniture, sits on small chair, stands on one foot.

- **2 years:** Walks with steady gait, runs with few falls, walks on toes, stands on one foot, walks up and down stairs, jumps, kicks ball, rides tricycle, throws ball overhand.

- **3 and 4 years:** Pedals tricycle, climbs and jumps well, walks up and down stairs with alternating feet, gains increased coordination and balance, hops on one foot, throws ball overhand proficiently.

- **5 and 6 years:** Hops; skips well; jumps rope; has improved coordination and control of muscles; active; throws and catches ball; runs without difficulty, hits nail on head.

- **7, 8, and 9 years:** Repeats activities for mastery; active; rhythm, smoothness, and control of muscular movements increases; displays motor skills; strength and endurance increase.

- **10, 11, and 12 years:** Has control of timing, graceful high level of energy, explores environment, participates in team sports, builds or constructs things, interested in physical skills.

FINE MOTOR

- **0 to 4 months:** Attempts to grab object but misses, brings object to mouth, holds hands in front and plays with hands and feet, grasps object with both hands; 1 month displays grasp reflex; 3 months, hands are usually open; 2 to 4 months, looks and plays with own fingers; 3 months, when object is placed in hands, will retain briefly; 4 months, reaches for objects and picks them up with a raking action of fingers.

- **4 to 8 months:** Grasps with thumb and fingers, explores objects, moves arms at sight of toy, reaches for object, picks up object with cupped hands, holds objects in both hands at same time, holds own bottle, puts nipple in mouth, feeds self a cookie; 5 months, able to voluntarily grasp an object; 6 to 7 months, able to transfer objects from one hand to another, enjoys banging objects together.

- **8 to 12 months:** Releases toy or object, locates hands for play, eats with fingers, uses spoon with assistance, drinks from cup with assistance, holds crayon and makes marks on paper; 10 months, pincer grasp is present, able to pick up small objects like a raisin; 11 months, able to put objects into a container and enjoys removing them; 12 months, displays interest in building a tower of two blocks, but it often falls down.

- **12 to 15 months:** Builds tower of 2 to 4 blocks, opens boxes, pokes finger in hole, turns pages of book, uses spoon with spilling.

- **15 to 24 months:** Drinks from cup with one hand, uses spoon without spilling, empties jar of contents, draws vertical line, scribbles, builds tower of 4 blocks.

- **2 years:** Builds tower of 5 to 8 blocks, turns knob to open door, drinks from glass held in one hand, makes train of cubes by manipulating play materials.

- **3 and 4 years:** Strings beads, builds tower of blocks, learns to use and masters use of scissors, copies a circle-and-cross figures, holds crayon with fingers, unbuttons buttons on side or front, laces shoes, brushes teeth, cuts out simple pictures.

- **5 and 6 years:** Copies letters of alphabet and prints name, dresses self with assistance, uses hammer and nails, knows right from left hand, cuts and pastes well, may tie shoes, uses fork.

- **7, 8, and 9 years:** Hand-eye coordination improves; enjoys video games; writes rather than prints words; may play musical instruments, sew, build models, work jigsaw puzzles; adds details to drawings and uses perspective in drawing, uses both hands independently.

- **10, 11, and 12 years:** Uses increased detail in work, handwriting skill improves, more refinement to motor activities, gradual improvement to adult level.

LANGUAGE

- **0 to 4 months:** Cries, whimpers; responds to sounds or activity; coos, gurgles, and babbles; smiles in response to adult sounds and makes sounds.

- **4 to 8 months:** Laughs out loud, vocalizes, uses two syllable sounds like da da without meaning, imitates expressions, cries if scolded.

- **8 to 12 months:** Responds to adult emotional tone, says one or two words, uses sounds to identify objects or persons, uses wide range of sounds, understands use of no, knows own name, communicates with others and self.

- **12 to 14 months:** Uses jargon, names for familiar pictures or objects; points to desired object or vocalizes wants, knows at least 10 words or more; uses short phrases; points to body parts.

- **2 years:** Uses about 300 words, uses pronouns, speaks 3 to 4 word sentences, enjoys stories, does not ask for help.

- **3 and 4 years:** Uses about 900 to 1500 words; talks in sentences; asks questions consistently; states own name; talks whether someone present or not; uses plural form of words; repeats words and sentences at will; may omit prepositions, adverbs, adjectives in speech; asks how and why; boasts and tattles; tells a story; counts to at least 3, understands simple questions.

- **5 and 6 years:** Identifies colors, uses 2,100 words, knows names of days of week, asks thoughtful questions, uses prepositions and conjunctions, uses complete sentences, shares experiences with others through language, expands vocabulary with exposure and stimulation, errors in sound disappear, begins to have a concept of abstract words.

- **7, 8, and 9 years:** Increases use of words to express self, increases use of words for exchange and communication, considers what others say, uses all parts of speech.

- **10, 11, and 12 years:** Uses 50,000 words, uses compound and complex sentences, understands abstract words.

PLAY AND SOCIALIZATION

- **0 to 4 months:** Stares at environment, smiles indiscriminately or responsively, enjoys having others around, recognizes familiar faces, determines that face is unfamiliar and freezes gaze, establishes cycle for sleep and awake periods; 0 to 1 month, prefers to look at faces, at black and white geometric designs, able to follow objects in line of vision; 2 to 4 months, follows objects 180°, turns head to look for voices and sounds.

- **4 to 8 months:** Self-centered, begins to be fearful of strangers; 4 to 6 months, watches the course of a falling object, responds readily to sounds, smiles at self in mirror, fascinated by own fingers and toes; 6 to 8 months, recognizes own name and responds by smiling when it is heard, seeks attention, imitates faces and sounds in play.
- **8 to 12 months:** Plays simple peek-a-boo, prefers mother, cries when upset, becomes anxious if separated, recognizes family members' requests if one at a time, displays various emotions.
- **12 to 24 months:** Plays pat-a-cake, is curious and gets into everything, has short attention span, enjoys solitary play or watching others play, has a favorite toy or object.
- **2 years:** Unable to distinguish right from wrong, imitates parents and others, enjoys parallel play, wants things own way, refuses to share, is possessive, sees self as a separate person, rituals important, benefits from transitional objects such as teddy bear.
- **3 and 4 years:** Able to share with peers and adults, interested in new activities and learning from them, may have an imaginary playmate, participates in imaginative play and imitation of adults.
- **5 and 6 years:** Likes achieving, wants to accept responsibilities, has strong feeling for family and home, identifies with parent of same sex, participates in fair play and cooperation, shows off.
- **7, 8, and 9 years:** Independently plays, able to reason and has a concept of right or wrong, likes rewards and praise, peer group gains in importance, short-lived interests, completes tasks.
- **10, 11, and 12 years:** Feels positive about self; is more tolerant; interested in rules and money;

relates well with peers, friends, relatives; likes conversation, change, and variety in activities; avoids doing tasks; develops conscience. Enjoys sports, games.

PLAY

Play is described as the work of childhood. Children use play to learn about themselves and the world and also to cope with new or stressful events. Child development experts recognize play as a significant coping strategy for children. For example, children may use play as an outlet for self-expression, to manipulate experience, and to attempt to master the environment. Play provides the child with a measure of control over events and settings. Children's play also promotes social, cognitive, and physical development.

Illness, treatment, and hospitalization create emotional stress for children. Reactions may include crying, clinging to parents, loss of sleep, and regression. Structured and/or medical play has been shown to be therapeutic in helping children preserve usual coping strategies and maintain emotional health. Therapeutic play has been identified as an effective intervention to help children prepare for, cope with, assimilate, and master painful procedures and the stress of hospitalization. A significant nursing intervention is to provide the child with a pleasurable play experience at the onset of hospitalization, that may ease the emotional distress associated with invasive procedures or with the hospitalization process itself. The nurse bases the choice of play activity offered on the child's developmental level, play preferences, and therapeutic goals.

PLAY

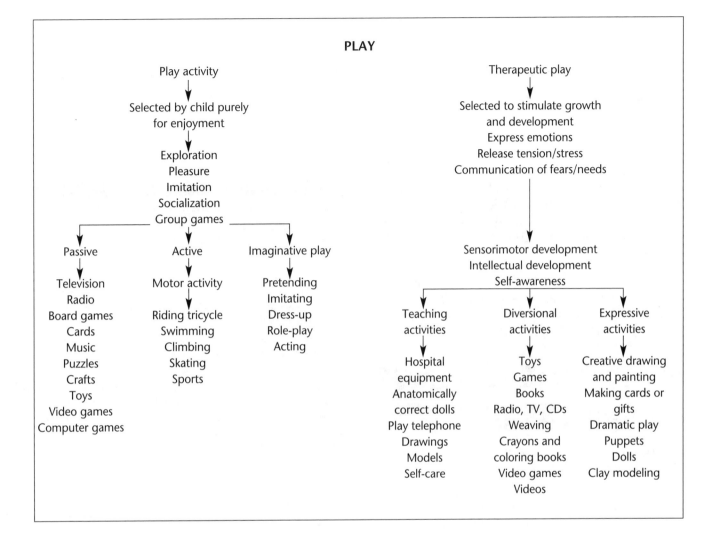

CHAPTER 1.1

BASIC CARE PLAN: WELL CHILD

Healthy children are assessed at regular intervals to monitor growth and development, prevent disease through immunization, promote wellness, and provide families with anticipatory guidance. The nursing care plan for a well child is based on a thorough nursing history, assessment, and review of medical and laboratory findings. The child's parent (or caretaker) is included in all aspects of the child's care. Specific client-related data should be inserted within parentheses and whenever possible.

NURSING DIAGNOSES

HEALTH-SEEKING BEHAVIORS: WELL-CHILD VISIT

Related to: Parent's belief in the benefits of health screening and health promotion for the child.

Defining Characteristics: Child is brought in for routinely scheduled well-child office visits (specify). Parent appears interested and asks appropriate questions related to the child's health and growth and development. (Specify, using quotes whenever possible.)

Goal: Parent will continue health-seeking behaviors.

Outcome Criteria

✔ The parent keeps all scheduled well-child appointments.
✔ The parent calls the health care provider for concerns related to the child's health and well-being.

NOC: *Knowledge: Health Promotion*

INTERVENTIONS	RATIONALES
Establish a comfortable environment for the child and parent: provide privacy, assume a position at the child's level without approaching too	Promoting comfort and a sense of safety for the child decreases the stress of health care visits.

INTERVENTIONS	RATIONALES
suddenly, listen attentively, and allow adequate time to address the parent and child's concerns.	
Establish the reason for health care visit (specify, e.g., 6-month well-baby checkup; high school physical exam). Elicit and address any concerns the parent or child (if age appropriate) might have.	Provides the framework for the health care experience and encourages information-sharing and giving.
Assess the child's growth and physical well-being based on developmental level (specify, e.g., an infant may be examined sitting in the parent's lap with auscultation the first technique. An adolescent may benefit from having the parent wait outside during the physical exam.)	The nurse's knowledge of growth and development allows the exam to be structured to cause the least stress for the child.
Provide health teaching as appropriate during and after the exam.	Teaching helps the parent and child to maintain optimal health.
Evaluate the child's competence on several appropriate developmental milestones (specify which parameters are appropriate for individual child).	More than one measure is necessary to gain an accurate evaluation of development.
Provide the parent (and child if appropriate) with anticipatory guidance related to expected development in the near future (specify).	Anticipatory guidance helps the parent to support the child's development.
Offer praise to parent and child for attempts to maintain a healthy lifestyle, including keeping health care appointments.	Positive reinforcement may help maintain the desired behavior.
Provide written information about growth and development.	Written information can be read at leisure and provides reinforcement of teaching.

INTERVENTIONS	RATIONALES
Encourage parent to call health care provider for concerns about the child's health and well-being. Provide appropriate phone numbers.	Encouragement helps the parent to seek information and care in a timely manner.
Make referrals as needed (specify, e.g., WIC, social services, etc.).	Describe rationale for specific referral.

NIC: *Health Screening; Health Education*

Evaluation

(Date/time of evaluation of goal)

(Has goal been met? Not met? Partially met?)

(Has the parent kept all scheduled well-child appointments?)

(Has the parent called the health care provider for concerns related to the child's health and well-being?)

(Revisions to care plan? D/C care plan? Continue care plan?)

READINESS FOR ENHANCED ORGANIZED INFANT BEHAVIOR

Related to: Increasing stability of autonomic, motor, and state responses to environmental cues.

Defining Characteristics: (Specify, e.g., parent reports that the infant has established a sleep/wake pattern; infant responds to visual and auditory cues; infant demonstrates ability to console self, etc.)

Goal: The infant will continue to adapt appropriately to environmental stimuli by (date/time to evaluate goal).

Outcome Criteria

✔ Infant exhibits smooth movements (specify, e.g., hand-to-mouth, suck, swallow).

✔ Infant exhibits organized behaviors (specify, e.g., maintains quiet alert states, engages in reciprocal interaction with parent; self-consoling, etc.)

NOC: *Child Development*

INTERVENTIONS	RATIONALES
Assess parent(s)' understanding of infant's current behavioral states and cues (specify).	Assessment provides baseline information.
Provide parents with information about expected infant development (specify if verbal discussion, written information, or video will be used). Help parents to identify their infant's behavioral states and individual cues.	Recognizing the infant's individual behaviors enhances the parent-infant relationship.
Assist parents to identify when the infant's behavior indicates stress caused by excess environmental stimuli (specify).	Identifying infant behaviors helps the parent to modify stressors.
Encourage parents to decrease stimuli when infant appears overstimulated.	Promotes infant development without excessive stress.
Teach parents to provide developmental interventions for their infant (specify interventions based on infant's age and ability).	Interventions foster development and enhance parent-infant relationship.
Provide parents with referrals or additional information as indicated (specify for clients).	Provides parents with additional information to foster infant development.

NIC: *Infant Care*

Evaluation

(Date/time of evaluation of goal)

(Has goal been met? Not met? Partially met?)

(Does infant exhibit smooth movements? (Specify)

(Describe infant's behavior organization; specify as listed in outcome criteria)

(Revisions to care plan? D/C care plan? Continue care plan?)

RISK FOR INFECTION

Related to: Lack of completed immunizations.

Defining Characteristics: Infant/child has not received all immunizations against childhood illnesses (specify age and appropriate immunizations for age).

Goal: Infant/child will not experience infection with preventable childhood illnesses by (date/time to evaluate).

Outcome Criteria

✔ Infant/child receives all immunizations appropriate for age (specify which immunizations and when they should be completed).

✔ Infant/child does not experience infection with preventable childhood illnesses.

NOC: *Immunization Behavior*

INTERVENTIONS	RATIONALES
Assess infant/child's current immunization status.	Provides baseline data about immunization needs.
Teach parent about the benefits of childhood immunization against preventable illnesses. Provide written information about immunization.	Informed parents are able to make good decisions for their child.
Administer immunizations as ordered by the caregiver (specify drug, dose, route, and timing) providing the least traumatic care (specify based on developmental level).	Specify action of particular agent in preventing infection. Relate principles of growth and development to method of giving immunization.
Observe for side effects and teach parent to provide relief as ordered by caregiver (specify, e.g., Tylenol as ordered for discomfort).	Specify side effects of particular agent and action of Tylenol or other relief measures.
Teach parent (and child if age-appropriate) to practice good hygiene (specify, e.g., hand-washing, bathing, kitchen hygiene, etc.).	Teaching empowers the parent and child to take responsibility for health. Specify how infection is prevented by specific teachings.
Encourage parent to provide optimal nutrition and a balance between rest and activity for the infant/child (specify).	A well-nourished and rested infant/child is less susceptible to infection and better able to respond effectively.
Offer praise and encouragement to parent and child for taking good care of the child's health.	Positive reinforcement helps ensure that behavior will continue.

NIC: *Immunization/Vaccination Administration*

Evaluation

(Date/time of evaluation of goal)

(Has goal been met? Not met? Partially met?)

(Has infant/child received all immunizations appropriate for age? Specify)

(Has infant/child experienced infection with preventable childhood illnesses? Specify)

(Revisions to care plan? D/C care plan? Continue care plan?)

DELAYED GROWTH AND DEVELOPMENT

Related to: Separation from significant others (specify, parents, siblings, peers and/or primary caretaker).

Defining Characteristics: Ages 6 to 30 months (specify, crying, screaming, withdraws from others, inactive, sad, detachment behaviors, regressive behaviors); 3 to 6 yrs. (specify, temper tantrums, refusal to comply with hospital routine/treatments, crying, refusal to eat); 6 to 12 yrs. (specify, express feelings of loneliness, boredom, isolation, depression, worry about absence from school); 13 to 18 yrs. (specify, may react with dependency, uncooperativeness, withdrawal behaviors, fear of loss of peer status/acceptance at school).

Related to: Decreased or increased environmental stimulation.

Defining Characteristics: Inability to perform self-care or self-control activities appropriate for age, decreased responses, listlessness, flat affect; delay or difficulty in performing developmental tasks/skills (specify, motor, social or language) typical for age group.

Related to: Chronic illness or disability, repeated hospitalizations.

Defining Characteristics: Inability to perform gross and fine motor tasks appropriate to age, altered physical growth (specify).

Goal: Child will exhibit age-appropriate growth and development by (date/time to evaluate).

Outcome Criteria

✔ Child exhibits age-appropriate growth and development activities (specify).

NOC: *Child Development*

INTERVENTIONS	RATIONALES
Provide or arrange for growth and development assessment with the administration of tools	Identifies developmental level or any lag in development to assist in plan of care or therapy;

INTERVENTIONS	RATIONALES
such as Washington Guide, Denver Developmental Screening Test (DDST), Denver Developmental Screening Test Revised (DDST-R), Denver II, Revised Denver Prescreening Developmental Questionnaire (R-PDQ), Denver Articulation Screening Exam (DASE) (specify).	information should include age-expected gross and fine motor development, language and social development, psychosocial and psychosexual development, interpersonal skills, cognitive and moral and spiritual development.
Reassess developmental levels at intervals appropriate for illness or other problem (specify).	Provides evidence of progress to evaluate program to correct any growth and developmental deficit.
Provide consistent caretaker and care.	Promotes trust and progress in development.
Depending on age and abilities, encourage to participate in goal-setting decision-making, participation in care (specify).	Promotes independence needed for control and development.
Provide visual, auditory, tactile stimulation, including mobiles with or without color, music, toys, books, television, games or other age-related activities; hold child and rock or pat on back, talk to child.	Promotes stimulation needed to maintain developmental status.
Provide time for child, either quiet or talking, to play with other children, time for parents that remain in hospital to interact with child.	Promotes independence and development or maintenance of motor skills to prevent regression.
Provide developmentally appropriate activities based on child's age-related abilities (specify).	To enhance child's adjustment to hospitalization and treatment and to enhance child's maximum growth and developmental abilities.
Explore the family's and child's feelings regarding child's health status and required treatments.	Promotes family communication and attitude of acceptance and adaptation to child's health status and abilities.
Encourage independence and choices in as many areas as possible (i.e., dressing, feeding, type of foods/drinks, or Band-Aids).	Fosters child's sense of control, adaptation, and developmental growth during their altered health state and hospitalization.
Encourage socialization (i.e., in the play room, with siblings, peers, phone calls, if possible).	To foster child's ability to develop and maintain peer relationships.

INTERVENTIONS	RATIONALES
Recognize and support ritualistic behaviors (especially in the young child).	Fosters child's need for autonomy.
Encourage mastery of self-care activities, required health care equipment, if appropriate.	Fosters child's need for initiative and purpose; fosters child's self-esteem.
Instruct parents on growth and development for child's age (specify).	Provides information about age-related growth and development to ensure realistic expectations.
Inform of age-related play and other activities that enhance growth and development and provide needed stimulation; include those that encourage gross and fine motor development, sensory and cognitive development, others as determined by testing and needs.	Provides guidance for proper, safe activities and stimulation to prevent frustration of child and to promote normal development.
Teach parents whether developmental and growth lag is the result of the child's illness (acute or chronic) or some other reason.	Promotes understanding and relief from anxiety and guilt.
Discuss test results with child and parents and possible plan to resolve any deficits, both shortterm during hospitalization and long-term during convalescence.	Promotes understanding of special needs and formulation of goals and actions based on findings.
Initiate referral to child development expert if appropriate.	Provides source of assistance to ensure proper age-related development.

NIC: *Developmental Enhancement*

Evaluation

(Date/time of evaluation of goal)

(Has goal been met? Not met? Partially met?)

(Does child exhibit age-appropriate growth and developmental activities? Describe)

(Revisions to care plan? D/C care plan? Continue care plan?)

CHAPTER 1.2

HOSPITALIZED CHILD

Hospitalization of the child, whether it involves a short-term hospital admission, surgery, a follow-up evaluation, or repeated hospitalizations for a chronic illness or episode, creates a crisis for the child and family. Responses to hospitalization are related to the developmental level of the child but generally include fear of separation, loss of control, injury, and pain. The ease of transition from home to the hospital depends on how well the child has been prepared for it and how the child's physical and emotional needs have been met. Supporting the family, providing them with information, and encouraging their participation in the child's care contributes to the adjustment and well-being of all concerned.

COMMON NURSING DIAGNOSES

See DISTURBED SLEEP PATTERN

Related to: Physiologic factors related to illness and psychological stress, external factors of environmental changes.

Defining Characteristics: Interrupted sleep, irritability, restlessness, lethargy, disorientation, fatigue, pain, separation anxiety, side effects of medication (nausea, vomiting, diarrhea) (specify for child).

See IMPAIRED PHYSICAL MOBILITY

Related to: Pain and discomfort; neuro or musculoskeletal impairment (specify).

Defining Characteristics: Imposed restrictions of movement or activity, imposed bed rest, limited strength, endurance, weakness, fatigue, drainage tubes and IV catheters; disturbances in gait, vision, equilibrium (specify).

See IMBALANCED NUTRITION: LESS THAN BODY REQUIREMENTS

Related to: Loss of appetite; lack of interest in food; alteration in taste; inability to ingest, digest or absorb nutrients; nausea; vomiting; diarrhea; constipation; abdominal pain; oral ulcers (specify).

Defining Characteristics: Weakness, fatigue, anxiety, anorexia, illness, lack of interest in eating (specify behavior).

See DELAYED GROWTH AND DEVELOPMENT

Related to: Separation from significant others; environmental and stimulation deficiencies; effects of repeated hospitalizations; social isolation; sensory and/or motor delays (specify).

Defining Characteristics: (Specify, e.g., inability to perform self-care or self-control activities appropriate for age; regressive behavior; fear of unfamiliar environment and treatments; feelings of inferiority; low self-esteem, or alterations to body image.)

ADDITIONAL NURSING DIAGNOSES

ANXIETY

Related to: Change in health status; change in environment; threat to self-concept; situational crisis (specify).

Defining Characteristics: Increased apprehension; fear; helplessness; uncertainty; distress over hospitalization; restlessness; expressed concern over procedures, pain, loss of control, separation from significant others; crying; clinging; refusal to interact with staff, changes in VS, financial stresses caused by required absence from employment (specify child's behavior).

Goal: Child and family will experience decreased anxiety by (date/time to evaluate).

Outcome Criteria

✔ Reduced anxiety expressed by child and family.

✔ (Specify behaviors to look for: e.g., child is not crying or clinging, facial features are relaxed, parents verbalize understanding of procedures and plan of care, etc.)

NOC: *Anxiety Control*

INTERVENTIONS	RATIONALES
Assess child's and parents' level of anxiety, child's developmental level, understanding of illness, and reason for hospitalization, and responses to this and previous hospitalizations during admission.	Provides information about sources and level of anxiety related to illness and hospitalization; sources of anxiety and responses vary with age of child and include separation, pain and bodily injury, loss of control, enforced dependence, fear of unknown, fear of equipment, unfamiliar environment and routines, guilt, fear and concern for child's recovery, feelings of powerlessness.
Assess social and emotional history of child and family for strengths and successful coping ability.	Provides information about strengths and about weaknesses to draw upon to cope with hospitalization.
Allow expression of feelings and concerns about illness and procedures and listen individually to child and parents.	Provides opportunity to vent feelings and fears to reduce anxiety and promote adaptation to hospitalization.
Provide a calm, accepting environment and avoid rushing through interactions and care.	Assists child and family in establishing trust and obtaining emotional stability.
Provide orientation to hospital environment and room, routines, meal and play time, introduction to staff members, forms to sign and hospital policies.	Familiarizes child and family with environment, promotes secure feeling, and reduces fear of unknown.
Have same personnel following written care plan, care for child; schedule personal contact with child within work day (specify).	Promotes continuity and consistency of care to support trusting relationship.

INTERVENTIONS	RATIONALES
Encourage involvement of child and parents in planning and interventions of care; allow parents to remain with child; allow to hold and cuddle the child.	Promotes participation in and adaptation to hospitalization, reduces anxiety; allows demonstration of love and affection for child.
Allow child and parents to incorporate home routines as much as possible; bring toys, tapes, photographs and favorite foods from home as appropriate (specify).	Promotes security and reduces anxiety associated with new experiences.
Maintain a quiet environment, control visitors and interactions.	Decreases stimuli that increase anxiety.
Allow child to play out feelings. Accept feelings and responses expressed by the child.	Permits child to express feelings without fear of punishment.
Approach child in a positive way; use child's proper name; avoid communicating, either verbally or nonverbally, any rejection, judgments, or negativism.	Promotes rapport and trust and maintains identity.
Identify and recognize regressive behavior as a part of the illness and assist child in dealing with dependency associated with the hospitalization.	Allows for behaviors common to hospitalizations and loss of control.
Provide support to child during any procedures or distressing features associated with care, including intrusive procedures, exposure of body parts, need for personal privacy and privacy of others.	Reduces anxiety and fear caused by possible bodily injury.
Inform and explain all treatments and procedures in simple, understandable language to child and parents according to their intellectual level and age; pace information according to child/parental needs.	Provides easily understood information, which decreases anxiety.
Inform parents and child that behavior caused by anxiety and fear is normal and expected.	Prevents feeling of inadequacy and fear of punishment.
Use therapeutic play to explain and prepare child for procedures; repeat any teaching as needed.	Permits child to understand and become familiar with articles used for care or procedure.
If surgery planned (specify) instruct in preoperative and	Prepares child for surgical intervention with minimal anxiety.

(continues)

(continues)

INTERVENTIONS	RATIONALES
post-operative care, surgical procedure to be done, reason for surgery, and length of hospitalization; answer questions about surgery.	

NIC: *Anxiety Reduction*

Evaluation

(Date/time of evaluation of goal)

(Has goal been met? Not met? Partially met?)

(Did child or family express decreased anxiety? Use quotes. Describe behavioral change associated with decreased anxiety, e.g., child is no longer clinging to parent.)

(Revisions to care plan? D/C care plan? Continue care plan?)

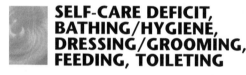

SELF-CARE DEFICIT, BATHING/HYGIENE, DRESSING/GROOMING, FEEDING, TOILETING

Related to: Impaired ability to perform ADL; pain and discomfort (specify).

Defining Characteristics: Inability to wash body, take off or put on clothing, feed self, positioning or mechanical restrictions, weakness, fatigue, imposed bed rest, inability to carry out toileting with use of bedpan or go to bathroom (specify for child).

Goal: Child will demonstrate increased ability to care for self by (date/time to evaluate).

Outcome Criteria

✔ Maximum self-care capability with or without use of aids (specify for child).

NOC: *Self-Care: Activities of Daily Living*

INTERVENTIONS	RATIONALES
Assess physical tolerance and abilities to perform ADL, and play activities and restrictions imposed by the illness and medical protocol.	Provides information about amount of energy and effect of illness on activity level.

INTERVENTIONS	RATIONALES
Anticipate child's needs for toileting, feeding, brushing teeth, bathing and other care if unable to manage on own; allow child to do as much as possible (specify).	Prevents embarrassing experiences with toileting and maintains comfort with personal cleanliness and appearance.
Provide personal care for infant and small child; assist child and encourage parent to assist child. Adjust times and methods to fit home routine.	Provides needed assistance where using patterns and articles that child is accustomed to using and doing.
Praise child for participation in own care according to age, developmental level, and energy (specify).	Promotes self-esteem and independence.
Provide assistive aids or devices to perform ADL, allow choices when possible (specify for child).	Assists child in performing self-care for ADL.
Balance activities with rest as needed; place needed articles and call light within reach if appropriate.	Prevents fatigue by conserving energy and promoting rest.
Instruct child in toileting, feeding, bathing, hygiene, dressing while in hospital environment and inform of differences from home care and methods as needed (specify).	Promotes performance of ADL skills already known by child.
Inform to rest when tired and to request quiet times.	Ensures proper rest and prevents fatigue.
Inform parents to assist child in ADL but to allow child as much independence as condition permits; inform parents that a place is provided for their personal needs in order to allow them to remain with the child.	Promotes independence and some control by the child without separating child from parents.
Instruct parents to interpret child's needs if child too young to talk.	Provides anticipatory care for child.

NIC: *Self-Care Assistance*

Evaluation

(Date/time of evaluation of goal)

(Has goal been met? Not met? Partially met?)

(Describe child's ability to attain behaviors specified under outcome criteria.)

(Revisions to care plan? D/C care plan? Continue care plan?)

 ## DEFICIENT DIVERSIONAL ACTIVITY

Related to: Environmental lack of diversion, long-term hospitalization.

Defining Characteristics: Boredom, desire for something to do because usual hobbies and activities cannot be done in hospital (specify, use quotes).

Goal: Child will engage in diversional activity by (date/time to evaluate).

Outcome Criteria

✔ Participation in age-appropriate activities within limitations imposed by illness (specify activity).

NOC: *Play Participation*

INTERVENTIONS	RATIONALES
Assess type of activities allowed and desired and amount of motor activity needed; check medical protocol for bed rest or limitations imposed by illness.	Provides information about type of activities and play to suggest.
Show playroom to child and introduce child and family to other children and families with similar illness (specify).	Provides a familiar environment for child.
Place child in a room with another child of same age if possible (specify).	Promotes interaction and diversion while hospitalized.
Schedule care and treatments to allow for play activities.	Provides opportunity for play and diversion.
Provide age-appropriate play activities according to amount of energy of child and activity allowed, including quiet play with games, television, reading, soft toys, favorite toys.	Prevents fatigue resulting from overactivity while ill and in need of rest and quiet.
Encourage family to play with child or interact with child.	Promotes diversion for child.
Provide play activities that include educational needs for school-age child; bring school-work from home if appropriate (specify).	Promotes therapy that includes educational needs.

INTERVENTIONS	RATIONALES
Suggest parents bring child's favorite toys or articles for play.	Promotes diversionary activity.
Teach parents and child of need to monitor activities and rest although still allowing for play and interactions with others.	Prevents fatigue during acute phase of illness.
Consult a play therapist for assistance in planning activities and assessing child's play needs as needed.	Promotes age-appropriate diversionary activities.

NIC: *Activity Therapy*

Evaluation

(Date/time of evaluation of goal)

(Has goal been met? Not met? Partially met?)

(Did child participate in diversional activity? Describe.)

(Revisions to care plan? D/C care plan? Continue care plan?)

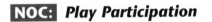 ## POWERLESSNESS

Related to: Health care environment, illness-related regimen.

Defining Characteristics: Expression of loss of control over situation, expression or behavior indicating dissatisfaction with inability to perform activities and dependence on others, reluctance to express true feelings, fear of alienation from others in the hospital environment (specify).

Goal: Client will experience less powerlessness by (date/time to evaluate).

Outcome Criteria

✔ Gains sense of control over situation

✔ (Specify how child and/or parent participates in plan of care: e.g., goal-setting, scheduling of treatments.)

✔ (Specify how child or parent verbalize increased sense of control—use quotes.)

NOC: *Family Participation in Professional Care*

INTERVENTIONS	RATIONALES
Encourage parents and child to verbalize feelings in an accepting environment.	Allows for venting of feelings about loss of control and frustrations over loss of ability to perform activities.
Allow for input from child and parents in care goals, care plan, and scheduling of activities, and integrate this input into routines as much as possible.	Allows for as much control as possible for child and family.
Encourage parents to participate in child's care as much as desired; and to visit or remains with child continuously.	Promotes support of child and allows family some control over the situation.
Provide encouragement and praise to child and parents for their participation; encourage and defend expression of their true feelings.	Promotes positive feedback and reduces fear of rejection by staff because of their behavior.
Allow child to perform simple tasks in hospital unit and for own care, such as pouring own water and marking amounts on record at bedside.	Promotes independence and control of the environment.
Inform parents and child of tasks that they can perform in care plan (specify).	Accommodates need for sense of control.

NIC: *Security Enhancement*

Evaluation

(Date/time of evaluation of goal)

(Has goal been met? Not met? Partially met?)

(Have child/parents participated in care? Specify how. Use quotes as applicable.)

(Revisions to care plan? D/C care plan? Continue care plan?)

RISK FOR TRAUMA

Related to: Developmental age, deficient knowledge and cognitive immaturity predisposing the child to safety hazards in the environment.

Defining Characteristics: Developmental age, developmental delays, disturbances in gait, vision, hearing, perceptual or cognitive functioning (specify).

Goal: Child will not experience any trauma by (date/time to evaluate).

Outcome Criteria

✔ Child engages in appropriate play (specify) without injury.

✔ Parents verbalize safety considerations related to toys/games (specify according to developmental level).

NOC: *Knowledge: Personal Safety*

INTERVENTIONS	RATIONALES
Assess age of child and reason for particular selection of type and article of play, and intended purpose of play (enjoyment, development, therapy).	Provides information needed to select appropriate toy or activity for play based on age: infants grasp and hold articles and stuffed toys; young child plays with replicas of adult tools and other toys, plays pretend, and later moves from toys to games, hobbies, sports; older child continues with games and sports and begins to daydream; play provides fun, diversion, and learning about procedures for the child who is hospitalized.
Select safe toys appropriate for age and amount of activity allowed (active or passive plays) and that suit the skills and interest of the child.	Provides guidelines for quiet play or play that involves motor activity.
Encourage play and allow parents to bring favorite toy, game or other play materials from home.	Promotes learning and skill development, and facilitates expression of feelings.
In a quiet environment, plan and implement an age-appropriate play activity to prepare the child for all invasive procedures, to observe child's behavior, or to allow child to reveal fears and concerns with or without someone in attendance (specify).	Promotes therapeutic play with a selection of toys and articles that include dolls or puppets (nurse, doctor, child, family members); hospital supplies (syringe, dressings, tape, tubes); paper, crayons, and paints; stuffed toys, toy telephone; prepares the child emotionally and cognitively for invasive procedures; fosters appropriate coping strategies.
Remove all unsafe, sharp, broken toys, toys with small parts that can be swallowed, toys inappropriate for age (specify).	Prevents trauma or injury to the child.
Allow child to communicate type of toy desired and to assist in the selection of toys and play activities.	Promotes independence and control over play situation.

INTERVENTIONS	RATIONALES
Teach parents to select toys, play equipment, and supplies that are labeled for intended age group; nontoxic and flame resistant with directions for use; that are durable and do not have sharp edges or points; that do not have small parts that can be swallowed; that do not contain any parts to be ejected; and that are not broken, rusted, or weak and need repairs.	Promotes safe play for the child.
Teach parents to store play materials meant for older children away from young child to provide a safe place for toys, to discard or repair broken toys.	Prevents accidents caused by toys in pathways or by toys meant for older, more mature play.

INTERVENTIONS	RATIONALES
Teach parent(s) to select play activity based on child's energy and tolerance level during an illness, and to evaluate toys given as gifts to the child.	Provides the enjoyment of active or passive play that is geared to child's condition.

NIC: *Parent Education: Child-Rearing Family*

Evaluation

(Date/time of evaluation of goal)

(Has goal been met? Not met? Partially met?)

(List appropriate play child engaged in without injury. Provide quotes from parents verbalization of safety considerations.)

(Revisions to care plan? D/C care plan? Continue care plan?)

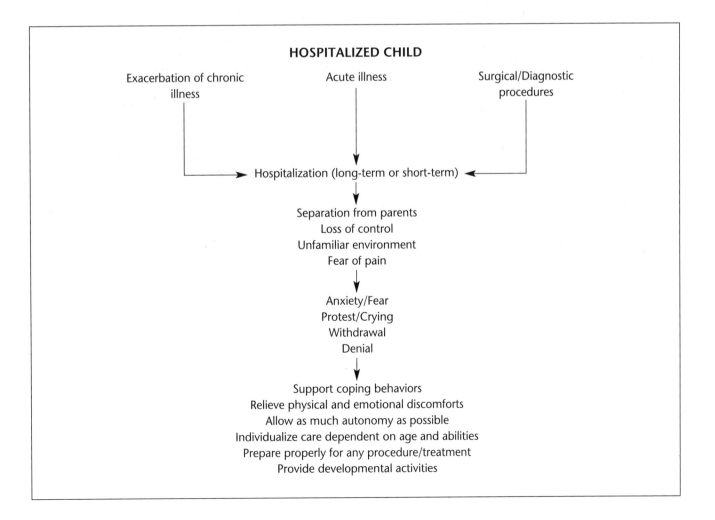

HOSPITALIZED CHILD

Exacerbation of chronic illness   Acute illness   Surgical/Diagnostic procedures

Hospitalization (long-term or short-term)

Separation from parents
Loss of control
Unfamiliar environment
Fear of pain

Anxiety/Fear
Protest/Crying
Withdrawal
Denial

Support coping behaviors
Relieve physical and emotional discomforts
Allow as much autonomy as possible
Individualize care dependent on age and abilities
Prepare properly for any procedure/treatment
Provide developmental activities

CHAPTER 1.3

CHILD ABUSE

The term child abuse is used to describe any neglect or mistreatment of infants or children including infliction of emotional pain, physical injury, or sexual exploitation. Neglect or abuse is most often inflicted by the child's biologic parents. Others who have been implicated include foster parents, babysitters, boyfriends, friends, and daycare workers. Nurses are legally and morally responsible to identify children who may be maltreated and to report findings to protect the child from further abuse.

Neglect is the most common form of abuse and may include deprivation of basic physical or emotional needs: food, clothing, shelter, health care, education, affection, love, and nurturing. Emotional abuse stems from rejection, isolation, and/or terrorizing the child. Physical abuse may result in burns, bruises, fractures, lacerations, or poisoning. Infants may suffer from "shaken baby syndrome" with severe or fatal neurologic injuries caused by violent shaking of the infant. Signs of shaken baby syndrome include retinal and subarachnoid hemorrhage. Signs of sexual abuse include bruising or bleeding of the anus or genitals, genital discharge, odor, severe itching or pain, and sexually transmitted diseases. A discrepancy between the nature of the child's injuries and the reported cause of injury is a frequent clue that abuse has occurred.

MEDICAL CARE

Complete Blood Count (CBC): reveals changes resulting from infection (increased WBC), blood loss (decreased RBC, Hgb).

Urinalysis: reveals blood, pus in urinary tract.

Vaginal/Anal Cultures: reveal sexually-transmitted disease.

X-ray: child abuse long bone series of X-rays are required to detect evidence of or to rule out healed fractures/current fractures.

C-scan: to rule out central nervous system damage caused by shaken baby syndrome.

COMMON NURSING DIAGNOSES

See IMBALANCED NUTRITION: LESS THAN BODY REQUIREMENTS

Related to: Inability to ingest food.

Defining Characteristics: (Specify, e.g., withholding of food by parent/caretaker, weight loss, malnutrition, lack of subcutaneous fat, failure to thrive, provides inadequate amount of food; knowledge of deficit regarding appropriate food preparations [i.e., cleaning bottles].)

See RISK FOR IMPAIRED SKIN INTEGRITY

Related to: External factor of trauma.

Defining Characteristics: (Specify, e.g., lacerations, burns, abrasions, skin trauma in different stages of healing, unclean skin, teeth, hair.)

See DELAYED GROWTH AND DEVELOPMENT

Related to: Inadequate caretaking, indifference, environmental and stimulation deficiencies.

Defining Characteristics: (Specify, e.g., delay or difficulty in performing skills [motor, social, or expressive] typical of age group, altered physical growth, inability to perform self-care or self-control activities appropriate for age, flat affect, decreased responses, withdrawal, antisocial behavior, fearfulness, poor relationships with peers, regressive behavior, acting out behavior.)

ADDITIONAL NURSING DIAGNOSES

ANXIETY

Related to: Threat to self-concept, change in health status, change in interaction patterns, situational crisis.

Defining Characteristics: Increased apprehension and uncertainty, fearfulness, feeling of powerlessness, fear of consequences, repeated episodes of maltreatment, mistrust, trembling, quivering voice, poor eye contact, lacks appropriate pain response, frozen watchfulness, developmental delays/regressive behaviors (specify).

Goal: Child will experience less anxiety by (date/time to evaluate).

Outcome Criteria

✔ (Specify measurable criteria, e.g., child makes eye contact, has relaxed facial features, reports decreased anxiety if age-appropriate.)

NOC: *Coping*

INTERVENTIONS	RATIONALES
Assess level of anxiety and fear in child and how it is manifested; identify the source of anxiety and observe reactions to staff and parents at each encounter.	Provides information about the source and level of anxiety and what might relieve it and basis to judge improvement.
Demonstrate affection and acceptance of the child even if not returned or ignored; avoid reinforcing any negative behavior.	Promotes trust of staff and positive behavior of the child.
Provide a play program with other children; set aside time to be alone with child or quiet time for child as well; praise child or reward with a special treat when appropriate (specify).	Modifies negative behavior by promoting interactions with others and rewarding desired behaviors; promotes self-esteem.
Provide consistent staffing for child, preferably those who seem to relate well to child.	Promotes familiarity and trusting relationship with staff.
Allow expression of concerns and fears of child about treatments, environment; allow questions and provide honest explanations and communication at child's age level.	Provides opportunity to vent feelings, which reduces anxiety.

INTERVENTIONS	RATIONALES
Provide treatment of injuries; avoid treating child as a victim, asking too many questions, or forcing any discussion.	Prevents increased anxiety and stress in child by discussion of abuse.
Explain all treatments and procedures to be done and the purpose for them and that someone will accompany them to a different department if needed (specify).	Provides preparation and information that will assist in preventing fear or anxiety.
Use therapeutic play kit to instruct child in any procedure to be done (dolls, syringe, tubing, dressing, other articles, specify).	Reduces anxiety by familiarizing child with what to expect to reduce anxiety.
Refer for counseling services for the child as indicated.	Reduces anxiety and supports child in dealing with abuse and negative behavior.

NIC: *Anxiety Reduction*

Evaluation

(Date/time of evaluation of goal)

(Has goal been met? Not met? Partially met?)

(Provide data about outcome criteria, e.g., does child make eye contact? Are facial features relaxed, does child report feeling "calmer," use quotes if possible.)

(Revisions to care plan? D/C care plan? Continue care plan?)

IMPAIRED PARENTING

Related to: (Specify: unmet social and emotional maturation needs of parental figures, ineffective role modeling, lack of knowledge, situational crisis or incident.)

Defining Characteristics: (Specify: lack of parental attachment behaviors, verbalization of resentment toward child and of role inadequacy, inattention to needs of child, noncompliance with health practices and medical care, inappropriate discipline practices, frequent accidents and illness of child, growth and development lag in child, history of child abuse or abandonment, multiple caretakers without regard for needs of child, evidence of physical and psychological trauma, actual abandonment of child.)

Goal: Parents will exhibit improved parenting skills by (date/time to evaluate).

Outcome Criteria

✔ Demonstration of appropriate parenting behaviors.

✔ Maintenance of safe environment for child.

✔ Establishment of positive relationship with child and realistic expectations for self and child.

✔ Acceptance of support for achievement of desirable parenting skills.

NOC: *Parenting*

INTERVENTIONS	RATIONALES
Assess parents for achievement of developmental tasks of self and understanding of child's growth and development; how they are bonded and attached to child; how they interpret and respond to child; how they accept and support child; how they meet child's social, psychological and physical needs.	Provides information about parent-child relationship and parenting styles that may lead to child abuse; identifies parents at risk for violence or other abusive behavior.
Provide a child nurturing role model for parents to emulate.	Promotes development of parenting skills by imitation.
Praise parents for their participation in child's care, tell them that they are giving good care to child.	Reinforces positive parenting behaviors and increases feeling of adequacy.
Include parents in planning care and setting goals.	Promotes participation of parents in meeting child's needs.
Provide an opportunity for parents to express their feelings, personal needs, and goals; avoid making judgmental remarks or comparing them to other parents.	Supports parents in meeting their own needs.
Teach parents developmental tasks for child and parents, difference in developmental level between child and parents, and appropriate tasks for age levels.	Provides information that assists parents in responding realistically and appropriately to child's needs at different age levels.
Discuss with parents methods to reduce conflict, to be consistent in approach to child's behavior and needs, to avoid siding with child or other parent.	Promotes a more positive child-parent relationship.

INTERVENTIONS	RATIONALES
Instruct parents to maintain their own health by getting adequate rest, nutrition, and exercise; and to participate in leisure activities and make social contacts.	Provides information on importance of parents meeting their own needs to enable them to better care for and cope with their children.
Refer to community agencies that offer parenting classes and support groups.	Provides education in parenting skills.
Initiate referrals to social services, parenting classes, or counseling as appropriate. Inform parents that child protection services have been contacted to investigate the child's health status and safety; keep the parents informed of the child's health status (unless or until custody of the child is removed from the parents.	Provides options if parenting is unsatisfactory or inadequate.

NIC: *Parent Education: Child-Rearing Family*

Evaluation

(Date/time of evaluation of goal)

(Has goal been met? Not met? Partially met?)

(Provide data about outcome criteria, e.g., parent attends to child's crying; feeds child; plays game with child; attends parenting classes or self-help groups; verbalizes child's developmental needs, etc., use quotes if possible.)

(Revisions to care plan? D/C care plan? Continue care plan?)

RISK FOR TRAUMA

Related to: Characteristics of child, caregivers, environment.

Defining Characteristics: (Specify: sexual assault of child, evidence of physical abuse of child, history of abuse of abuser, social isolation of family, low self-esteem of caretaker, inadequate support systems, violence against other members of the family.)

Goal: Child will not experience trauma by (date/time to evaluate).

Outcome Criteria

✔ Absence of violence or maltreatment of the child by parents or other offenders.

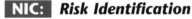 **NOC:** *Risk Detection*

INTERVENTIONS	RATIONALES
Assess the abuser for violent behavior or other abusive patterns, use of alcohol or drugs, or other psychosocial problems.	Provides information to determine warning signs of child abuse.
Assess behavior of parents toward child, including responses to the child's behavior, ability to comfort the child, feelings and perceptions toward the child, expectations for the child, overprotective or concern for the child.	Reveals characteristics that may indicate risk for abuse.
Communicate information and needs of child to those on the abuse team (or to new caretakers if child being placed with a foster parent or someone other than parents); provide written instruction for care and child's needs (specify).	Provides care plan for child based on court decision to caretakers working with the family based on court decision for child's care.
Maintain factual and objective documentation of all observations, including: child's physical condition, child's behavioral response to parents, health care workers, other visitors, parent's response to child, and interviews with family members.	Provides information that may be used in legal action regarding abuse.

INTERVENTIONS	RATIONALES
Inform parents of followup care and needs of child, need to evaluate child's progress.	Promotes emphasis on child's care and prevention of recurrence of abuse.
Instruct parents in identifying events that lead to child abuse and in methods to deal with behavior without harming the child.	Prevents further abusive behavior directed at the child.
Inform of Parents Anonymous and other child protective groups to contact for assistance.	Provides self-help group activities, information, and support based on type of abuse and parental needs.
Inform parents of child's placement in a foster home, allow them to meet and speak to new caretaker.	Prepares parents for court order of alternate placement to ensure a safe environment.
Initiate referral to social worker, public health nurse, psychological counselor before discharge to home (specify).	Provides support to child and family, and monitors behaviors following discharge.

NIC: *Risk Identification*

Evaluation

(Date/time of evaluation of goal)

(Has goal been met? Not met? Partially met?)

(Has the child suffered maltreatment or violence? Provide specifics if indicated.)

(Revisions to care plan? D/C care plan? Continue care plan?)

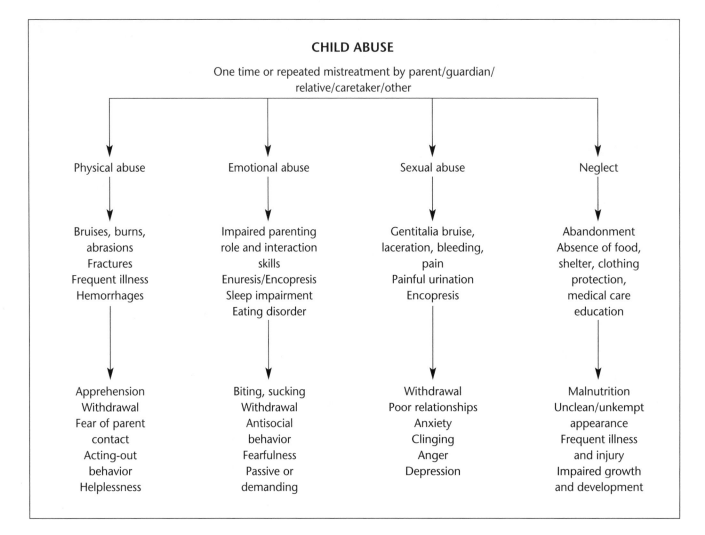

CHILD ABUSE

One time or repeated mistreatment by parent/guardian/
relative/caretaker/other

Physical abuse	Emotional abuse	Sexual abuse	Neglect
Bruises, burns, abrasions Fractures Frequent illness Hemorrhages	Impaired parenting role and interaction skills Enuresis/Encopresis Sleep impairment Eating disorder	Gentitalia bruise, laceration, bleeding, pain Painful urination Encopresis	Abandonment Absence of food, shelter, clothing protection, medical care education
Apprehension Withdrawal Fear of parent contact Acting-out behavior Helplessness	Biting, sucking Withdrawal Antisocial behavior Fearfulness Passive or demanding	Withdrawal Poor relationships Anxiety Clinging Anger Depression	Malnutrition Unclean/unkempt appearance Frequent illness and injury Impaired growth and development

CHAPTER 1.4

DYING CHILD

Care of the dying child includes the physical and emotional interventions necessary to support the totally dependent child and grieving family. Nursing considerations involve the dissemination of information to the child, whose perceptions of death and responses to death and dying are age-related, and family with sensitivity, caring, and honesty. The nurse also helps the child move through the stages of awareness and acceptance, and helps the family move through the stages of grieving. An additional role of the pediatric nurse, when caring for dying children, is to direct the child and family to appropriate age-related information about death and dying.

MEDICAL CARE

Medications that promote comfort, prevent/manage pain, rest and proper body functions specific to the child's needs.

COMMON NURSING DIAGNOSES

See DISTURBED SLEEP PATTERN

Related to: Illness and stressors, side effects of medications.

Defining Characteristics: (Specify: fatigue, lethargy, irritability, restlessness, pain, psychological stress [anxiety, fear], nausea and vomiting, increased voiding patterns.)

See IMPAIRED PHYSICAL MOBILITY

Related to: Pain and discomfort, side effects of medications.

Defining Characteristics: (Specify: weakness, inability to purposefully move, fatigue, limited strength, changes in consciousness, neuropathy, foot drop,

amputation, gait disturbances; muscle wasting; contractures.)

See IMBALANCED NUTRITION: LESS THAN BODY REQUIREMENTS

Related to: Loss of appetite, fatigue, oral ulcers, (specify).

Defining Characteristics: (Specify: weakness, anorexia, poor feeding, lack of interest in food, anorexia-cachexia syndrome, nausea and vomiting, chronic constipation or diarrhea; dryness and cracking of lips; alterations in taste.)

See RISK FOR IMPAIRED SKIN INTEGRITY

Related to: Immobilization, side effects of medications; invasive procedures/IV infiltration; radiation treatments (specify).

Defining Characteristics: (Specify: redness, disruption of skin surface.)

See DISTURBED THOUGHT PROCESSES

Related to: Physiologic changes, side effects of medication (specify).

Defining Characteristics: (Describe: disorientation, changes in consciousness, fatigue, hallucinations, mood changes.)

See INEFFECTIVE AIRWAY CLEARANCE

Related to: (Specify) decreased energy and fatigue, tracheobronchial secretions, oral ulcers; decreased gag reflex.

Defining Characteristics: (Describe: increasing secretions, changes in respiratory rate or depth [stridor, irregularity], inability to cough and remove secretions, shortness of breath.)

See CONSTIPATION

Related to: Less than adequate physical activity and intake, side effects of medications, food allergy, secondary to disease process (specify).

Defining Characteristics: (Specify: frequency less than usual pattern, hard-formed stool, decreased bowel sounds, abdominal pain, firm/hard abdomen; fecal impaction.)

ADDITIONAL NURSING DIAGNOSES

PAIN

Related to: Biologic, physical, psychological injuring agents (specify).

Defining Characteristics: (Specify, e.g., communication [verbal or coded] of pain descriptors, guarding, protective behavior, facial mask of pain, crying, moaning, withdrawal, changes in VS, irritability, restlessness, age-related expression of pain behaviors, facial grimacing, tension or flexion of muscles.)

Goal: Child will experience less pain by (date/time to evaluate).

Outcome Criteria

✔ Child verbalizes decreased pain (use a pain scale appropriate for age).

✔ VS return to baseline (provide range).

✔ Child appears relaxed and is not crying, grimacing, moaning.

NOC: *Pain Control*

INTERVENTIONS	RATIONALES
Assess severity of pain, fear of receiving pain medication, anxiety and coping mechanisms associated with pain, ability to rest and sleep (specify frequency and pain scale used).	Provides information as a basis for analgesic administration. Developmentally-based pain scales provide accurate assessment of child's discomfort.

INTERVENTIONS	RATIONALES
Administer analgesic intermittently or continuously as ordered, depending on pain severity, and administer before any painful procedure or care is performed(specify drugs, route, times).	Provides coverage of pain medications to ensure freedom from any type of pain and discomfort including administration of analgesic for prompt relief if given intermittently.
Teach child and parents of route of medication administration and effect to expect; that pain will be assessed continuously and medication adjusted as needed to control pain.	Provides assurance that pain will be controlled continuously whether or not child is able to express pain.
Provide position changes as tolerated, use pillows to support position, move slowly with gentle handling, give backrub.	Reduces pain by nonpharmacologic measures.
Provide companionship for child, familiar toys (specify).	Reduces fear and supports comfort of child.
Support coping mechanisms of child and family and adjust analgesic accordingly, with input from child, parents, and physician.	Promotes child's comfort, supports coping abilities, and includes parents and child in decision making regarding care.
Dim lights, avoid noise, maintain clean, comfortable bed with loose sheets and clothing, disturb for care only when needed to promote comfort.	Provides environment free of stimuli that increases anxiety and pain.
Provide nonpharmacologic pain management strategies: soothing baths; massage therapy to painful areas; education on possible (and encourage parent/child to use) distraction techniques (i.e., music, aroma, humor, reading, journal writing, art work, pets, prayer, hypnosis, relaxation techniques. Specify).	Reduces pain perceptions and may foster a sense of control.
Discuss with child and parents that fear of pain is common and that it is all right to express fear and feelings about pain and its control.	Reduces anxiety by recognizing fear of pain and encouraging to vent feelings and concerns about methods of control.
Teach parents and child that only palliative care and treatments will be administered.	Reduces anxiety and stress caused by anticipation of painful interventions.

NIC: *Medication Management*

Evaluation

(Date/time of evaluation of goal)

(Has goal been met? Not met? Partially met?)

(Provide data on pain scale rating, vital signs, muscle tension, and behavior such as crying, grimacing, or moaning.)

(Revisions to care plan? D/C care plan? Continue care plan?)

ANTICIPATORY GRIEVING

Related to: Potential loss of a child.

Defining Characteristics: (Specify: expression of distress at potential loss of child, denial of loss, guilt, anger, sorrow, choked feelings, change in need fulfillment, crying, self-blame, shock and disbelief, overprotectiveness, loss of hope and depression, withdrawal and avoidance of ill child.)

Goal: Clients will begin the grief process by (date/time to evaluate).

Outcome Criteria

✔ Child, parents, and family are able to verbalize feelings about their grief in a culturally relevant manner.

✔ Clients are able to share their grief with each other.

NOC: *Family Coping*

INTERVENTIONS	RATIONALES
Assess stage of grief process, problems encountered, feelings regarding terminal nature of illness and potential loss of child.	Provides information about need for grieving, which varies with individual members of a family when child's death is expected.
Provide emotional and spiritual comfort in an accepting environment, and avoid conversations that cause guilt or anger.	Provides for emotional need of parents and family and helps them to cope with dying child without adding stressors that are difficult to resolve.
Provide opportunities for family to express feelings and respond to child commensurate with stage of grieving.	Promotes progression through grieving and ability to express desires for themselves and their child.

INTERVENTIONS	RATIONALES
Allow parents and family members to be with child as much as they feel a need to, and help them understand the child's behavior and needs.	Promotes feeling that they are helping and supporting their child.
Assist child and family in identifying and use effective coping mechanisms and in understanding situation over which they have no control.	Promotes effective coping that is positive for the family.
Provide privacy when needed, while being available to the family.	Promotes a helping relationship with the family.
Arrange for clergy, social services, hospice care, or return to home for dying as appropriate; support choices made by the family (specify).	Provides for and assists with alternative care and preferences for that care.
Encourage parents to express their thoughts and feelings about the possible death of their child; to share memories of their child's life; to create memories (now, if possible); to take family pictures, and create a memory box of their child's memory.	Promotes parent coping, acceptance of grief process, and may minimize sense of guilt.
Encourage parents to be involved with child's care (i.e., procedures, how to help with nausea, pain control).	Reduces parent feelings of powerlessness and helplessness.
Reassure child, parents, and family that their grief response is normal.	Promotes understanding of grief reaction and may enhance coping abilities.
Educate parents regarding child's developmental understanding of death; educate and encourage parents to utilize children's books to aid in a discussion about the child's understanding/fears of death.	Promotes family communication; promotes family coping abilities.
Inform (child, if appropriate) parents, and family of stages of grieving and acceptable behaviors during the grief process.	Promotes understanding of feeling and behaviors manifested by the grieving process.
Provide information about child's condition, including appearance of the child, and reactions to expect.	Allows parents to follow course of terminal condition and change to expect.

(continues)

(continued)

INTERVENTIONS	RATIONALES
Instruct parents in care and procedures they want to participate in and in those they will carry out if the child is taken home to die; suggest resources to contact for assistance.	Involves parents involvement in child's care and allows them to share their sadness with child.
Encourage family to ask questions and to be honest about their feelings and acceptance of information about death and dying.	Promotes honest and realistic view of situation to enhance grieving.
Teach family to maintain own needs and health during this difficult time.	Allows family to better cope with child's needs if own needs are fulfilled, since terminal period may be prolonged.

NIC: *Grief-Work Facilitation*

Evaluation

(Date/time of evaluation of goal)

(Has goal been met? Not met? Partially met?)

(Specify, e.g., parents and child are able to verbalize the grief process, use quotes; parents and child identify coping mechanisms to assist with grief work (specify); parents and child make decisions regarding care, death, and funeral.)

(Revisions to care plan? D/C care plan? Continue care plan?)

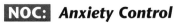 ANXIETY

Related to: Specify: diagnosis, tests, treatments, pain, side effects of medication and prognosis.

Defining Characteristics: (Specify, e.g., states: fear of death, loss of control, loneliness; increased feelings of helplessness and hopelessness; poor prognosis of terminal illness.)

Goal: Client will experience lessened anxiety by (date/time to evaluate).

Outcome Criteria

✔ Specify, e.g., child and parents verbalize decreased anxiety.

✔ Child and parents identify at least two coping mechanisms for anxiety.

NOC: *Anxiety Control*

INTERVENTIONS	RATIONALES
Assess anxiety level, fears and concerns, ability to express needs, and how anxiety is manifested.	Reveals information needed for interventions to relieve anxiety and increased comfort.
Ask clients to rank their anxiety as mild, moderate, severe, or incapacitating.	Ranking allows assessment of improved or worsening levels of anxiety.
Assist child and family to identify at least two coping mechanisms to use for coping with anxiety (specify suggestions such as music, exercise, talking to spiritual advisor, use of humor).	Coping mechanisms help relieve the stress of anxiety. Humor is not always out of place and may be helpful to diffuse tension if judiciously used.
Allow family friend to stay with child or remain with child during stressful periods if family not able to be there.	Promotes comfort of child and provides support during anxious and fearful times.
Allow expressions of fears and concerns about terminal stage of illness, answer all questions honestly based on what family has been told about prognosis.	Provides opportunity to vent feelings and fears to reduce anxiety.
Provide appropriate pain control and preparation prior to invasive procedures (specify, i.e., application of EMLA cream before bone marrow aspiration, or before restarting IV sites).	Promotes comfort and minimizes emotional distress related to invasive procedures (action of EMLA).
Provide calm reassurance and kindness, be available to child at all times as needed for support.	Promotes comfort and love of child to reduce anxiety.
Involve child and parents in as much planning and care as possible without forcing participation.	Promotes interactions and attitude of caring within family.
Inform child and parents of all anticipated care and activities.	Promotes understanding of physical needs of dying child, limiting activities to those that are essential.
Inform family members, with honesty and openness, of physical changes in child as death nears.	Prepares them for the changes and assists in the recognition of impending death.
Reassure child and parents that they are not to blame for illness and its consequences.	Reduces fear and guilt caused by terminal nature of the illness.
Encourage parents to talk to the child and sit or lie near the child as desired.	Reduces possibility of additional stress for child; reduces child's fear of being alone.

INTERVENTIONS	RATIONALES
Provide parents and family members telephone numbers and methods of acquiring information about the child.	Provides a source of communication about the child's condition.

NIC: *Anxiety Reduction*

Evaluation

(Date/time of evaluation of goal)

(Has goal been met? Not met? Partially met?)

(Specify, e.g., are parents and child able to verbalize lessened anxiety? use quotes. List coping mechanisms parents and child identified to assist with anxiety. Have parents and child made decisions regarding terminal illness?)

(Revisions to care plan? D/C care plan? Continue care plan?)

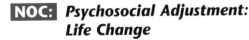 DYSFUNCTIONAL GRIEVING

Related to: Loss of child as result of (specify: accident, SIDS, absence of anticipatory grieving).

Defining Characteristics: (Specify: expressed distress; anger; guilt over loss; difficulty in expressing loss; sadness; crying; sudden, unexplained and unexpected death of infant; shock; grief; denial; social isolation.)

Goal: Parents will resolve dysfunctional grieving.

Outcome Criteria

✔ Parents verbalize understanding about the cause of the death (specify).

✔ Parents acknowledge that their grief is unresolved and seek assistance.

NOC: *Psychosocial Adjustment: Life Change*

INTERVENTIONS	RATIONALES
Assess feelings of parents and what they perceive happened to infant; listen to any feelings expressed.	Allows feelings of anger, guilt, and sorrow to be expressed following death of infant.

INTERVENTIONS	RATIONALES
Provide privacy and remain with parents; avoid conversation and questions that may place any blame or cause guilt; (explain cause of death; reinforce that the cause of SIDS is unknown, with no absolute means to prevent or predict it).	Provides support without adding to grief and feelings of guilt.
Prepare child for parents to view and hold; stay with parents during this experience.	Allows parents to say good-bye to their child.
Allow parent to determine the length of time they hold their infant or child; this varies by culture and individual parent needs.	Promotes positive grief resolution if parents hold/see the infant and spend time saying good-bye on their own terms.
Notify clergy or other support if requested; offer baptism/prayer to parents; arrange for clergy to be present, if applicable.	Provides support and comfort.
Provide parents the opportunity to call significant others; if unable, staff member should call.	Presence of other family members and significant others often serves as support for grieving family.
(Answer any questions about SIDS and explain need for autopsy to verify diagnosis.)	Reinforces physician's explanation of disorder.
Take pictures of infant and offer to parents; saving clothing infant was wearing, ID bracelets, hats, as part of a "memento packet" to be given to parents; if parents refuse packet, save for future retrieval (if appropriate).	Promotes positive grief resolution.
Assist parents to inform and help siblings understand loss; answer children's questions honestly and appropriately for age level.	Children's concept of death develops with age, and help is needed to avoid feelings of blame and guilt by siblings.
Assist to identify and use effective coping mechanisms applicable to situation.	Promotes movement through grieving process by utilizing defense mechanisms that have worked in the past.
Reassure parents that they are not responsible for the death of their child.	Reinforces that SIDS is an unpreventable, unexplainable sudden death of an infant and that no one can be blamed.
Obtain thorough history from parents, including parental resuscitation efforts and illness history (experienced or trained member of staff recommended because of sensitive nature of information).	Provides optimal level of accurate information for medical examiner.

(continues)

(continued)

INTERVENTIONS	RATIONALES
Contact the infant's primary care provider.	Enhances the parental support system and enhances communication.
Inform of stages and importance of grieving and of behavior that is expected in resolving grief.	Allows, in a nonjudgmental environment, for the initial shock and disbelief that are expected behaviors of grief.
Use therapeutic communication techniques, especially active listening. Encourage parents to verbalize their understanding of the cause of death, their feelings of grief, and any concerns about seeking assistance with grieving.	Therapeutic communication assists the parents to express their feelings and identify dysfunctional aspects of their grief.
Refer family to counseling services, local SIDS chapter, community health nursing agency, grief support groups.	Provides support and assistance during bereavement or chronic grief which may affect family relationships, presence of infertility or other problems.

INTERVENTIONS	RATIONALES
Correct any misinformation or misconceptions regarding the death.	Assists with resolution of guilt and grieving.

NIC: *Grief Work Facilitation*

Evaluation

(Date/time of evaluation of goal)

(Has goal been met? Not met? Partially met?)

(What are the parents' understandings about the cause of death? Did parents acknowledge their grief and seek assistance? Use quotes.)

(Revisions to care plan? D/C care plan? Continue care plan?)

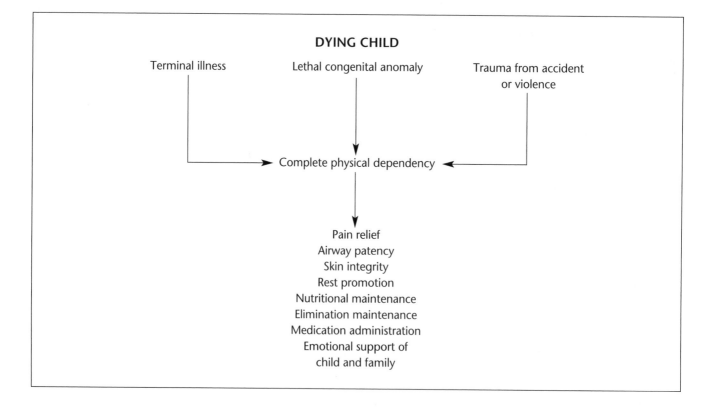

DYING CHILD

Terminal illness   Lethal congenital anomaly   Trauma from accident or violence

Complete physical dependency

Pain relief
Airway patency
Skin integrity
Rest promotion
Nutritional maintenance
Elimination maintenance
Medication administration
Emotional support of
child and family

UNIT 2

CARDIOVASCULAR SYSTEM

CHAPTER 2.0

CARDIOVASCULAR SYSTEM: BASIC CARE PLAN

The cardiovascular system consists of the heart and a network of blood vessels: arteries, veins, and capillaries. The heart is an efficient pumping mechanism that circulates oxygenated blood and nutrients to all parts of the body and provides a path for removal of wastes. Alteration in the function of the system may interfere with the client's well-being, thereby causing physical and psychosocial problems for both the affected child and family. Diseases of the cardiovascular system are classified as either congenital malformations or acquired disorders that result from infection, autoimmune responses, or environmental insult. The degree of alteration in function determines the acuity or chronicity of the condition, the interference with growth and development, and the preferred treatment.

Before birth, fetal structures allow the blood to bypass the nonfunctional lungs and circulate through the placenta for gas, nutrient, and waste exchange. Shortly after birth, fetal circulation converts to postnatal circulation, which continues throughout life.

CARDIOVASCULAR GROWTH AND DEVELOPMENT

HEART AND BLOOD VESSEL STRUCTURE

- Circulation changes at birth involve the closure of the fetal shunts (foremen ovale at birth, ductus arteriosus by the fourth day after birth, and eventually the ductus venosus).
- Size of the heart in the infant is large in relation to total body size and occupies more space in the chest surrounded by the lungs.
- The heart lies at a transverse angle in infancy and gradually changes to a lower and more oblique angle as the lungs grow until maturity is reached.

- The weight of the heart doubles by 1 year of age, and increases four times by 5 years of age.
- The walls of the ventricle are of equal thickness at birth but become thicker on the left side as the demand of peripheral circulation increases.
- Arteries and veins become longer as the body grows, and the walls of the vessels thicken as blood pressure increases.
- The apical pulse is located laterally and to the left of the fourth intercostal space and to the right of the midclavicular line in infants and small children; it changes laterally to the left of the fifth intercostal space and midclavicular line after 7 years of age; the point of maximal intensity (PMI) may be noted at these same areas.

CARDIOVASCULAR ASSESSMENT

- Blood pressure increases and pulse decreases with growth in heart size.
- Heart rate (pulse), resting and awake:

1 to 3 months:	100 to 180/min
3 months to 2 years:	80 to 120/min
2 to 4 years:	80 to 110/min
4 to school-aged:	75 to 100/min
Adolescents:	60 to 90/min

- Pulse pressure: 10 to 15 mm Hg during infancy; 20 to 50 mm Hg throughout childhood.
- Blood pressure (varies with age and position):

	Systolic (average)	Diastolic (average)
Infant	65 to 90 mm Hg	55 to 56 mm Hg
1 to 5 years	90 to 95 mm Hg	54 to 56 mm Hg
5 to 10 years	14 to 102 mm Hg	56 to 62 mm Hg
Over 10 years	102 to 121 mm Hg	62 to 70 mm Hg

COMMON NURSING DIAGNOSES

DECREASED CARDIAC OUTPUT

Related to: Mechanical factors—alterations in preload; alterations in afterload; alterations in inotropic function of heart.

Defining Characteristics: Variations in hemodynamic readings (BP, CVP); hypovolemia; jugular vein distention; oliguria; decreased peripheral pulses; cold, clammy skin; crackles; dyspnea (specify).

Related to: Electrical factors—alterations in rate; alterations in rhythm; alterations in conduction.

Defining Characteristics: Arrhythmias, ECG changes, bradycardia, changes in contractility resulting from preload or afterload abnormalities (specify).

Related to: Structural factors.

Defining Characteristics: Murmurs, fatigue, cyanosis, pallor of skin and mucous membranes, dyspnea, clubbing, activity intolerance (specify).

Goal: Client will experience increased cardiac output by (specify date and time to evaluate).

Outcome Criteria

✔ Client's BP, heart rate, and respirations will return to or remain within (specify appropriate ranges for each).

✔ Absence of cardiac dysrhythmias.

✔ Skin color and mucous membranes pink; tolerates activity (specify level).

NOC: *Cardiac Pump Effectiveness*

INTERVENTIONS	RATIONALES
Assess cardiac output by monitor—heart rate (apical and peripheral pulses) for 1 minute, noting quality, rate, rhythm, intensity; pulse deficiency; use radial site with gentle palpation in child over 2 years of age, and use apical site with stethoscope and correct size diaphragm in infant and young child; grade pulse on a range from 0 to +4 (specify).	Cardiac output is the amount of blood pumped from the heart in 1 minute and is determined by multiplying the heart rate by the stroke volume (amount of blood ejected with 1 contraction), which depends on heart contractility, preload and afterload; pulse easily obliterated by compression.

INTERVENTIONS	RATIONALES
Assess blood pressure using proper size cuff; diaphragm on stethoscope of proper size; and aneroid or mercury instrument, Doppler method, or electronic device. Approximate cuff width sizes are 4 to 6 cm for infant, 8 to 9 cm for child 2 to 10 years of age; BP cuff bladder should completely encircle extremity circumference and cuff width should cover 2/3 of upper arm/thigh. Take BP of infant with infant supine; take child BP with child sitting and arm supported at heart level; sites for BP determinations may be (radial), leg (popliteal), or ankle (dorsalis pedis) (specify).	Doppler method transmits audible sounds through a transducer in the cuff caused by ultrasound frequency caused by blood flow in the artery; the use of oscillometry transmits pressure changes through the arterial wall to the pressure cuff which are detected by an indicator that prints out the readings for BP and pulse.
Assess BP when infant/child is at rest (give expected range).	Crying or other activity can increase BP 5 to 10 mm Hg; BP elevations that are considered abnormal are: >110/70 in 3 to 6 year olds, >120/75 in 6 to 9 year olds, and >130/80 in 10 to 13 year olds.
Assess existence of dysrhythmias per ECG tracings.	Device that measures and records the heart's electrical activity and provides information about heart rate and rhythm, hypertrophy, effects of electrolyte imbalances, conduction problems and cardiac ischemia.
Administer cardiac (specify drug, dose, route, and times as ordered) glycosides, vasodilators; monitor for digoxin toxicity by symptoms of anorexia, nausea, vomiting, bradycardia, arrhythmias and digoxin level within 0.8 to 2.0 mcg/L range (therapeutic level) potassium level; take apical pulse for 1 minute before administering digoxin, and withhold if pulse below desired level for age of child.	Vasodilators decrease pulmonary and systemic vascular resistance, which decrease afterload and BP; cardiac glycoside strengthens and decreases the heart rate, which decreases the workload of the heart by more efficient cardiac performance; decreased potassium level enhances risk for digoxin toxicity.
Position for comfort and chest expansion in Fowler's, provide quiet environment, pace any activity to allow for rest.	Promotes ease of breathing and rest; reduces stress and workload of the heart.

(continues)

(continued)

INTERVENTIONS	RATIONALES
Monitor temperature for increases q 4 hours.	Pulse increased at rate of 8 to 10/minute with every degree of elevation on F scale.
Attach cardiac monitor to infant/child if prescribed.	Reveals changes in heart rate and respirations.
Inform about heart condition's effect on pulse and blood pressure, and the need for rest and reduction of stress.	Provides information to promote compliance with medical regimen and realization of importance of reducing workload of the heart.
Instruct in correct taking of peripheral and apical pulses and when to take them.	Encourages caretaker, parents to correctly monitor changes in heart function.
Instruct in administration of cardiac glycoside (specify form, dosage, how to take, frequency and time of day), to give 1 hour before or after feedings and not with food, to avoid second dose if child vomits, to avoid making up missed doses when less than 4 hours have passed, and to maintain careful records of administration and effects or adverse signs/symptoms.	Ensures correct administration of cardiac glycoside to prevent toxicity and improve cardiac performance.
Inform to report changes in pulse, blood pressure, digoxin toxicity, change in breathing pattern, edema, presence of infection.	Allows for prompt treatment to prevent complications like dysrhythmias or heart failure.
Instruct in application, settings and alarms in use of cardiac monitor.	Monitoring may be advised and prescribed for cardiac and respiratory changes.

NIC: *Cardiac Care*

Evaluation

(Date/time of evaluation of goal)

(Has goal been met? Not met? Partially met?)

(What are BP, heart rate, and respirations?)

(Describe cardiac rhythm.)

(What color are skin and mucous membranes? What activity does the child tolerate?)

(Revisions to care plan? D/C care plan? Continue care plan?)

EXCESS FLUID VOLUME

Related to: Compromised regulatory mechanisms.

Defining Characteristics: (Specify: periorbital usually but may be dependent on weight gain, effusion, shortness of breath, orthopnea, crackles, change in respiratory pattern dyspnea, tachypnea, oliguria, specific gravity changes, altered electrolytes.

Goal: Client will return to a state of fluid balance by (date/time to evaluate).

Outcome Criteria

✔ Intake equals output.

✔ Lung sounds clear.

✔ Absence of periorbital edema.

✔ (Specify others if appropriate for client.)

NOC: *Fluid Balance*

INTERVENTIONS	RATIONALES
Assess presence of edema in periorbital tissue or dependent areas, such as extremities when standing; in sacrum and scrotum when in lying position; or generalized in an infant; neck vein distension in child (specify frequency).	Increased sodium and water retention result in increased systemic vascular pressure and fluid overload, which lead to edema; gravity determines the site of dependent edema.
Weigh (specify: daily BID or as needed) on same scale, at same time, and with same clothing.	Weight gain from fluid retention is an early sign of fluid retention.
Assess for plueral effusion by presence of dyspnea, tachypnea, crackles, orthopnea, acites; for hepatomegaly by measuring abdominal girth (specify frequency).	Indication of gross fluid retention which causes impaired organ function (pulmonary and system venous congestion) is associated with some cardiac or renal conditions.
Assess for oliguria, increased specific gravity, electrolyte imbalances.	Indicates decreased renal perfusion, which activates the renin-angiotensin and aldosterone mechanism, resulting in water, sodium, and potassium retention.
Administer diuretic therapy early in the day (specify drug, dose, route, and times for client), and monitor resulting diuresis by accurate I&O and weight.	Diuretics prevent reabsorption of water, sodium and potassium by tubules in the kidneys, resulting in excretion of excess.

INTERVENTIONS	RATIONALES
Note and document I&O (including losses from breathing and diaphoresis) and intake from all fluids IV or orally taken with medications and meals (if child not toilet trained, weigh diaper to calculate output at 1 gm = 1 ml).	Intake and output ratio should normally be 2:1 or 1 to 2 ml/kg/h.
Restrict fluid intake as ordered (specify amount calculated for this child); schedule over 24 hours with most given during the day hours; use small cups and allowing older child to keep track of daily amounts.	Supports possible need for additional loss of fluid based on age and using possible limit of 65 ml/kg/24 hrs as a guideline.
Limit sodium intake as ordered by removing salt shaker, foods high in salt.	Sodium intake is necessary for normal growth and development, and to offset diuretic therapy.
Maintain bed rest, and position and support edematous body parts; change position (q 2h or specify) provide sheepskin, eggcrate mattress.	Protects and supports edematous parts from pressure and trauma.
Instruct caregiver in taking weights, noting and reporting gains and losses; and in measuring I&O, and reporting excessive outputs from diuretic therapy or decreases in comparison or intake.	Monitors weight to determine fluid accumulation and I&O to prevent imbalances (fluid overload or dehydration).
Instruct caregiver in correct administration of diuretic early in the day for a child (specify amount, frequency, side effects, and amount of output to expect in relation to intake).	Promotes excretion of fluid to prevent accumulation.
Instruct and assist caregiver to schedule fluid intake over 24 hours, with major portion administered during day hours.	Promotes compliance if fluids are restricted.

NIC: *Fluid Management*

Evaluation

(Date/time of evaluation of goal)

(Has goal been met? Not met? Partially met?)

(Specify intake and output and time frame.)

(Are lung sounds clear?)

(Is there any periorbital edema?)

(Provide data released to other outcomes criteria that were identified.)

(Revisions to care plan? D/C care plan? Continue care plan?)

INEFFECTIVE TISSUE PERFUSION: (CARDIOPULMONARY, CEREBRAL, GASTROINTESTINAL, RENAL, PERIPHERAL)

Related to: Interruption of arterial or venous flow, exchange problems, hypovolemia.

Defining Characteristics: (Specify: Cardiopulmonary—BP and pulse changes, dyspnea, tachypnea, changes in ABGs, cyanosis, changes in cardiac output, ventilation perfusion imbalances, crackles;

Cerebral—changes in mentation, restlessness, lethargy;

Gastrointestinal—vomiting, inability to digest and absorb nutrients, gastric distention;

Renal—oliguria, anuria, periorbital edema, electrolyte imbalance;

Peripheral—skin cold, mottled, or pale; decreased peripheral pulses).

Goal: Client will exhibit effective tissue perfusion by (date/time to evaluate).

Outcome Criteria

✔ Based on specific defining characteristics. Specify for client: (ABG values—specify ranges).

✔ Client is alert, not restless or lethargic.

✔ Bowel sounds present, abdomen soft, non-distended.

✔ Urine output > (specify cc/hr).

✔ Skin warm, pink, and dry, without edema.

NOC: *Tissue Perfusion*

INTERVENTIONS	RATIONALES
Assess organ functional abilities in relation to disease and its effect on a particular system (specify how).	Interrelationships of systems cause an overlapping of signs and symptoms associated with tissue perfusion causing changes in elimination, oxygenation, nutrition, and mental function.

(continues)

(continued)

INTERVENTIONS	RATIONALES
Assess pulse, blood pressure, presence of peripheral pulses, capillary refill time, skin color and temperature; oxygenation saturation as measured by pulse oximetry; urinary output, mentation, anorexia, gastric distention (specify when).	Provides information about cardiac output, which, if decreased, will reduce blood flow and tissue perfusion.
Provide O$_2$ by hood, cannula, or face mask, depending on age and at rate determined by ABGs as ordered (specify route and rate).	Provides oxygen to organs for proper functioning.
Administer vasodilator, cardiac glycoside as ordered (specify drugs, doses, routes, and times).	Promotes cardiac output and slows and strengthens heart rate for a more efficient pump action and increased return flow of blood to the heart and decreased heart workload
Position change q 2–4h (specify) to avoid pressure on susceptible body parts, perform ROM if needed.	Promotes circulation and prevents breakdown of tissue from further perfusion decreases associated with pressure.
Position in Fowler's at height of comfort if respiratory status compromised by pulmonary perfusion.	Decreases blood volume returning to heart by pooling of blood in lower dependent parts of the body.
Inform caregiver of causes of decreased circulation and its effect on body organs.	Promotes understanding of condition and risk to organ function.

INTERVENTIONS	RATIONALES
Demonstrate positions that enhance comfort and circulation, such as cardiac chair or infant seat (specify), which alleviate pressure on body parts; use of pillows to maintain Fowler's position.	Promotes comfort and prevents tissue breakdown.
Inform caregiver to avoid tight and restrictive clothing, such as belts, elastic waists on pajamas, diapers.	Constricts circulation.

NIC: *Cardiac Care*

Evaluation

(Date/time of evaluation of goal)

(Has goal been met? Not met? Partially met?)

(What are ABG values?)

(Is client alert, not restless or lethargic?)

(Are bowel sounds present? Is abdomen soft and nondistended?)

(Specify cc/hr of urine output/time frame.)

(Is skin warm, pink, and dry, without edema?)

(Revisions to care plan? D/C care plan? Continue care plan?)

CHAPTER 2.1

CARDIAC CATHETERIZATION

Cardiac catheterization is the insertion of a flexible catheter through a blood vessel (most often the femoral vein) into the heart for diagnostic and therapeutic purposes. It is usually combined with angiography when radiopaque contrast media is injected through the catheter and circulation is visualized on fluoroscopic monitors. Catheterization allows measurement of blood gases and pressures within chambers and great vessels; measurement of cardiac output; and detection of anatomic defects such as septal defects or obstruction to blood flow. Therapeutic, or interventional, cardiac catheterizations use balloon angioplasty to correct such defects as stenotic valves or vessels, aortic obstruction (particularly recoarctation of the aorta), and closure of patent ductus arteriosus.

MEDICAL CARE

Chest X-ray: to determine condition of lung fields and cardiac size.

ECG: to detect any cardiac conduction changes or abnormalities.

Complete Blood Count: to provide baseline data and ensure the child is not in an infectious state.

Blood Coagulation Time: to provide baseline data for comparison after the procedure.

Type and Cross-match: obtained for interventional cardiac catheterizations as risk of hemorrhage is greater; not usually obtained for diagnostic procedures.

Analgesics: precatheterization sedation given on-call to the catheterization laboratory.

Intravenous Fluids: IV access is essential for additional medications during catheterization and may be started on the nursing unit or after arrival at the laboratory. Ringer's lactate or 5% Ringer's lactate are routine.

COMMON NURSING DIAGNOSES

See DEFICIENT FLUID VOLUME

Related to: NPO status, blood loss during the catheterization, and diuretic effect of the contrast media.

Defining Characteristics: Elevated temperature, increased heart rate and respiratory rate, decreased blood pressure, decreased skin turgor, pallor, dry mucous membranes (specify).

See PAIN

Related to: Percutaneous puncture site, numerous needle sticks from local anesthesia during procedure, positioning during procedure.

Defining Characteristics: Crying, guarding or refusal to move, verbal expression of pain, increased heart rate and respiratory rate. Cardiac catheterization is described by most children as painful, but there should be minimal pain postcatheterization (puncture site described as sore). Severe pain needs further investigation (specify).

ADDITIONAL NURSING DIAGNOSES

FEAR

Related to: Invasive, painful procedure, risk of harm, separation from parents, fear of needles, and fear of exposure.

Defining Characteristics: (Specify: Apprehension, expressed concern over impending procedure. In children: increased motor activity, inattention, withdrawal, crying, clinging to parent(s), verbal protests).

Goal: Child (and parents) will exhibit decreased anxiety by (date/time to evaluate).

Outcome Criteria

✔ Child will not cry, cling to parents, or protest.

✔ Parent(s) will verbalize decreased anxiety/concern.

NOC: *Anxiety Control*

INTERVENTIONS	RATIONALES
Assess parents' and child's understanding of catheterization and any special fears.	Provides information on parents' and child's knowledge, misunderstanding and particular concerns; sources of anxiety for the parents include fear and uncertainty over the procedure, fear of complications, guilt and anxiety over the child's pain, and uncertainty over the outcome; for the child, fears may include: fear of mutilation and death, separation from parents, fear of the unknown (if the first catheterization), or remembered fear and pain (if repeat catheterization).
Allow expression of fears, clarify any misconceptions or lack of knowledge.	Allows parents and child to express feelings and provides them correct, complete information.
Encourage the child to take along a familiar, comforting item (specify stuffed animal, pillow, taped music).	A familiar object provides comfort and security to the child experiencing unfamiliar events and surroundings.
Encourage parents to accompany child and be with child immediately following the procedure.	Children cope with stressful events best when in the presence of their parents.
Prepare the child using age-appropriate guidelines; (specify) use concrete explanations just prior to an event for younger children. Include information on what the child will experience through all senses (sights, smells, sounds, feel).	Age-appropriate information given to the child allows for greater understanding and reassurance; young children process information through all their senses and need to know what to expect to better cope.
Explain reason for each pre- and postcatheterization procedure.	Knowledge of rationale for all treatments provides greater understanding and acceptance.
Inform parents that the child may temporarily act differently at home: may need to stay close to parents, have nightmares, and be less independent; encourage parents to comfort and reassure child, to allow child to "re-live"	Stressful events may cause the child to need extra reassurance and may cause a temporary regression in development as the child reverts to comfortable, familiar "safe" activities; children, like adults, have a need to replay

INTERVENTIONS	RATIONALES
the experience through stories or play, and to accept temporary setbacks in development.	stressful events in order to understand and cope, and this is often accomplished through play activities.
Inform parents about, and demonstrate how to care for the child's catheterization site; leave Steri-Strips in place until they fall off, do not place child in a tub bath for 3 days; immediately report any bleeding, bruising, redness or swelling to physician.	Information provides parents the knowledge they need to feel comfortable and confident in caring for their child.

NIC: *Anxiety Reduction*

Evaluation

(Date/time of evaluation of goal)

(Has goal been met? Not met? Partially met?)

(Describe child's behavior: does child cry, cling to parents, or protest?)

(Specify what parents said to indicate decreased anxiety/concern; use quotes whenever possible.)

(Revisions to care plan? D/C care plan? Continue care plan?)

RISK FOR INJURY

Related to: Altered hemostasis and trauma from percutaneous puncture.

Defining Characteristics: Increased apical heart rate and decreased blood pressure, bleeding from catheterization site, bruising, decreased level of consciousness (specify).

Goal: Child will not experience injury by (date and time to evaluate).

Outcome Criteria

✔ No bleeding from puncture site.

✔ BP and heart rate remain within (specify ranges appropriate for child).

NOC: *Risk Control*

INTERVENTIONS	RATIONALES
Obtain baseline laboratory values from precatheterization assessment.	Provides comparative data for postcatheterization assessment.

INTERVENTIONS	RATIONALES
Assess vital signs (apical HR, respiratory rate and BP) every 15 minutes × 4, every 30 minutes × 3 hours, then every 4 hours.	Changes in vital signs may indicate blood loss and with internal bleeding may be the first indicator of problems.
Maintain pressure dressing on catheterization site and check every 30 minutes for bleeding. If bleeding does occur, apply continuous direct pressure 1″ above puncture site and notify physician immediately.	Constant pressure on site is needed to prevent bleeding; no bleeding, even oozing, should occur.
Maintain bed rest for 6 hours postcatheterization as ordered.	Bed rest prevents strain to catheterization site which otherwise might precipitate bleeding; a 45-degree head elevation and slight bend at the knees are acceptable; young children may be held by parents: this is beneficial in decreasing agitation.
Inform parents and child of need for frequent assessments and for bed rest.	Promotes understanding and cooperation.
Encourage parents and child to engage in quiet activities (i.e., reading stories, music).	Allows for expression and interaction without physical stress; provides distraction for comfort.
Encourage parents of infants and young children to hold their children as an acceptable alternative to resting in bed.	Allows parents to touch and comfort their child in a more normal manner; this decreases the child's agitation, thereby promoting more rest.
Instruct parents to immediately report any sign of bleeding. Teach parents that pressure dressing will be removed after 24 hours and that they should continue to monitor the site and report to the physician if any bleeding is seen.	Increases close monitoring of the site.

NIC: *Bleeding Precautions*

Evaluation

(Date/time of evaluation of goal)

(Has goal been met? Not met? Partially met?)

(Is there any bleeding from puncture site?)

(Specify child's BP and heart rate.)

(Revisions to care plan? D/C care plan? Continue care plan?)

INEFFECTIVE TISSUE PERFUSION: PERIPHERAL

Related to: Clot formation at puncture site.

Defining Characteristics: Cool, mottled appearance of involved extremity, decreased or absent pulses distal to catheterization site, pain, tingling or numbness in involved extremity (specify).

Goal: Child will experience adequate peripheral tissue perfusion.

Outcome Criteria

✔ Affected extremity will be pink and warm.

✔ Pulses present distal to the catheterization site and equal bilaterally.

✔ Child responds to sensation in extremities equally bilaterally.

NOC: *Tissue Perfusion: Peripheral*

INTERVENTIONS	RATIONALES
Assess temperature, color and capillary refill of affected extremity and assess distal pulses by palpation and Doppler every 15 minutes × 4, every 30 minutes × 3 hours, then every 4 hours.	Clots form at puncture site and the child is at risk of the clots seriously obstructing distal blood and resulting in tissue damage. Assessing the extremity frequently for adequate perfusion allows for early intervention as needed.
Maintain bed rest with extremity straight or slight bend in knee (10 degrees) for 6 hours.	Bed rest and slight, or no flexion, allows for greater blood flow and decreases risk of further trauma which could increase clot formation.
Apply warmth to the opposite extremity.	Improves circulation without causing risk of increased bleeding at site.
Inform parents and child of need for frequent assessment of vital signs and need for bed rest with extremity extension.	Promotes understanding and cooperation.
Teach parents and child to avoid tub baths for three days after procedure.	May help decrease risk of infection.

NIC: *Bleeding Precautions*

Evaluation

(Date/time of evaluation of goal)

(Has goal been met? Not met? Partially met?)

(Describe pulses distal to the catheterization site and compared to other extremity.)

(Describe how child responds to sensation in extremities bilaterally.)

(Revisions to care plan? D/C care plan? Continue care plan?)

HYPERTHERMIA

Related to: Reaction to radiopaque contrast material used in catheterization.

Defining Characteristics: Elevated body temperature (specify) within a few hours of procedure.

Goal: Child will not be hyperthermic by (date and time to evaluate).

Outcome Criteria

✔ Child's axillary temperature will be <100° F.

NOC: *Thermoregulation*

INTERVENTIONS	RATIONALES
Assess body temperature every hour × 6 hours and then routine (specify route).	Provides information on which action to take.
Continue IV fluids (specify) while child is drowsy, and when fully awake, encourage PO intake (specify fluids).	Increased fluid intake promotes more rapid excretion of the dye.
Administer age-appropriate dose of acetaminophen every 4 hours (specify dose).	Acetaminophen will help decrease fever and associated discomfort.
Record hourly I&O.	Assesses routine adequacy of fluid intake and elimination.
Instruct parents to encourage PO fluids.	Involving parents in care increases the likelihood of achieving the goal.
Teach parents to take child's temperature and report any elevations after discharge.	Teaching empowers parents to care for child and helps monitor for hyperthermia.

NIC: *Fever Treatment*

Evaluation

(Date/time of evaluation of goal)

(Has goal been met? Not met? Partially met?)

(Specify child's temperature.) (Revisions to care plan? D/C care plan? Continue care plan?)

CHAPTER 2.2

CONGENITAL HEART DISEASE

Congenital heart disease results from malformations of the heart that involve the septums, valves, and large arteries. They are classified as acyanotic or cyanotic defects. Acyanotic defects occur when a left-to-right shunt is present that allows a mixture of oxygenated and unoxygenated blood to enter the systemic circulation. The most common consequences of these defects in children are growth retardation and congestive heart failure (CHF).

Common cyanotic defects include tetralogy of Fallot and transposition of the great vessels. Tetralogy of Fallot involves four defects that include pulmonic stenosis, ventricular septal defect, right ventricular hypertrophy, and an aorta that overrides the ventricular septal defect. Transposition of the great vessels is a condition in which the aorta arises from the right ventricle instead of the left ventricle, and the pulmonary artery arises from the left ventricle instead of the right ventricle, thereby causing a reversal of the normal position of these arteries. Transposition of the great vessels is incompatible with life unless septal defects are also present to allow mixing of blood from the two circulations.

Acyanotic defects include coarctation of aorta, patent ductus arteriosus, and ventricular septal defect. Coarctation of the aorta is the narrowing of the aorta proximal to the ductus arteriosus (preductal), distal to the ductus arteriosus (postductal), or level with the ductus arteriosus (auxtaductal). The position of the narrowing during fetal development determines circulation to the lower body and development of collateral circulation. Patent ductus arteriosus is the failure of the structure needed for fetal circulation to close after birth. Ventricular septal defect is the incomplete development of the septum that separates the right and left ventricles, and it often accompanies other defects.

Congenital heart defects vary in severity, symptoms, and complications, many of which depend on the age of the infant/child and the size of the defect. Treatment may include management with medications, open heart surgery to repair or resect, or to temporarily correct the defect until the child is older and growth takes place.

MEDICAL CARE

Diuretics: chlorothiazide (Diuril), spironolactone (Aldactone) PO, or furosemide (Lasix) PO or IV, depending on acuity of condition and need to promote fluid excretion by decreasing reabsorption of water, potassium, and sodium by the kidneys.

Cardiac Glycosides: digoxin (Lanoxin) tablets or elixir PO or IV-form; administered to prevent or treat congestive heart failure resulting from congenital heart defect by increasing the force of and decreasing the rate of cardiac contractions.

Antibiotics: penicillin G potassium (Pentids solution or tablets) PO, or erythromycin (Ilosone tablets, chewables, suspension) PO if patient is penicillin-sensitive as prophylaxis for bacterial endocarditis.

Prostaglandin Synthesis Inhibitors: indomethacin (Indocin) IV to close PDA.

Prostaglandin Hormones: alprostadil (Prostin VR Pediatric) IV to maintain open PDA when needed for blood flow.

Electrolytes: potassium chloride tablet (Klorvess), elixir (Pan-Kloride) PO as potassium replacement with use of diuretic therapy.

Chest X-ray: reveals cardiomegaly involving left side of heart, no enlargement depending on defect or cardiomegaly involving right ventricle, increased pulmonary blood flow or congested lungs, egg-shaped heart and narrowed mediastinum.

Electrocardiography (ECG): reveals abnormal changes associated with right ventricular and/or atrial hypertrophy, possible abnormal changes associated with left ventricular hypertrophy in older children, may not reveal any abnormality depending on specific defect; identifies arrhythmias.

Echocardiography (contrast, two-dimensional or real time, M-mode): reveals cardiomegaly, atrial or ventricular changes and location and size, great vessel location and size, valve function and any abnormalities or obstructions of the valves, increase in left atrial to aortic ratio, location of shunting in heart.

Doppler: reveals circulation abnormalities and congested lung areas, done with or without echocardiography.

Cardiac Catheterization: reveals abnormalities in communication between chambers, oxygen, and pressure levels in the chambers; location and number of septal defects.

Angiography: reveals cardiac defect by revealing detailed heart structure.

Electrolyte Panel: reveals possible decreased potassium and increased sodium.

Complete Blood Count (CBC): increased WBC with infection, decreased Hgb and Hct with anemia, increased RBC, decreased platelet count.

Prothrombin or Partial Thromboplastin Times (PT, APPT): reveals bleeding tendency and evaluates components of the blood-clotting mechanisms.

Blood Urea Nitrogen (BUN): reveals increase when heart is not able to perfuse kidneys.

Arterial Blood Gases (ABG): reveals decreased pH and PO_2 and increased PCO_2 resulting from changes in pulmonary blood flow.

Surgical Shunt: increases blood flow to the lungs for severely hypoxic newborns creating an artificial connection between the right or left subclavian artery and the pulmonary artery on the same side (modified Blalock-Taussig shunt).

COMMON NURSING DIAGNOSES

See DECREASED CARDIAC OUTPUT

Related to: Structural factors of congenital heart defect.

Defining Characteristics: Variations in hemodynamic readings (hypertension, bounding, pulses, tachycardia, specify values), ECG changes, arrhythmias, fatigue, dyspnea, oliguria, cyanosis or absence of cyanosis, murmur, decreased peripheral pulses,

widened pulse pressure, squatting or knee-chest position.

See INEFFECTIVE BREATHING PATTERN

Related to: Decreased energy and fatigue, pulmonary complications.

Defining Characteristics: Dyspnea, hypoxia (blue baby), tachypnea, abnormal ABGs, cyanosis (specify).

See IMBALANCED NUTRITION: LESS THAN BODY REQUIREMENTS

Related to: Inability to ingest, digest, or absorb nutrients because of biologic factors.

Defining Characteristics: Poor feeding, fatigue, slow growth, lack of interest in food, prolonged impaired cardiac function, decreasing perfusion to gastrointestinal organs (specify).

See DELAYED GROWTH AND DEVELOPMENT

Related to: Effects of acute or chronic illness or disability (specify).

Defining Characteristics: Altered physical growth, delay or difficulty in performing motor or social skills typical of age, dependence and isolation (specify).

ADDITIONAL NURSING DIAGNOSES

ACTIVITY INTOLERANCE

Related to: Generalized weakness.

Defining Characteristics: (Specify: presence of circulatory/respiratory problem, verbal complaint of fatigue or weakness, needs to rest after short period of play.)

Related to: Imbalance between oxygen supply and demand.

Defining Characteristics: Abnormal heart rate or blood pressure response to activity, exertional dyspnea (specify).

Goal: Child will tolerate increased activity.

Outcome Criteria

✔ (Specify for this child the activity level that is optimal within the limitations of the congenital heart disease.)

NOC: *Activity Tolerance*

INTERVENTIONS	RATIONALES
Assess level of fatigue, ability to perform ADL and other activities in relation to severity of condition.	Provides information about energy reserves and response to activity.
Assess dyspnea on exertion, skin color changes during rest and when active.	Indicates hypoxia and increased oxygen need during energy expenditure.
Allow for rest periods between care; disturb only when necessary for care and procedures.	Promotes rest and conserves energy.
Avoid allowing infant to cry for long periods of time, use soft nipple for feeding; cross-cut nipple; if unable for infant to ingest sufficient calories by mouth, gavage-feed infant.	Conserves energy. Cross-cut nipple requires less energy for infant to feed.
Provide toys and games for quiet play and diversion appropriate for age of child (specify), allow to limit own activities as much as possible.	Promotes growth, diversion, and physical and mental development.
Provide neutral environmental temperature; when bathing infant, expose only the area being bathed and keep the infant covered to prevent heat loss.	Avoids hot or cold extremes which increase oxygen and energy needs.
Explain to parents need to conserve energy and encourage rest.	Avoids fatigue.
Inform of activity or exercise restrictions and to set own limits for exercise and activity (specify for child).	Prevents fatigue while engaging in activities as nearly normal as possible.
Inform to request assistance when needed for daily activities.	Prevents overtiring and fatigue.
Assist parents to plan for care and rest schedule.	Provides for rest and prevents overexertion, minimizes energy expenditure.

NIC: *Cardiac Precautions*

Evaluation

(Date/time of evaluation of goal)

(Has goal been met? Not met? Partially met?)

(Describe child's ability to engage in the activity level that was specified as criteria.)

(Revisions to care plan? D/C care plan? Continue care plan?)

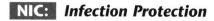 RISK FOR INFECTION

Related to: Chronic illness.

Defining Characteristics: Debilitated condition, IV-site contamination, susceptibility to bacterial endocarditis, immobility, change in VS (specify).

Goal: Child will not experience any infection by (date and time to evaluate).

Outcome Criteria

✔ Temperature <100° F

✔ Absence of inflammation of IV site: no swelling, redness, or increased tenderness.

NOC: *Risk Control*

INTERVENTIONS	RATIONALES
Assess temperature, IV site if present, increased WBC, increased pulse and respirations (specify when).	Provides information indicating potential infection.
Provide adequate rest and nutritional needs for age (specify for child).	Protects against potential infection by increasing body resistance and defenses.
Wash hands before giving care.	Prevents transmission of microorganisms to infant/child.
Avoid allowing those with infections to have contact with infant/child.	Prevents transmission of infectious agents to infant/child with compromised defense.
Administer antibiotics as ordered (specify drug, dose, route, and times).	Describe action of specific antibiotic ordered.
Use sterile technique for IV maintenance if present.	Prevents contamination, which causes infection.
Inform to avoid contact with those in family or friends that have an infection.	Infections are easily transmitted to a debilitated child.
Instruct parents and child in personal hygiene and practices (rest, nutrition, activity, bathroom for elimination, bathing).	Prevents reduced defenses or exposure to possible contaminants.

NIC: *Infection Protection*

Evaluation

(Date/time of evaluation of goal)

(Has goal been met? Not met? Partially met?)

(What is temperature?) (Describe assessment of IV site.)

(Revisions to care plan? D/C care plan? Continue care plan?)

▨ RISK FOR INJURY

Related to: Cardiac function compromised by congenital defects and medication administration.

Defining Characteristics: (Specify: digoxin toxicity (vomiting, dysrhythmia), hypokalemia (muscle weakness, hypotension, irritability, drowsiness), congestive heart failure (tachycardia, dyspnea fatigue, restlessness, cough, cyanosis, orthopnea, edema, weight gain, neck vein distention, decreased BP, cardiomegaly), hypoxemia, possible cardiac surgery.)

Goal: Child will not experience injury by (date/time to evaluate).

Outcome Criteria

✔ Specify, e.g., digoxin level <2.5 ng/mL.

✔ Parent correctly administers medications.

✔ Parent verbalizes signs and symptoms of complications to report (specify).

NOC: *Risk Control*

INTERVENTIONS	RATIONALES
Assess for risk of drug toxicity, cardiac complication of heart failure.	Early identification of signs and symptoms of complications allows preventive measures and adjustments to be made.
Monitor orders for diagnostic tests and procedures.	Allows for preparation and support of parents and infant/child.
Administer digoxin or indomethacin in correct dosages (specify), check dosages, take apical pulse for a full minute before administering digoxin, assess for drug responses.	Promotes safe administration of cardiotonic to decrease and strengthen heart rate (digoxin), or to promote closing of ductus (indomethacin).
Assist and support family's feelings and decision regarding surgery.	Provides needed support to allay anxiety and promote caring attitude.

INTERVENTIONS	RATIONALES
Instruct in administration of cardiotonic, taking apical pulse, when to withhold (less than 70–80 in child and 90–100 in infant), to notify physician of low pulse or irregular pulse, signs of toxicity.	Ensures safe and accurate administration of cardiac glycoside.
Prepare parents and child (use play doll) for diagnostic procedures and/or surgery; should be extensive, consistent, and comprehensive, including surgical procedure to be performed and expected results, prognosis and whether corrective, palliative, temporary, or permanent.	Assists in allaying anxiety and understanding that diagnostic tests are usually done before surgery.
Teach actions to take if child becomes cyanotic (knee-chest or squatting position, elevating head and chest), when to call physician.	Encourages calmness during attack and teaches actions that will relieve episode and associated fear.

NIC: *Medication Administration*

Evaluation

(Date/time of evaluation of goal)

(Has goal been met? Not met? Partially met?)

(What is digoxin level? Describe parent ability to administer medication safely. Did parent verbalize complications signs to report? Use quotes.)

(Revisions to care plan? D/C care plan? Continue care plan?)

▨ COMPROMISED FAMILY COPING

Related to: Situational and developmental crises of family and child.

Defining Characteristics: (Specify: family expresses concern and fear about infant/child's disease and condition, displays protective behavior disproportionate to need to grow and develop, chronic anxiety and possible hospitalization and surgery.)

Goal: Family will cope more effectively by (date/time to evaluate).

Outcome Criteria

✔ (Specify signs of increased development of coping skills with infant/child's illness and changes in family coping.)

NOC: *Family Coping*

INTERVENTIONS	RATIONALES
Observe for erratic behaviors (anger, tension, disorganization), perception of crisis situation.	Information affecting ability of family to cope with infant/child's cardiac condition.
Assess usual family coping methods and effectiveness.	Identifies need to develop new coping skills if existing methods are ineffective in changing behaviors exhibited.
Assess need for information and support.	Provides information about need for interventions to relieve anxiety and concern.
Encourage expression of feelings and provide factual information about infant/child.	Reduces anxiety and enhances family's understanding of condition.
Assist in identifying and using techniques to cope with and solve problems and gain control over the situation (specify).	Provides support for problem solving and management of situation.
Provide anticipatory guidance for crisis resolution and allow for grieving process.	Assists family in adapting to situation and developing new coping mechanisms.
Suggest and reinforce appropriate coping behaviors, support family decisions.	Promotes behavior change and adaptation to care of infant/child.
Teach that overprotective behaviors may hinder growth and development during infancy/childhood.	Knowledge will enhance family understanding of condition and of adverse effects of behaviors.
Encourage to maintain health of family members and social contacts.	Chronic anxiety, fatigue, and isolation as result of infant care will affect health and care capabilities of family.

INTERVENTIONS	RATIONALES
Teach family about the disease process and behaviors, physical effects, and symptoms of condition.	Relieves tension when they know what to expect.
Clarify any misinformation and answer questions regarding disease process.	Prevents unnecessary anxiety resulting from inaccurate knowledge or beliefs.
Encourage parents to include ill infant/child in family activities rather than family revolving around needs of infant/child.	Promotes normal growth and development of family and infant/child.
Encourage to maintain consistent behavior limits and modification techniques.	Prevents behavioral problems and child control over family, which interfere with child's growth and family relationships.
Instruct parents in nutritional and activity needs and/or limitations and approaches that will assist in establishing an effective pattern.	Assists in coping with effects and special needs of infant/child with cardiac defect.
Refer family for additional support and counseling if indicated (specify where to refer family).	Referral supplies more assistance with coping than is available from nursing personnel.

NIC: *Family Therapy*

Evaluation

(Date/time of evaluation of goal)

(Has goal been met? Not met? Partially met?)

(Describe increased coping skills of family.)

(Revisions to care plan? D/C care plan? Continue care plan?)

CONGENITAL HEART DISEASE

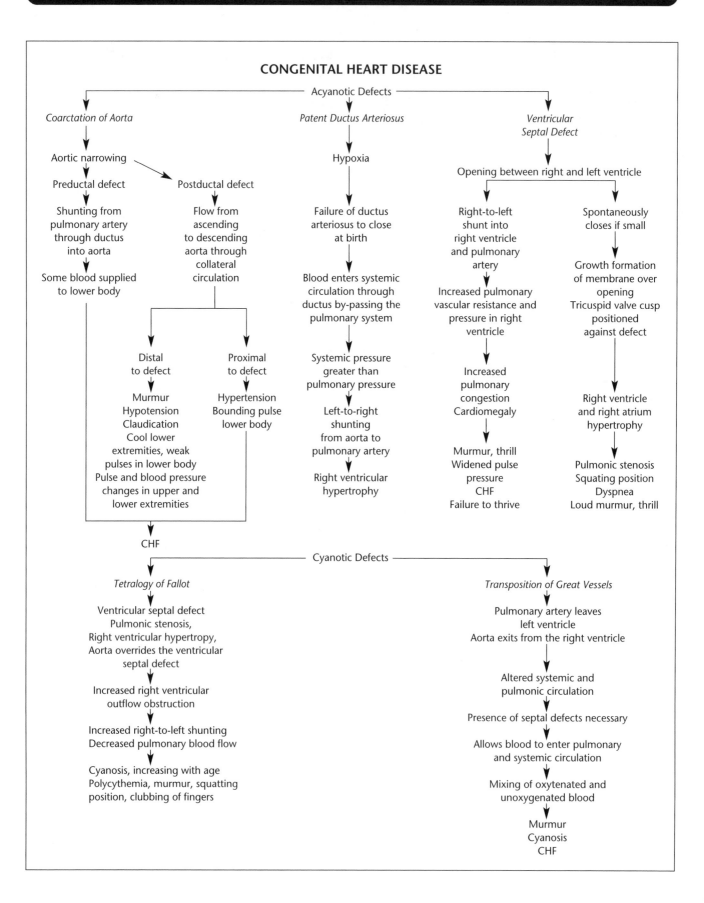

Acyanotic Defects

Coarctation of Aorta

Aortic narrowing

Preductal defect → Postductal defect

Shunting from pulmonary artery through ductus into aorta

Flow from ascending to descending aorta through collateral circulation

Some blood supplied to lower body

Distal to defect

Murmur
Hypotension
Claudication
Cool lower extremities, weak pulses in lower body
Pulse and blood pressure changes in upper and lower extremities

Proximal to defect

Hypertension
Bounding pulse lower body

CHF

Patent Ductus Arteriosus

Hypoxia

Failure of ductus arteriosus to close at birth

Blood enters systemic circulation through ductus by-passing the pulmonary system

Systemic pressure greater than pulmonary pressure

Left-to-right shunting from aorta to pulmonary artery

Right ventricular hypertrophy

Ventricular Septal Defect

Opening between right and left ventricle

Right-to-left shunt into right ventricle and pulmonary artery

Increased pulmonary vascular resistance and pressure in right ventricle

Increased pulmonary congestion
Cardiomegaly

Murmur, thrill
Widened pulse pressure
CHF
Failure to thrive

Spontaneously closes if small

Growth formation of membrane over opening
Tricuspid valve cusp positioned against defect

Right ventricle and right atrium hypertrophy

Pulmonic stenosis
Squating position
Dyspnea
Loud murmur, thrill

Cyanotic Defects

Tetralogy of Fallot

Ventricular septal defect
Pulmonic stenosis,
Right ventricular hypertropy,
Aorta overrides the ventricular septal defect

Increased right ventricular outflow obstruction

Increased right-to-left shunting
Decreased pulmonary blood flow

Cyanosis, increasing with age
Polycythemia, murmur, squatting position, clubbing of fingers

Transposition of Great Vessels

Pulmonary artery leaves left ventricle
Aorta exits from the right ventricle

Altered systemic and pulmonic circulation

Presence of septal defects necessary

Allows blood to enter pulmonary and systemic circulation

Mixing of oxytenated and unoxygenated blood

Murmur
Cyanosis
CHF

CHAPTER 2.3

CONGESTIVE HEART FAILURE

Congestive heart failure is the inability of the heart to maintain the workload necessary to pump blood throughout the circulatory system of the body because of ineffective contractions. In children, cardiac heart failure occurs as a result of changes associated with congenital heart defects, such as those resulting in left-to-right shunts (volume overload) or obstructive lesions within the heart (pressure overload), of cardiomyopathy affecting the myocardium or dysrhythmias (decreased contractility), or of disorders such as anemia or sepsis (high cardiac output needs). In infants and children, failure of one side of the heart generally causes failure in the other side. Normally, any predisposing problem that blocks the effective flow of blood causes the heart to respond by compensatory mechanisms that maintain the workload of the heart. Congestive heart failure occurs when the compensatory mechanisms are not able to maintain the workload of the heart, and the body tissues and organs are deprived of the oxygen and nutrients they need to function properly.

MEDICAL CARE

Diuretics: chlorothiazide (Diuril), spironolactone (Aldactone) PO, which promotes fluid excretion by acting on the distal and proximal tubules or blocks action of aldosterone to decrease water, sodium chloride, and potassium absorption; furosemide (Lasix) PO or IV for acute failure, which acts to block reabsorption of water and sodium in the proximal, distal tubules and loop of Henle.

Cardiac Glycosides: digoxin (Lanoxin) tablets or elixir PO or IV form, depending on treatment, for acute or maintenance therapy to increase the force of and decrease the rate of cardiac contractions. Digoxin has a narrow therapeutic serum level of 0.8 to 2.0 g/L.

Angiotensin-Converting Enzyme (ACE) Inhibitors: captopril (Capoten), enalapril (Vasotec), PO to inhibit conversion of angiotensin I to II by reducing the production of renin; ultimately the result is to reduce vasoconstriction and aldosterone secretion, which lowers blood pressure and the work of the heart.

Electrolytes: potassium chloride tablet (Klorvess), elixir (Pan-Kloride) PO as a potassium replacement with use of diuretic therapy.

Humidified Oxygen: relaxes pulmonary vasculature and decreases cardiac workload.

Analgesics/Sedatives: morphine sulfate SC or IV to relax smooth muscle.

Chest X-ray: for cardiac dilatation and hypertrophy.

Electrocardiography: reveals ventricular hypertrophy and arrhythmias.

Echocardiography: for abnormal valve function via ultrasound.

Digoxin Level: for serum level, to prevent toxicity, and regulate dosage.

Electrolyte Panel: for hypokalemia caused by diuretics or hyperkalemia resulting from K^+ supplements and/or Vasotec. May result in cardiac dysrhythmias.

Complete Blood Count: decreased Hgb and Hct in anemia.

Arterial Blood Gases: for decreased PO_2 and pH and increased PCO_2 leading to acidosis with pulmonary changes.

COMMON NURSING DIAGNOSES

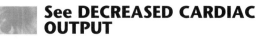 **See DECREASED CARDIAC OUTPUT**

Related to: Mechanical factors with alterations in (specify: preload, afterload, and inotropic changes in heart).

Defining Characteristics: (Specify: fatigue; oliguria; decreased peripheral pulses; pale, cool extremities; tachycardia; decreased BP; dyspnea, crackles.)

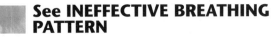
See INEFFECTIVE BREATHING PATTERN

Related to: Decreased lung expansion; pulmonary congestion.

Defining Characteristics: (Specify: dyspnea, tachypnea, orthopnea, cough, nasal flaring, respiratory depth changes, altered chest excursion, use of accessory muscles with retractions, abnormal arterial blood gases, wheezing, crackles, grunting, cyanosis.)

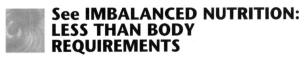
See FLUID VOLUME EXCESS

Related to: Compromised regulatory mechanisms.

Defining Characteristics: (Specify: edema [periorbital, peripheral], effusion, weight gain, dyspnea, orthopnea, crackles, blood pressure changes, oliguria, jugular vein distention, hepatomegaly, restlessness and anxiety, altered electrolytes, change in mental status.)

See IMBALANCED NUTRITION: LESS THAN BODY REQUIREMENTS

Related to: (Specify, e.g., fatigue.)

Defining Characteristics: (Specify, e.g., percentage of meals eaten, weight loss, weight percentile, laboratory values.)

See RISK FOR DEFICIENT FLUID VOLUME

Related to: Medication (diuretics).

Defining Characteristics: (Specify, give values: output greater than intake, weight loss, hypokalemia, hypernatremia.)

See INEFFECTIVE TISSUE PERFUSION: CARDIOPULMONARY, PERIPHERAL

Related to: Hypervolemia, prolonged cardiac failure

Defining Characteristics: (Specify: edema, dyspnea, change in color, temperature of extremities [mottled, cold], decreased peripheral pulses, effusion, changes in BP (specify), tachypnea, orthopnea, tachycardia, cough.)

ADDITIONAL NURSING DIAGNOSES

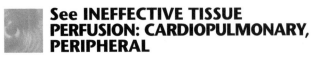
ANXIETY

Related to: (Specify: threat of death, threat of or change in health status, threat of change in environment [hospitalization].)

Defining Characteristics: (Specify: parent—increased apprehension that condition might worsen into life-threatening situation, increased concern and worry about possible hospitalization, increased tension and uncertainty, chronic worry. Child—unhappy and sad attitude; withdrawn or aggressive behavior; somatic and fatigue complaints; failure to thrive and participate in school, play, or social activities.)

Goal: Client will experience decreased anxiety by (date/time to evaluate).

Outcome Criteria

✔ (Specify, e.g., display relaxed facial features, engage in relaxation exercises, express feeling in control of anxiety.)

NOC: *Anxiety Control*

INTERVENTIONS	RATIONALES
Assess level and manifestations of anxiety in parents and child at each visit.	Provides information needed for interventions and clues to severity of anxiety.
Allow expression of fears and concerns and time to ask questions about disorder and what to expect.	Provides opportunity to vent feelings and secure information to reduce anxiety.
Provide supportive, nonjudgmental environment and individualized, consistent care.	Promotes trust and reduces anxiety.
Hold and cuddle infant when crying/tense.	Promotes comfort and security.
Inform parents and child of all procedures and treatments, anticipate needs.	Relieves anxiety caused by fear of the unknown.
Allow parents to stay and provide open visitation and telephone communication; encourage to participate in care and to plan care similar to usual home patterns.	Reduces anxiety by allowing presence and involvement in care and provides familiar persons and routine for child.

INTERVENTIONS	RATIONALES
Keep parents informed of changes in condition, progress made.	Promotes understanding and reduces anxiety about whether child is improving.
Explain why hospitalization became necessary (specify).	Promotes understanding of disorder and underlying disease that causes this complication.
Clarify any misinformation with simple, understandable language and honesty.	Promotes knowledge and prevents anxiety caused by inaccurate information or beliefs.
Instruct in signs and symptoms indicating possible heart failure (fatigue, tachycardia, anorexia, dyspnea, tachypnea) and measures to take (specify).	Provides information of what might be expected and what to report in order to allay anxiety.

NIC: *Anxiety Reduction*

Evaluation

(Date/time of evaluation of goal)

(Has goal been met? Not met? Partially met?)

(Did parent/child verbalize decreased anxiety? Describe facial tension; did parent/child do relaxation exercises? What did parent/child say about feeling in control? Use quotes whenever possible.)

(Revisions to care plan? D/C care plan? Continue care plan?)

ACTIVITY INTOLERANCE

Related to: Imbalance between oxygen supply and demand.

Defining Characteristics: (Specify: abnormal heart rate or blood pressure response to activity, exertional dyspnea, fatigue, weakness, respiratory/circulatory problem, provide data.)

Goal: Child will engage in tolerable levels of activity by (date/time to evaluate).

Outcome Criteria

✔ Engages in stimulating activities appropriate for developmental needs and energy level (specify). Balances periods of activity and rest.

✔ Controls level of activity to prevent fatigue or cardiac symptoms.

NOC: *Activity Tolerance*

INTERVENTIONS	RATIONALES
Assess level of fatigue, V/S, and responses to activity.	Provides information about change in vital signs and energy level.
Allow for rest periods between care, disturb only when necessary and then perform care and treatments during one period of time.	Promotes rest, conserves energy and reduces heart workload.
Avoid allowing infant to cry for long periods of time; use soft nipple with large opening for feeding and feed frequently, slowly, and in small amounts (specify).	Conserves energy and prevents fatigue.
Provide small, frequent meals for child.	Conserves energy.
Provide toys and quiet, age-appropriate play (specify).	Allows for play without depleting energy reserves.
Provide neutral environmental temperature.	Extremes of temperature increase oxygen and energy needs, which increase work of heart.
Explain reason for need to conserve energy and encourage rest.	Promotes compliance with activity restrictions.
Discuss activities allowed, type of play recommended, and rationale.	Prevents fatigue while still allowing activities as near normal as possible.
Assist in planning for rest and activity schedule.	Provides for rest, prevents over-exertion and symptoms, minimizes energy expenditure.
Inform of continued stimulation-type activities (visual, auditory, tactile, mental, and physical; Specify).	Promotes normal growth and development.

NIC: *Activity Therapy*

Evaluation

(Date/time of evaluation of goal)

(Has goal been met? Not met? Partially met?)

(Describe activity child engaged in; provide information about balance of activity and rest; describe how child controls activity in response to fatigue or cardiac symptoms.)

(Revisions to care plan? D/C care plan? Continue care plan?)

DEFICIENT KNOWLEDGE

Related to: Lack of information about disorder and treatments/care.

Defining Characteristics: (Specify: verbalization of need for information about disease, medications, dietary restrictions.)

Goal: Parents will gain knowledge about disorder and treatment by (date/time to evaluate).

Outcome Criteria

✔ Parents verbalize understanding of child's disorder, causes, and risk factors.

✔ Parents participate in treatment planning.

✔ Parents correctly administer medications to child.

✔ Parent verbalizes signs of medication side effects and signs of congestive heart failure to report.

NOC: *Knowledge: Diseases Process*

INTERVENTIONS	RATIONALES
Assess knowledge of disease, causes and methods to prevent or control condition, willingness and interest to implement care to reduce work of heart, ability and readiness to learn.	Promotes plan of instruction that is realistic to ensure compliance of medical regimen, prevents repetition of information.
Provide information about disorder causes and risk factors; use clear, understandable language, pictures, pamphlets, models, video tapes, anatomic doll in teaching (specify).	Ensures understanding and aids in reinforcement of learning.
Teach to plan menus that include sodium restriction, fluids if prescribed, additional calories (specify for child).	Allows input, control over planning for sodium; fluid restriction may be needed to prevent fluid retention; additional calories provided for higher metabolic needs.

INTERVENTIONS	RATIONALES
Teach about administration of cardiac glycosides and diuretics, including dosage, frequency, route, side effects to report, expected results (specify).	Ensures correct administration of drugs to prevent heart failure and drug toxicity.
Instruct in taking pulse for 1 minute and allow return demonstration.	Apical pulse taken before administration of cardiac glycoside.
Discuss effects of disorder on infant/child (growth and physical development).	Disorder slows growth and development for age.
Teach to report infection or changes in breathing, pulse, irritability, restlessness, edema, temperature (increase), or weight.	Reduction in body defenses predisposes to infectious process, signs and symptoms reported to prevent progressive heart failure.
Ask parent to verbalize or return-demonstrate all teaching that has been done.	Parents may be overwhelmed with too much information. Allows the nurse to identify areas for additional instruction.
Provide additional written or video information for parents.	Allows parent to review information at home; allows for varied learning styles.

NIC: *Teaching: Disease Process*

Evaluation

(Date/time of evaluation of goal)

(Has goal been met? Not met? Partially met?)

(Did parents verbalize understanding of child's disorder, causes, and risk factors? Did parents participate in treatment planning? Do parents correctly administer medications? Can parent verbalize signs of medication side effects and signs of congestive heart failure to report?)

(Revisions to care plan? D/C care plan? Continue care plan?)

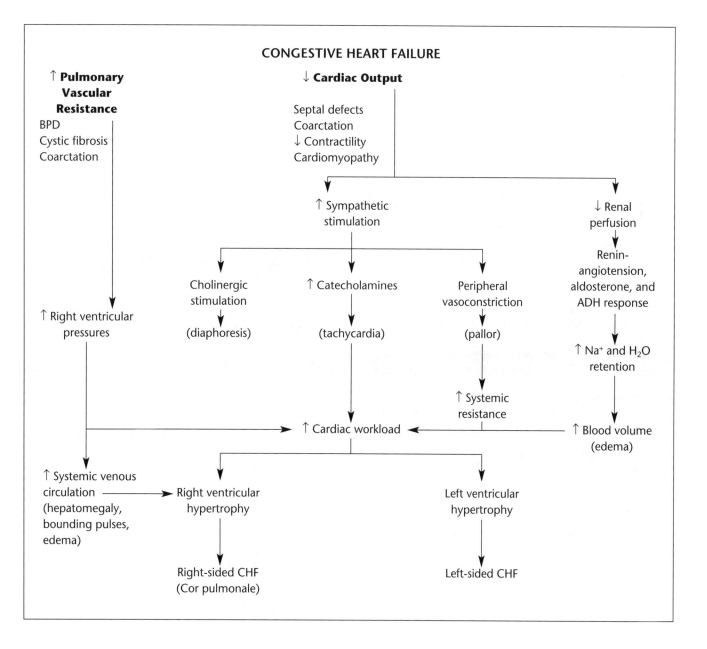

CONGESTIVE HEART FAILURE

↑ **Pulmonary Vascular Resistance**

BPD
Cystic fibrosis
Coarctation

↓ **Cardiac Output**

Septal defects
Coarctation
↓ Contractility
Cardiomyopathy

↑ Sympathetic stimulation

↓ Renal perfusion

Renin-angiotension, aldosterone, and ADH response

Cholinergic stimulation

↑ Catecholamines

Peripheral vasoconstriction

↑ Right ventricular pressures

(diaphoresis)

(tachycardia)

(pallor)

↑ Na+ and H₂O retention

↑ Systemic resistance

↑ Cardiac workload

↑ Blood volume (edema)

↑ Systemic venous circulation (hepatomegaly, bounding pulses, edema)

Right ventricular hypertrophy

Left ventricular hypertrophy

Right-sided CHF (Cor pulmonale)

Left-sided CHF

CHAPTER 2.4

CARDIAC DYSRHYTHMIAS

Dysrhythmia is a term used to describe cardiac rate and rhythm abnormalities or irregularities. They may originate from any site in the heart, as any cell in the myocardium has the ability to discharge an impulse. In children, they may occur as the result of cardiac surgery or congenital heart defects and are less common than in adults. Treatment consists of medications, and in some cases, a permanent pacemaker to manage conduction disturbances in the heart.

MEDICAL CARE

Antidysrhythmics: verapamil (Isoptin) PO or IV, depending on acuteness of condition, to slow SA and AV node conduction in tachyarrhythmias.

Cardiac Glycosides: digoxin (Lanoxin) PO to slow and strengthen heart beat.

Cardiac Pacemaker: to initiate or supplement conduction in the myocardium.

Chest X-ray: reveals correct placement of pacemaker catheter.

Electrocardiography/Holter Monitoring: reveals deviations suggesting dysrhythmias that assist in diagnosis of cardiac conditions and provide rhythm strips to monitor pacer function; test to determine pharmacologic treatment of dysrhythmias; similar to cardiac catheterization, which artificially induces a dysrhythmia and administers different drugs IV to see which will terminate the dysrhythmia.

COMMON NURSING DIAGNOSES

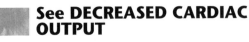 **See DECREASED CARDIAC OUTPUT**

Related to: Electrical factors with alteration in rate, rhythm, and conduction.

Defining Characteristics: (Specify: dysrhythmias, ECG changes, changes in apical and peripheral pulses, fail-

ing batteries or break in pacemaker catheter, provide data.)

ADDITIONAL NURSING DIAGNOSES

RISK FOR INFECTION

Related to: Inadequate primary defenses (broken skin) (specify where).

Defining Characteristics: (None, as this is a potential diagnoses.)

Goal: Child will not experience any infection by (date/time to evaluate).

Outcome Criteria

✔ Site will be clean and dry, without redness, edema, drainage, or odor.

✔ Child's temperature will be <101° F.

NOC: *Risk Detection*

INTERVENTIONS	RATIONALES
Assess temperature q 4 hours. Monitor lab work as obtained.	Temperature >101° F or ↑ WBC may indicate development of an infection.
Wash hands before and after providing care for patient. Teach family and child to wash hands frequently.	Handwashing prevents the spread of microorganisms that may cause infection.
Assess site for warmth, redness, pain, drainage, and odor q 4 hours.	Indicates infectious process at site of wound.
Assess IV site for edema, infiltration, redness, and warmth q hour.	Indicates phlebitis or dislodgement of infusion catheter for administration of fluids and IV medications.

INTERVENTIONS	RATIONALES
Assess skin under ECG electrodes for erythema, irritation, or rash (if cardiac monitoring present).	Infection can result from skin irritation and breakdown caused by electrode gel and adhesive pads.
Maintain sterile technique for dressing changes, IV site changes, and care of any breaks in skin.	Prevents contamination by pathogenic microorganisms.
Change IV site and tubing every 24 to 72 hours according to protocol.	Prevents bacterial growth and prolonged irritation to vein.
Gently wash and dry electrode sites when removed and before reapplication.	Prevents prolonged irritation to skin.
Administer antibiotic therapy as ordered by physician (specify).	Prevents irritation to vein and phlebitis (action of drug).
Teach parents to take oral or axillary temperature.	Monitors for infection.
Instruct on care of site during and after healing.	Maintains sterility or cleanliness of site.

NIC: *Infection Control*

Evaluation

(Date/time of evaluation of goal)

(Has goal been met? Not met? Partially met?)

(Describe wound. What is child's temperature?)

(Revisions to care plan? D/C care plan? Continue care plan?)

RISK FOR INJURY

Related to: Chemical or mechanical insult.

Defining Characteristics: (Specify: negative response to medications [digoxin toxicity]; pacemaker or catheter malfunction; failure of pacemaker to capture or sense arrhythmias.)

Goal: Child will not experience any injury by (date/time to evaluate).

Outcome Criteria

✔ Proper functioning and maintenance of pacemaker system with pulse rate, rhythm, and duration occurring as programmed.

✔ Digoxin level maintained at therapeutic level (specify); K$^+$ levels within normal ranges (specify).

NOC: *Risk Detection*

INTERVENTIONS	RATIONALES
Assess pulse, changes in cardiac output, changes in ECG (specify when).	Decreases in pulse and cardiac output indicate battery depletion; ECG changes may indicate loss of capture, arrhythmias from malpositioning of pacing catheter.
Assess digoxin, potassium and calcium levels as obtained.	Electrolyte imbalance may result in arrhythmias, too high or too low dosages, or cardiotonic causes arrhythmias.
Monitor effect of antidysrhythmics by taking pulse rate and rhythm; carefully administer correct dosage at correct rate (specify).	Ensures desired effect of medications (action of drugs).
Instruct parents in administration of antidysrhythmics; cardiac glycosides; diuretics, including name, actions, dosage, frequency, side effects, how to take, expected results.	Ensures proper dosage, frequency, and knowledge of when to report side effects.
Describe to parents and child the device and its parts, how it functions, and type of lead used; use manufacturer's instruction pamphlet, drawing, and models.	Provides understanding of type and function of pacemaker; parts include the generator with the battery and electronic circuitry, which produces the impulse to the heart, and a lead, which operates as a conductor of the impulse to the heart; lead may be epicardial or transvenous.
Teach parents the method of taking pulse (apical) for 1 minute.	Monitors effect of medication and changes to report.
Describe procedure for transmission of ECG by telephone to parents.	Transmits ECG strips by phone to monitor for dysrhythmias, pacemaker function, and battery depletion.
Review activity limitations, types of activities to avoid that might affect pacemaker function (contact sports).	Activity tolerance usually improved with pacemaker.
Stress the importance of wearing identification with pacemaker type, site of insertion, physician name and number.	Provides information for emergency care.

(continues)

(continued)

INTERVENTIONS	RATIONALES
Inform to avoid electrical interferences, microwave ovens, and to request hand scanner at airports.	Some pacemakers are still affected by electrical interference of current leakage.
Stress the importance of follow-up visits to physician.	Ensures monitoring of condition and pacemaker function.
Refer to cardiopulmonary resuscitation (CPR) classes.	May be needed as an emergency measure to maintain normal rhythm.

NIC: *Dysrhythmia Management*

Evaluation

(Date/time of evaluation of goal)

(Has goal been met? Not met? Partially met?)

(Is pacemaker functioning properly? Specify; what is digoxin level? What is potassium level?)

(Revisions to care plan? D/C care plan? Continue care plan?)

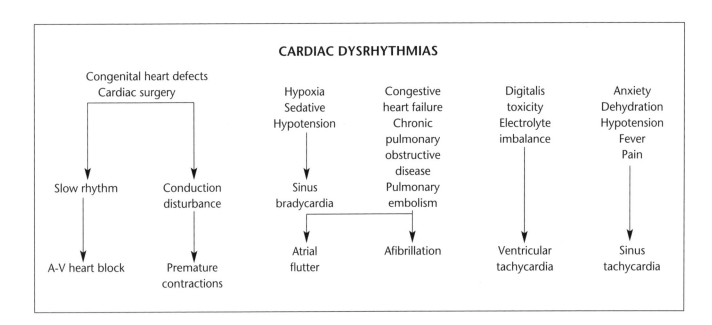

CARDIAC DYSRHYTHMIAS

CHAPTER 2.5

HYPERTENSION

Hypertension in children is reflected by the consistent readings of the systolic and/or diastolic blood pressure at the level of or above the 95th percentile for age and sex. It may be primary or secondary. Fifty to 80% of secondary hypertension is caused by renal parenchymal disease; therefore, infants and children with hypertension and adolescents with severe hypertension need to be evaluated for renal pathology. Hypertension in children is of particular concern because of its close association with adult hypertension. Children with increased blood pressure usually do not display any overt symptoms. Blood pressure determinations are a part of routine examination in children 3 years and older. Children under 3 who have been diagnosed with a heart condition are also screened for hypertension.

MEDICAL CARE

Diagnosis and Treatment of Underlying Cause: preferred over use of drug therapy in children.

Chest X-ray: hypertrophy of left ventricle in sustained hypertension.

Electrocardiography: cardiac abnormalities.

Urinalysis: renal disease or infection.

Electrolytes: hypokalemia, hypernatremia during diuretic therapy.

Lipid Panel: increases in lipoproteins, cholesterol, and triglyceride levels.

Blood Urea Nitrogen: increases in impaired renal function in secondary hypertension.

Creatinine: increases in impaired renal function in secondary hypertension.

Complete Blood Count: increased WBC in presence of infection.

Diuretics: chlorothiazide (Diuril and Hydrochlorothiazide Chydrodiuril) PO promotes diuresis and elimination of sodium by preventing reabsorption; it also decreases cardiac output, which reduces peripheral vascular resistance.

Beta-Blockers: propranolol (Inderal), PO to lower cardiac output, which decreases blood pressure.

Angiotension-Converting Enzyme (ACE) Inhibitors: captopril (Capoten), PO to lower total peripheral resistance by inhibiting angiotensin-converting enzyme.

Vasodilators: hydralazine (Apresoline), PO to relax smooth muscle of arterioles, resulting in reduced peripheral resistance.

COMMON NURSING DIAGNOSES

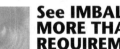 See FLUID VOLUME EXCESS

Related to: (Specify: compromised regulatory mechanisms, excessive sodium intake.)

Defining Characteristics: (Specify: edema, weight gain, intake greater than output, blood pressure changes, altered electrolytes—give data.)

See IMBALANCED NUTRITION: MORE THAN BODY REQUIREMENTS

Related to: Excessive intake in relationship to metabolic need.

Defining Characteristics: (Specify: weight 10% over ideal for height and frame, dysfunctional eating pattern, hereditary predisposition—provide data.)

See INEFFECTIVE TISSUE PERFUSION: RENAL

Related to: (Specify: interruption in renal, arterial, or venous flow.)

Defining Characteristics: (Specify: edema, oliguria, hypertension.)

 ## See RISK FOR DEFICIENT FLUID VOLUME

Related to: Medications (diuretic).

Defining Characteristics: (Specify: increased urinary output, sudden weight loss, hypokalemia, dry skin and mucous membranes.)

ADDITIONAL NURSING DIAGNOSES

RISK FOR INJURY

Related to: Internal regulatory function.

Defining Characteristics: (Specify: uncontrolled hypertension; neurologic status [blurred vision, headache, irritability, dizziness, papilledema]; future renal, heart, circulatory problems.)

Goal: Child will not experience injury by (date/time to evaluate).

Outcome Criteria

✔ Blood pressure will remain within appropriate range for child (specify range).

✔ Child denies headache, dizziness, or visual changes.

NOC: *Symptom Control*

INTERVENTIONS	RATIONALES
Assess BP (using a Doppler method on an infant and proper size cuff on child). Use a cuff that covers 2/3 of the upper arm and inflatable bladder that encircles the child's arm circumference (take an infant's BP in a supine position; take a child's BP with the child seated and the arm supported at the level of the heart); obtain readings when infant/child is at rest q 2h.	Provides accurate systolic and diastolic readings to establish a pattern of elevations, although no definite readings are used to diagnose hypertension in children.
Assess for headache, dizziness, nose-bleed, visual changes.	Indicates increased BP, although symptoms in children are varied and some or none of the symptoms may be present.

INTERVENTIONS	RATIONALES
Provide quiet environment and reduce activities, stress and stimuli.	May increase BP by sympathetic stimulation.
Administer antihypertensives and diuretics as prescribed (specify drug, dose, route, and time).	Drug therapy is given diuretics as prescribed when BP does not respond to nonpharmacologic methods of reducing it; control is managed with the use of one drug and cautious addition of another drug, depending on side effects produced and achieved reduction of BP (action).
Teach medication administration including action, dosage, frequency, side effects, importance of long-term therapy, physical and behavioral changes to report (specify).	Pharmacologic intervention to control hypertension.
Demonstrate and have parents return the demonstration of taking BP correctly and of maintaining a log of readings.	Offers correct monitoring of BP for changes that might indicate need for initiation and/or changes in treatments for children with chronic hypertension.
Instruct parents to report any sustained elevation of BP or neurologic symptoms.	Provides opportunity to prevent neurologic impairment or other complications.
Reinforce that therapy is long term and of consequences of noncompliance (specify).	Provides realistic support and rationale to encourage compliance of drug therapy.
Praise child and family for compliance with regimen.	Positive reinforcement enhances compliance and self-esteem.

NIC: *Teaching: Prescribed Medication*

Evaluation

(Date/time of evaluation of goal)

(Has goal been met? Not met? Partially met?)

(What is child's BP? Does child deny headache, dizziness, and visual disturbances?)

(Revisions to care plan? D/C care plan? Continue care plan?)

DEFICIENT KNOWLEDGE: HYPERTENSION

Related to: Lack of information or experience about disease and treatment.

Defining Characteristics: (Specify: parents, child verbalize need for information about nonpharmacologic treatments for hypertension.)

Goal: Parents (and child) will gain information about hypertension.

Outcome Criteria

✔ Parents (and child) verbalize correct understanding of underlying cause of hypertension.

✔ Parents (and child) verbalize understanding of treatment plan for hypertension (specify, e.g., drugs, diet, etc.).

NOC: *Knowledge: Treatment Regimen*

INTERVENTIONS	RATIONALES
Assess knowledge of disease, causes and methods to control disease.	Provides baseline information.
Provide information and explanations in clear language; use pictures, pamphlets, video tapes, models in teaching about disorder, causes and risk factors.	Ensures understanding based on readiness, aids reinforce learning.
Instruct and assist in planning dietary menu that includes restrictions that help reduce BP (specify).	Weight reduction and restricted sodium, fat, and cholesterol intake may be part of the medical regimen.

INTERVENTIONS	RATIONALES
Suggest activity and exercise plan specific to child's needs and interests (swimming, cycling).	Assists in weight reduction and contributes to lowering BP.
Teach relaxation techniques, such as breathing, biofeedback (specify).	Reduces stress that raises BP.
Reinforce importance of follow-up visits to physician.	Provides early detection of complication and evaluation therapy.
Discuss long-term nature of medical regimen and potential for cardiac, cerebral, and renal damage or complications that result from htn.	Provides rationale for acceptance of long-term care.
Refer to stress, weight reduction, nutritional or support groups or counseling as needed (specify).	Provides specialized guidance if needed to ensure compliance and success.

NIC: *Teaching: Disease Process*

Evaluation

(Date/time of evaluation of goal)

(Has goal been met? Not met? Partially met?)

(Specify what parents/child said about understanding of the cause and treatment of the hypertension. Use quotes.)

(Revisions to care plan? D/C care plan? Continue care plan?)

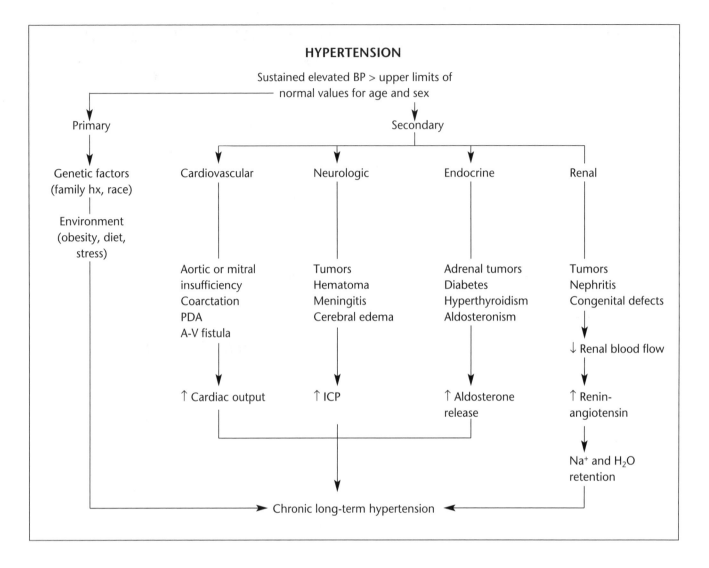

HYPERTENSION

Sustained elevated BP > upper limits of normal values for age and sex

Primary

Genetic factors (family hx, race)

Environment (obesity, diet, stress)

Secondary

Cardiovascular

Aortic or mitral insufficiency
Coarctation
PDA
A-V fistula

↑ Cardiac output

Neurologic

Tumors
Hematoma
Meningitis
Cerebral edema

↑ ICP

Endocrine

Adrenal tumors
Diabetes
Hyperthyroidism
Aldosteronism

↑ Aldosterone release

Renal

Tumors
Nephritis
Congenital defects

↓ Renal blood flow

↑ Renin-angiotensin

Na^+ and H_2O retention

Chronic long-term hypertension

CHAPTER 2.6

KAWASAKI DISEASE

Kawasaki Disease, or mucocutaneous lymph node syndrome, is an acute vasculitis of unknown cause. Most cases occur in children less than 5 years of age. The disease is self-limiting, but about 20% of those affected will develop cardiac sequelae (most commonly dilatation of the coronary arteries resulting in coronary aneurysms). The disease occurs in 3 phases: the acute phase is characterized by progressive inflammation of small blood vessels accompanied by high fever, inflammation of the pharynx, dry, reddened eyes, swollen hands and feet, rash, and cervical lymphadenopathy. In the subacute phase, the manifestations disappear, but there is inflammation of larger vessels and the child is at greatest risk for the development of coronary aneurysms. In the convalescent phase (6–8 weeks after onset), the clinical signs are resolved, but lab values are not completely normal. There are no diagnostic tests for Kawasaki disease, so the diagnosis is made on the basis of the child exhibiting at least 5 of 6 criterion manifestations.

MEDICAL CARE

Hgb/Hct: the child with KD is often anemic at the time of diagnosis.

WBC: may show leukocytosis with a "shift to the left" (increased immature white blood cells during the acute phase).

Sedimentation Rate: elevated, reflecting inflammation, and lasts 6 to 8 weeks.

Platelet Count: thrombocytosis and hypercoagulability occur in the subacute phase and gradually return to normal.

Liver Enzymes: usually elevated during the acute phase.

Echocardiogram: baseline and to monitor changes in myocardium and coronary arteries.

Gamma Globulin: IV gamma globulin is given during the first 10 days of the illness; usually given as a single dose of 2g/kg over 10 to 12 hours.

Aspirin (ASA): used for its anti-inflammatory and anti-coagulant actions; given in large doses (80 to 100 mg/kg/day) while the child is febrile, and then 3 to 5 mg/kg/day until the platelet count returns to normal.

COMMON NURSING DIAGNOSES

See HYPERTHERMIA

Related to: Inflammatory disease process.

Defining Characteristics: High fever (specify degrees, not responsive to antipyretics or antibiotics.)

See RISK FOR DEFICIENT FLUID VOLUME

Related to: (Specify: decreased PO intake during uncomfortable acute phase, fluid losses through fever and increased metabolic rate.)

Defining Characteristics: (Specify, e.g., refusal to take PO fluids, oliguria, poor skin turgor, dry mucous membranes, weight loss, provide data.)

ADDITIONAL NURSING DIAGNOSES

PAIN

Related to: Inflammatory process (dry mucous membranes, conjunctivitis, pharyngitis, fever, joint pain, swollen hands and feet).

Defining Characteristics: (Specify: crying, extreme irritability, refusal to play, cries when being touched or moved, increased rating on pain scale.)

Goal: Child will experience less pain by (date/time to evaluate).

Outcome Criteria

✔ (Specify, e.g., client is not crying, is playing, has relaxed facial features, allows touch, pain rating is less than before interventions [give number].)

NOC: *Pain Control*

INTERVENTIONS	RATIONALES
Assess level of pain by observation (crying, grimacing, vocal expressions of pain), using pain assessment scales, and by obtaining relevant pain information from parents about child's expression of pain.	Provides information upon which accurate assessments of pain and treatment effectiveness can be based.
Apply cool cloths to skin, lotion, and soft, loose clothing on child.	Decreases skin discomfort.
Apply lubricating lip ointments and glycerin swabs to the oral mucosa; offer cool liquids and soft foods.	Moistens dry oral mucosa to decrease discomfort and promote oral intake.
Keep child's room quiet and semidark.	Promotes rest; darkness decreases eye discomfort caused by conjunctivitis.
Disturb child as little as possible; when necessary, handle gently and avoid unnecessary handling.	Movement causes discomfort.
Administer IV gamma globulin and high dose ASA therapy as directed (specify doses, routes times).	Decreases inflammatory process and helps decrease fever.
Explain to parents reason for child's discomfort/irritability; ask parents for information on child's expression of pain.	Promotes understanding and cooperation; provides valuable assessment data.
Explain to parents that irritability may persist for up to 2 months; that peeling skin on hands and feet is normal and not painful.	Promotes understanding and allows parents to anticipate needs.
If child has joint pain, explain to parents that it may persist for several weeks; passive ROM exercises in a warm bath may help.	Persistent joint pain is not uncommon; ROM with heat helps increase flexibility.

NIC: *Pain Management*

Evaluation

(Date/time of evaluation of goal)

(Has goal been met? Not met? Partially met?)

(Specify: Is child crying? Describe activity of child; what is pain ranking? Use quotes if possible.)

(Revisions to care plan? D/C care plan? Continue care plan?)

ANXIETY

Related to: Acute, serious illness of unknown origin with possible cardiac sequelae.

Defining Characteristics: (Specify: verbalization of anxiety, use quotes.)

Goal: Client will experience decreased anxiety by (date/time).

Outcome Criteria

✔ Parents verbalize decreased anxiety levels.

NOC: *Anxiety Control*

INTERVENTIONS	RATIONALES
Assess anxiety level of parents. Ask them to rank their anxiety on a scale from 1 to 5 with 1 being no anxiety.	Assessment provides baseline information for the design of interventions.
Encourage parents to express their feelings freely. Reassure parents that some anxiety is appropriate when their child is ill.	Encouragement and reassurance help the parents to identify and regain control of their emotions.
Provide information about the disease (the unknown etiology, the disease phases and manifestations, diagnostic tests and treatments).	Ensures understanding; the unknown etiology helps allay any guilt parents may have concerning the child contracting the disease.
Support parents in their efforts to comfort their irritable child; encourage them to "take a break" while the nurse cares for the child; reassure parents that irritability is a manifestation of Kawasaki disease and that they should not feel embarrassed or guilty.	Provides support to parents during a stressful event.

INTERVENTIONS	RATIONALES
Monitor child closely during IV gamma globulin administration (temperature, pulse, BP). Stop the infusion and report immediately any signs of reaction (chills, fever, dyspnea, nausea/vomiting).	Gamma globulin is a blood product and requires the same close observation for safe administration to prevent a reaction; this reassures parents that their child is receiving appropriate care.
Explain to parents that touching the child may cause pain; demonstrate gentle handling of child as needed.	Provides information parents need to give comfort to their child.
Explain to parents that the child may have recurrent fever at home and demonstrate how to take the child's temperature and when to notify physician (temp. greater than 38.4° C/101° F).	Helps ensure child will receive needed care at home. Empowers the parent and decreases anxiety associated with uncertainty.
Demonstrate ASA administration to parents and instruct them to report any signs of toxicity (tinnitus, headache, dizziness, or confusion). Explain that ASA may	Helps ensure safe, proper administration of ASA at home. Empowers parents.

INTERVENTIONS	RATIONALES
cause easy bruising and that the ASA should be stopped and the physician notified if child exposed to chickenpox or influenza (risk of Reye's syndrome).	
Assist parents to make any referral (specify) and follow-up appointments for child.	Assistance helps decrease anxiety.

NIC: *Anticipatory Guidance*

Evaluation

(Date/time of evaluation of goal)

(Has goal been met? Not met? Partially met?)

(Did parents specify decreased levels of anxiety? Use quotes if possible.)

(Revisions to care plan? D/C care plan? Continue care plan?

KAWASAKI DISEASE

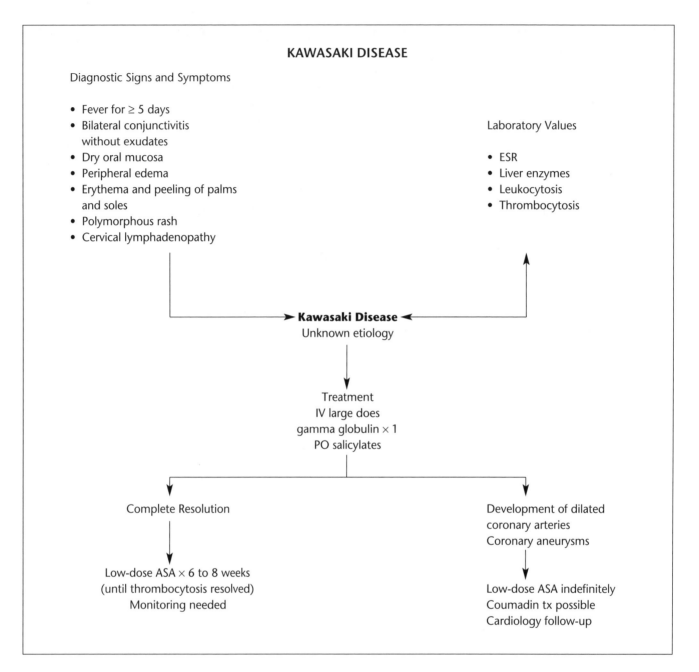

Diagnostic Signs and Symptoms

- Fever for ≥ 5 days
- Bilateral conjunctivitis
  without exudates
- Dry oral mucosa
- Peripheral edema
- Erythema and peeling of palms
  and soles
- Polymorphous rash
- Cervical lymphadenopathy

Laboratory Values

- ESR
- Liver enzymes
- Leukocytosis
- Thrombocytosis

Kawasaki Disease
Unknown etiology

Treatment
IV large does
gamma globulin × 1
PO salicylates

Complete Resolution

Low-dose ASA × 6 to 8 weeks
(until thrombocytosis resolved)
Monitoring needed

Development of dilated
coronary arteries
Coronary aneurysms

Low-dose ASA indefinitely
Coumadin tx possible
Cardiology follow-up

CHAPTER 2.7

ACUTE RHEUMATIC FEVER

Acute rheumatic fever is an autoimmune disease responsible for cardiac valve disease or rheumatic heart disease. It is associated with infections caused by the group A streptococcus and occurs about 2 to 6 weeks following a streptococcal upper respiratory infection. It is prevented by adequate treatment of the infection with appropriate antibiotic therapy within 9 days of onset of streptococcal infection before further complications can occur. Because rheumatic heart disease does not occur after only one attack and children are susceptible to recurrent attacks of rheumatic fever, it is vital that an initial episode is diagnosed and treated, and that long-term prophylactic therapy (5 years or more) is given following the acute phase. There is no specific test for rheumatic fever; the diagnosis is based upon the manifestations using the revised Jones criteria as a guideline. Jones criteria consist of major manifestations (polyarthritis, carditis, chorea, subcutaneous nodules, and erythema marginatum) and minor manifestations (fever, arthralgia, ECG and laboratory changes). The presence of 2 major manifestations, or 1 major and 2 minor manifestations, supported by evidence of a preceding group a streptococcal infection is indicative of acute rheumatic fever.

MEDICAL CARE

Antibiotics: benzathine penicillin G IM, penicillin G potassium (Pentids solution), ampicillin (Amcill tablets, suspension or pediatric drops) PO or erythromycin (Ilosone tablets, chewables, suspension PO if penicillin-sensitive). Followed by: penicillin G benzathine (Bicillin) IM monthly or penicillin G potassium (Pentids) PO daily as long-term therapy.

Anti-inflammatory/Antipyretic/Analgesic: aspirin (acetylsalicylic acid tablets, suspension or liquid) PO to reduce temperature and reduce inflammatory process by inactivating the enzyme required for prostaglandin synthesis, that contributes to inflammatory process.

Electrocardiogram: reveals prolonged P-R interval.

Antistreptolysin-O Titer: reveals increase 7 days after streptococcal infection with elevation above 330 Todd units, indicating recent infection.

Complete Blood Count: reveals increased WBC in presence of infectious process.

Erythrocyte Sedimentation Rate: reveals increase in presence of inflammatory process in rheumatoid disease.

C-reactive Protein: reveals increase during inflammatory process and may be done in place of ESR.

Throat Culture: reveals presence of streptococci, Group A.

COMMON NURSING DIAGNOSES

See HYPERTHERMIA

Related to: Illness or inflammatory disease.

Defining Characteristics: (Low-grade increase in body temperature above normal range, temperature tends to spike in late afternoon, specify for child.)

See IMBALANCED NUTRITION: LESS THAN BODY REQUIREMENTS

Related to: Inability to ingest food because of anorexia, increased metabolic rate and/or chores (specify).

Defining Characteristics: (Specify: anorexia, fatigue, weight loss, abdominal pain, give figures.)

See IMPAIRED PHYSICAL MOBILITY

Related to: Pain and discomfort.

Defining Characteristics: (Specify: verbalizes joint pain of polyarthritis.)

Related to: Neuromuscular impairment from chorea.

Defining Characteristics: Decreased muscle control and strength, clumsiness, uncoordination, sudden and aimless movement of extremities, bed rest protocol (describe activity).

ADDITIONAL NURSING DIAGNOSES

PAIN

Related to: Inflammation, arthralgia.

Defining Characteristics: (Specify: verbal description of pain, use scale, guarding and protective behavior of painful joints, edema, redness, heat at affected joints.)

Goal: Child will experience less pain by (date/time to evaluate).

Outcome Criteria

✔ Child verbalizes pain less than (specify) on scale of 1 to 10.
✔ Child appears relaxed without guarding.
✔ Joints are not swollen, red, or warm.)

NOC: *Pain Control*

INTERVENTIONS	RATIONALES
Assess child's perception of pain using an appropriate scale (specify) q 2 to 3 hours.	Provides data about degree of pain the child is experiencing.
Assess behavior changes, such as crying, restlessness, refusal to move, irritability, aggressive or dependent behavior.	Nonverbal responses to pain that are age-related as child or infant may be unable to describe pain; fear and anxiety associated with pain causes changes in behavioral responses.
Assess severity of pain, joints involved, level of joint movement.	Provides information regarding pathologic changes in joints; joint involvement is reversible, usually affecting large joints, such as knees, hips, wrists, and elbows; an increase in numbers of affected joints occurs over a period of time.
Administer analgesic and anti-inflammatory agents as ordered (specify drugs, dose, route, and times), and inform child that the medication will decrease the pain;	Relieves pain, edema in joints and promotes rest and comfort (action of drugs).

INTERVENTIONS	RATIONALES
administer a sustained-action analgesic before bedtime or 1 hour before anticipated movement.	
Maintain bed rest during the acute stage of disease.	Promotes comfort and reduces joint pain caused by movement.
Elevate affected extremities above level of heart.	Promotes circulation to the heart to relieve edema.
Change position q 2h while maintaining body alignment.	Prevents contractures and promotes comfort.
Move gently and support body parts; minimize handling of affected parts as much as possible.	Prevents additional pain to affected parts.
Apply bed cradle under outside covers over painful parts.	Prevents pressure on painful joints.
Provide toys, games for quiet, sedentary play (specify for child).	Provides diversionary activity to distract from pain.
Use nonpharmacologic measures to decrease pain (distraction, cutaneous stimulation, imagery, relaxation, heat application).	Provides additional measures to decrease pain perception.
Inform of limited activity or amount of joint movement allowed.	Prevents increase or exacerbation of pain.
Teach parents and child of need for analgesia and that it will help him/her to feel better.	Controls pain, and allows for uninterrupted sleep and activity within tolerance level.
Reassure parents and child that joint involvement is temporary, that pain and edema will subside, and that joints will return to normal size.	Reduces anxiety associated with fear of permanent damage.
Teach parents in body positioning and handling of affected parts.	Promotes comfort and prevents pain and contractures while on enforced bed rest.

NIC: *Pain Management*

Evaluation

(Date/time of evaluation of goal)

(Has goal been met? Not met? Partially met?)

(Specify pain-rating on scale of 1 to 10; does child appear relaxed without guarding? Are joints not swollen, red, or warm? Describe.)

(Revisions to care plan? D/C care plan? Continue care plan?)

RISK FOR INFECTION

Related to: Chronic recurrence of disease.

Defining Characteristics: None, as this is a potential diagnosis.

Goal: Child will not experience recurrence of infection.

Outcome Criteria

✔ Absence of occurrence of reinfection.
✔ Child is afebrile; no complaints of discomfort.
✔ Child takes medications as ordered.

NOC: *Risk Control*

INTERVENTIONS	RATIONALES
Assess parents' ability to provide long-term treatment with pre-scribed antimicrobials; daily oral administration or monthly intra-muscular injections.	Long-term antibiotic therapy (as long as 5 years) as a preventive measure may be difficult.
Assess for chest pain, dyspnea, cough, tachycardia during sleep, friction rub, gallop during acute stage of disease.	Signs and symptoms of carditis, which may lead to endocarditis causing vegetation that becomes fibrous at the valve areas that is at increased risk with repeated infections.

INTERVENTIONS	RATIONALES
Administer antibiotic therapy during acute phase of disease as ordered (specify drugs, dose, route, and times).	Inhibits cell wall synthesis of microorganisms, destroying causative agent.
Instruct in long-term antibiotic regimen, need for protection before dental work or any invasive procedure, and inform of importance to prevent recurrence.	Therapy starts after acute phase and medical supervision is needed for life as rheumatic fever may recur; a large percentage of children who have had the disease have heart disease later in life.
Teach to report to physician any upper respiratory infections, elevated temperature, joint pain, or inability to continue antibiotic therapy.	May indicate recurrence of the disease or need to change or adjust medication.

NIC: *Infection Protection*

Evaluation

(Date/time of evaluation of goal)

(Has goal been met? Not met? Partially met?)

(What is child's temperature? Does child complain of discomfort? Is child taking the medications as ordered?)

(Revisions to care plan? D/C care plan? Continue care plan?)

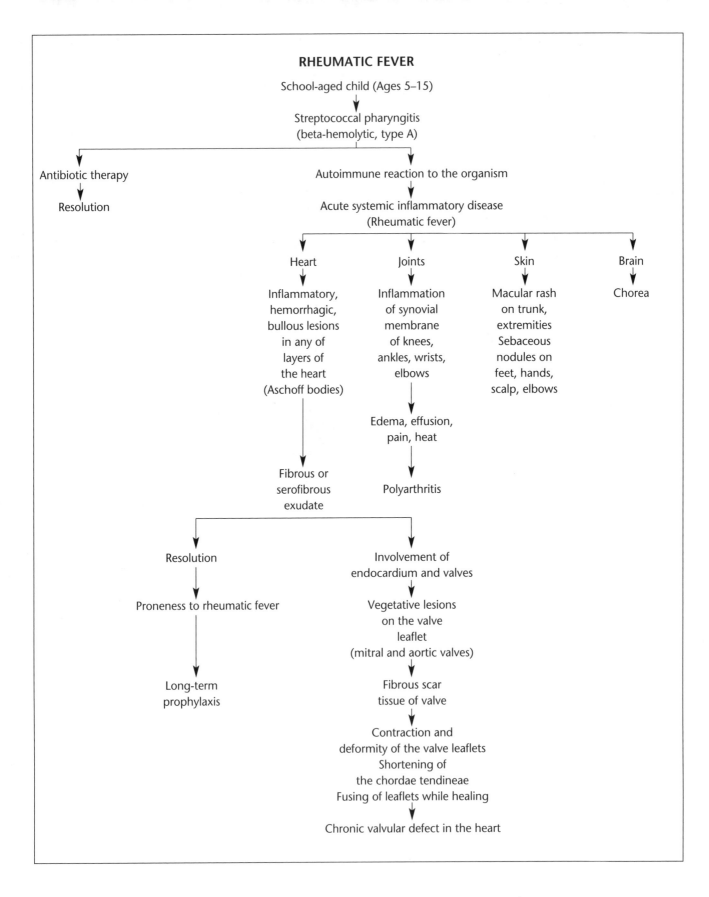

RHEUMATIC FEVER

School-aged child (Ages 5–15)

↓

Streptococcal pharyngitis
(beta-hemolytic, type A)

Antibiotic therapy → Resolution

Autoimmune reaction to the organism

↓

Acute systemic inflammatory disease
(Rheumatic fever)

Heart	Joints	Skin	Brain
Inflammatory, hemorrhagic, bullous lesions in any of layers of the heart (Aschoff bodies)	Inflammation of synovial membrane of knees, ankles, wrists, elbows	Macular rash on trunk, extremities Sebaceous nodules on feet, hands, scalp, elbows	Chorea

Heart → Fibrous or serofibrous exudate

Joints → Edema, effusion, pain, heat → Polyarthritis

Resolution → Proneness to rheumatic fever → Long-term prophylaxis

Involvement of endocardium and valves

↓

Vegetative lesions on the valve leaflet
(mitral and aortic valves)

↓

Fibrous scar tissue of valve

↓

Contraction and deformity of the valve leaflets
Shortening of the chordae tendineae
Fusing of leaflets while healing

↓

Chronic valvular defect in the heart

UNIT 3
RESPIRATORY SYSTEM

CHAPTER 3.0

RESPIRATORY SYSTEM: BASIC CARE PLAN

The respiratory tract is a common site of major and minor disorders in infants and children, and any alteration in respiratory structure or function has a profound effect on the ability to supply the body with oxygen and remove carbon dioxide. A constant supply of oxygen is necessary to sustain organ function and survival, and any decrease in or cessation, obstruction, and infection, can compromise airway patency and pattern. This in turn changes the respiratory rate and efficiency. This tendency gradually decreases after the age of five. Each stage of life and its associated changes resulting from growth and developmental patterns establish different pulmonary parameters and susceptibility to diseases. Although the system generally functions the same as in an adult, anatomic changes that occur with growth influence the way that the infant or child responds to acute or chronic illnesses related to this system.

GROWTH AND DEVELOPMENT

CHEST STRUCTURE AND BRONCHOPULMONARY MOVEMENT

- Chest shape and anteroposterior diameter:

  Infant: rounded chest where diameter equals transverse diameter;

  School-age: changes gradually to lateral diameter ratio of 1:2 or 5:7 as chest assumes a more flattened anteroposterior diameter with growth.

- Narrow, smaller lumen of airway system with increased airway resistance until age of five years.

- Ability to respond to irritating stimuli by age 4 to 5 months as smooth muscle develops in airways, gradually reaching smooth muscle development of an adult by age of one year.

- Glottis has more cephalad location in the infant than in the child; epiglottis is longer, and the narrowest part of the larynx located at the same level as the cricoid cartilage; larynx grows slowly during infancy and childhood, with a spurt of growth after childhood phase during preadolescence (voice change).

- Airways grow faster than cervical and thoracic spine, causing a descent of the larynx and trachea; the tracheal bifurcation gradually descends from opposite T3 in the infant to T4 by the end of the growth period, and the cricoid cartilage descends from C4 in the infant to C6 by the end of the growth period.

- Diaphragm in the infant is attached higher in front and is longer, causing a decreased ability to contract with the same force of an older infant or child.

- Lung growth changes from globular to lobular shape by 12 years of age.

- Lung growth produces an increase in alveoli numbers and size as septa in the alveoli develop, divide, and increase their numbers at each terminal airway.

- Branching of terminal bronchioles is increased as alveoli are increased as the child grows.

- Collateral pathways develop between bronchioles and growth pores in alveolar walls during child's growth.

BREATHING PATTERN AND VENTILATORY FUNCTION

- Respiratory rate (ratio to pulse is 1:4)

Infant:	30 to 60/minute
Toddler:	25 to 40/minute
Preschool:	22 to 34/minute
School age:	18 to 30/minute

  Rate decreases as metabolic needs decrease.

- Respiratory depth (chest expansion)

Infant:	2 to 4 inches
Toddler:	4 to 6 inches
Preschool:	6 to 8 inches
School age:	9 to 10 inches

- Respiratory pattern:

  Infant: obligate nasal and diaphragmatic breathing during first year of life;

  School age: changes gradually from infancy through childhood to a more thoracic breathing for girls and a more abdominal breathing for boys—volume of inspired air increases as lungs grow in size, which results in a decreased amount of oxygen taken in and an increased amount of carbon dioxide expired.

- Increased surface area available for gas exchange as alveoli increase in numbers and size.

- Changes in compliance with age, from high compliance in the infant with a more pliant rib cage to gradually decreasing to normal compliance level; chest structure changes with growth.

- Arterial blood gas values:

  pH: 7.35 to 7.45

  pO_2: 80 to 100 mm Hg (pressure of dissolved oxygen in the blood)

  pCO_2: 35 to 45 mm Hg (pressure of dissolved carbon dioxide in the blood)

  HCO_3: 22 to 28 mEq/L (bicarbonate level in the blood to reveal buffering effect on acid)

NURSING DIAGNOSES

INEFFECTIVE AIRWAY CLEARANCE

Related to: (Specify: tracheobronchial infection, obstruction, secretions.)

Defining Characteristics: (Specify, e.g., abnormal breath sounds: fine or coarse crackles, rhonchi, wheezes, changes in rate or depth of respirations, tachypnea, cyanosis, fever, provide data.)

Related to: Decreased energy and fatigue.

Defining Characteristics: (Specify, e.g., ineffective cough with or without sputum, labored respirations, inability to feed self, sleeplessness, lack of activity, weakness.)

Goal: Infant/child will experience improved airway clearance by (date/time to evaluate).

Outcome Criteria

✔ Return of respiratory status to baseline parameters for rate, depth and ease (specify).

✔ Breath sounds clear bilaterally.

✔ Ability to cough up and remove secretions that are thin and clear.

NOC: *Respiratory Status: Airway Patency, Ventilation*

INTERVENTIONS	RATIONALES
Assess respirations for rate (count for one full minute), depth and ease, presence of tachypnea (specify), dyspnea and if it occurs during sleep or quiet time; note panting, nasal flaring, grunting, retracting, slowing, deep (hyperpnea) or shallow (hypopnea) breathing, stridor on inspiration, head bobbing during sleep (specify frequency).	Reveals rate and type of respirations (baselines or deviations) that are related to age and size of the infant/child, changes that indicate obstruction and consolidation of airways and lungs resulting in a decrease in lung surface for gas diffusion, extreme changes in depth are abnormal, head bobbing indicates dyspnea in the infant and fatigue causing neck flexion, grunting indicates respiratory distress.
Assess breath sounds by auscultation, consolidation by percussion and fremitus (specify when).	Provides indication of patent airways by auscultation, revealing crackles heard in the presence of secretions (fine and coarse), rhonchi (audible and palpable) in larger airway obstruction and wheezes in small bronchiolar narrowing (inspiration and expiration), diminished breath sounds in presence of decreased airflow and lung consolidation; indication of consolidation by presence of dullness on percussion and increased fremitus, decreased functional lung area by presence of tympany on percussion.
Assess skin color changes, distribution and duration of cyanosis (nail beds, skin, mucous membranes, circumoral) or pallor (specify frequency).	Reveals presence and degree of cyanosis, indicating an uneven distribution of gas and blood in the lungs, and alveolar hypoventilation resulting from airway obstruction, the weakness of muscles used in respiration or respiratory center depression.
Assess cough (moist, dry, hacking, paroxysmal, brassy, or croupy): onset, duration, frequency, if occurs at night, during day, or during activity; mucus production: when produced, amount,	Reveals characteristics of cough as an indication of a respiratory condition that may be produced by infection or inflammation; small and narrow airways of an infant/child and the difficulty to

(continues)

(continued)

INTERVENTIONS	RATIONALES
color (clear, yellow, green), consistency (thick, tenacious, frothy); ability to expectorate or if swallowing secretions, stuffy nose or nasal drainage.	cough up secretions cause obstruction from the stasis of secretions, which lead to infection and change in respiratory status.
Elevate head of bed at least 30° for child and hold infant and young child in lap or in an upright position with head on shoulder; older child may sit up and rest head on a pillow on overbed table (specify); check child's position frequently to ensure child does not slide down in bed.	Positioning facilitates chest expansion and respiratory efficiency by reducing pressure of abdominal organs on diaphragm.
Reposition on sides q 2h; position child in proper body alignment.	Prevents accumulation and pooling of secretions.
Provide fluids at frequent intervals over 24-h time periods, specify amounts; encourage clear liquids, and avoid milk.	Maintains hydration status, and clear liquids liquefy and mobilize secretions; milk tends to thicken secretions.
Provide for periods of rest by organizing procedures and care and disturbing infant/child as little as possible in acute stages of illness.	Prevents unnecessary energy expenditure resulting in fatigue.
Perform postural drainage between meals using gravity, percussion, and vibration unless contraindicated; hold infant on lap; support child with pillows. Teach parents.	Promotes removal of secretions and sputum from airways; percussion and vibration loosen and dislodge secretions, and gravity drains the airways and lung segments through positioning.
Assist to perform deep breathing and coughing exercises in child when in a relaxed position for postural drainage unless procedures are contraindicated; use incentive spirometer in older child, blowing up balloon, blowing bubbles, blowing a pinwheel or blowing cotton balls across the table in younger child (specify).	Promotes deeper breathing by enlarging tracheobronchial tree and initiating cough reflex to remove secretions.
Suction nasal and/or oropharyngeal passages, if needed and appropriate, using correct catheter and method, amount of negative pressure, and time limits (specify); orotracheal with the administration of oxygen before	Removes secretions when cough is nonproductive (older child if unable to regulate cough or breathe through mouth); if nose obstructed by mucus (infant or young child); type of suctioning dependent on amount, ability to

INTERVENTIONS	RATIONALES
and after suctioning if needed; use bulb syringe to suction mucus from infant's nose; catheter size is age dependent (specify), maximum negative pressure of 60 to 90 cm H_2O with time limit of 5 seconds for infant, and 90 to 110 cm H_2O with 5 second time limit for child.	drain or cough up, breath sounds in upper airways; prolonged suctioning causes vagal stimulation, oxygen desaturation, and bradycardia, and the use of high pressure damages the mucous membrane lining of airways.
Administer pain medications as ordered (specify drug, dose, route, and time); assess level of pain using appropriate pain assessment tools (specify).	Promotes comfort during deep breathing exercises and coughing to aid in the removal of secretions.
Provide mouth care qid and after suctioning.	Prevents drying of oral mucous membranes.
Provide toys, games for quiet play, and a quiet environment (specify).	Prevents excessive energy expenditure and need for additional oxygen consumption, which changes respiratory status while still providing moderate activity and diversion of play.
Place airway maintenance equipment and supplies at bedside (resuscitation bag, oxygen and suction equipment, endotracheal tube, tracheostomy tube, and supplies).	Provides immediate access to emergency equipment for interventions to treat airway obstruction if needed.
Administer medications (mucolytics, bronchodilators, antibiotics, expectorants, decongestants, and/or antihistamines) orally, parenterally, via aerosol therapy with hand-held measured-dose inhaler, small volume nebulizer, IPPB according to physician order (provides specifics).	(Specify drug action, e.g., treats conditions affecting secretions, infection by liquefying secretions and enhancing outflow and removal of secretions (mucolytics, expectorants), relieving bronchospasms (bronchodilators), destroying infectious agents by interfering with cell way synthesis (antibiotics), reducing allergic responses and discomfort of nose stuffiness (decongestant, antihistamines), and by suppressing cough (cough suppressants) unless cough is desired to bring up secretions.)
Instruct parents/child in handwashing techniques.	Prevents transmission of microorganisms from touching or handling supplies, touching face of child by parent(s)/child without handwashing.
Instruct parents/child to avoid contact with those who have respiratory infections.	Prevents transmission of microorganisms via airborne droplets.

INTERVENTIONS	RATIONALES
Inform parents of need to maintain or increase fluids, type of fluids to include and avoid, to offer small amounts (q 1h to infant and 50 to 100 ml to child q 2h) during waking hours using small cup or straw.	Maintains hydration.
Teach the importance of physical exercise; activities with short burst of energy (baseball, sprinting, skiing) are recommended.	Promotes better tolerance than endurance exercises.
Recommend swimming as a form of physical exercise.	Promotes saturation of inhaled air with moisture; exhaling underwater prolongs expiration and improves end expiratory pressures.
Teach parents to use bulb syringe to remove mucus from infant's nose, demonstrate and instruct in oropharyogeal suctioning if appropriate; allow return demonstration.	Removes secretions in those too weak or unable to cough up secretions, removing mucus from nose of infant enhances breathing (obligate breather).
Teach parents and possibly older child (specify) administration of medications via proper route with name and action of each drug: dosage; why given; frequency; time of day or night; side effects to report; how to administer in food—crushed, chewable, by measured dropper, or other recommended form; and method (nose drops, inhaler).	Ensures compliance with correct drug dosage and other considerations for administrations for desired results, and what to do if side effects occur.
Instruct parents and child to administer aerosols with use of hand-held inhaler, small volume nebulizer using oral or mask breathing apparatus; assembling of devices, cleaning and care of reusable supplies and equipment (specify).	Promotes proper administration and independence of child depending on age and ability.

NIC: *Airway Management*

Evaluation

(Date/time of evaluation of goal)

(Has goal been met? Not met? Partially met?)

(What is respiratory rate, depth, and ease? Are breath sounds clear bilaterally? Is child able to cough, are secretions thin and clear?)

(Revisions to care plan? D/C care plan? Continue care plan?)

INEFFECTIVE BREATHING PATTERN

Related to: Inflammatory process.

Defining Characteristics: (Specify: shortness of breath, tachypnea, fremitus.)

Related to: Decreased lung expansion.

Defining Characteristics: (Specify: apnea, dyspnea, respiratory depth changes.)

Related to: Tracheobronchial obstruction.

Defining Characteristics: (Specify: dyspnea, head bobbing in infant, drooling, tachypnea, abnormal arterial blood gases, cyanosis (skin, circumoral, mucous membranes), nasal flaring, respiratory depth changes, use of accessory muscles and retractions, altered chest excursion, prolonged expiratory phase, grunting, apnea during sleep, anxiety, air hunger, sitting up with mouth open to breathe, stridor on inspiration, persistent cough, throat edema.)

Goal: Infant/child will experience an effective breathing pattern by (date/time to evaluate).

Outcome Criteria

✔ Return of respiratory status to baseline parameters for pattern rate, depth, and ease (specify).

✔ Effective breathing effort and improved chest expansion.

NOC: *Respiratory Status: Airway Patency, Ventilation*

INTERVENTIONS	RATIONALES
Assess respirations for rate (count for one full minute), pattern, depth, and ease; presence of tachypnea (specify), dyspnea and use of accessory muscles and retractions (intercostal, subcostal, substernal, suprasternal), nasal flaring; note expiratory phase, chest expansion, periods of apnea, head bobbing in infant during sleep.	Reveals rate and type of respirations (baselines or deviations) that are related to age and size of the infant/child and presence of anxiety and disease processes, changes in patterns indicate the acuteness of a condition and the respiratory function that result from infection and obstruction; retractions that become severe are responses to a decrease in intrathoracic pressure that may

(continues)

(continued)

INTERVENTIONS	RATIONALES
	extend to suprasternal area if lung consolidation is severe, nasal flaring occurs as the work of breathing increases, head bobbing occurs with dyspnea in infants.
Assess configuration of chest by palpation; auscultate for breath sounds that indicate a movement restriction (absent or diminished, crackles or rhonchi).	Reveals an increased antero-posterior ratio common in children with chronic respiratory disease that results from hyper-expansion of the airways.
Assess skin for pallor or cyanosis, distribution and duration of cyanosis (nail beds, skin, mucous membranes, circumoral).	Reveals presence of hypoxemia causing cyanosis from an uneven distribution of gases and blood in the lungs, and alveolar hypoventilation caused by air-way obstruction, weakness of muscles used in respirations.
Assess for cough, pain when coughing, characteristics of cough and sputum, ability to mobilize and bring up secretions when amounts increase.	Cough is an indication of a respiratory condition and if excessive may cause chest pain and interfere with respirations, accumulation of mucus in air-ways affects respiration if obstruction is present.
Position with head elevated at least 30° or seated upright with head on pillows; position on side if more comfortable; tripod position for the child with epiglottitis; avoid tight clothing or bedding; for child with low muscle tone, use pillows and/or padding to maintain positioning.	Facilitates chest expansion and respiratory efficiency by reducing pressure of abdominal organs on diaphragm; position of comfort is age-related and dependent on degree of dyspnea.
Perform deep breathing exercises and upper body exercises (isometric).	Strengthens intercostal and abdominal muscles, and diaphragm, which enhances breathing and prolongs expira-tory phase.
Assess child's pain and administer analgesics as prescribed (specify drug, dose, route, and time); use a pain assessment tool appropriate to the child's age (specify) and developmental level; assess and record child's response to pain control measures; provide age-appropriate diversional activities as tolerated (specify).	Promotes improved oxygenation.
Pace activities and exercises, and allow for rest periods and energy conservation.	Prevents changes in respiratory pattern brought about from exertion and fatigue.

INTERVENTIONS	RATIONALES
Monitor blood gas levels and provide supplemental oxygen via hood, tent, cannula, or face mask as needed if hypoxia results from inadequate breathing pattern and ventilation; if an infant is apneic, provide access at bedside at all times.	Maintains oxygen level in blood to maintain tissue and organ function, amount and type of oxygen administration dependent on hypoxia and changes in mentation.
Administer bronchodilators via oral, subcutaneous, or aerosol therapy; antibiotics, or sedatives (cautiously) via oral therapy if respiratory efficiency is not reduced; antiasthmatics and steroids via oral or aerosol therapy as ordered (specify).	Relieves bronchospasms that affect respirations (tachypnea, rhonchi), prevents or treats infection, promotes rest and reduces anxiety to enhance breathing; prevents asthmatic attack and reinforces body defenses against allergic reac-tions (action of drug).
Assess family's responses to child's illness and/or hospital-ization; utilize the principles of family-centered caregiving, which encourages the parents to participate in their child's illness within their comfort level.	Parents know their child's behaviors, temperament, and reactions to previous illnesses and treatments better than the health care professionals; utilizing the parent's knowledge will promote understanding and improved caregiving.
Teach parents and child in hand-washing and when to perform; disposal of tissues; covering mouth and nose when coughing to avoid those with respiratory infections.	Prevents transmission of microorganisms to child from inanimate objects or airborne droplets.
Demonstrate and instruct to parents and child in possible positions for comfort and venti-lation during activities and sleep.	Facilitates ease of breathing.
Inform parents and child of activ-ity restrictions and to avoid any activities beyond tolerance and energy level.	Reduces potential dyspnea and fatigue.
Instruct child in relaxation exercises, quiet play, and controlled breathing.	Reduces anxiety in older child which increases respiratory rate.
Inform parents and child to avoid allergens, changes in environ-mental temperatures, humidity, and pollutants, effect of pets, dust, dirty filters, plant odors, and other irritants in the home.	Prevents responses that change respiratory pattern.
Teach parents about oxygen administration (correct rate and method specify) and safety measures (fire prevention).	Supplies oxygen when needed in a correct and safe manner.

INTERVENTIONS	RATIONALES
Instruct and demonstrate medication regimen to parents (and older child) and include route, dosage, time, action, what to expect, and how to administer according to form prescribed (specify).	Ensures accurate and safe administration for medications for optimal effect.
Teach parents to avoid giving child over-the-counter medications unless advised by physician.	Prevents any undesirable interactions with prescribed drugs.
Instruct parents in disinfection, care of reusable supplies, and care of equipment used to administer medications.	Reduces potential for infection and preserves equipment and supplies for long-term use.
(Teach and demonstrate use of apnea monitor to parents (application, setting, alarms, electric source) and how to perform cardiopulmonary resuscitation on infant if needed).	Provides alert system for parents to monitor changes in respirations and heart rate of infant with apnea episodes.

NIC: *Airway Management*

Evaluation

(Date/time of evaluation of goal)

(Has goal been met? Not met? Partially met?)

(What is respiratory rate, depth, and ease? Are breath sounds clear bilaterally? Is child able to cough, are secretions thin and clear?)

(Revisions to care plan? D/C care plan? Continue care plan?)

IMPAIRED GAS EXCHANGE

Related to: Ventilation perfusion imbalance.

Defining Characteristics: (Specify: ABGs.)

Goal: Child will experience improved gas exchange by (date/time to evaluate).

Outcome Criteria

✔ Arterial blood gases within normal ranges for age (specify).

NOC: *Respiratory Status: Gas Exchange*

INTERVENTIONS	RATIONALES
Assess respiratory rate, depth, and ease, (count for one minute), presence of dyspnea, tachypnea, chest movement, periods of apnea (specify frequency).	Reveals respiratory effort, rate and depth (baselines or deviations), symmetry of movements, and use of accessory muscles, which affect the amount of air that reaches the alveoli for ventilation process and diffusion of oxygen (external respiration).
Monitor SaO_2 continuously with pulse oximeter alarms turned on (specify if using TCM to obtain $TcPaO_2$ and $TcPaCO_2$ levels). Assess ABGs for ↓ pH, ↓ PaO_2, ↑ $PaCO_2$ as obtained. Observe nail beds, circumoral area, and mucous membranes for development of cyanosis.	Reveals status of hypoxemia and hypercapnia and potential for respiratory failure: cyanosis in children results from hypoventilation or an uneven distribution of gas and circulation through the lungs, usually caused by disease and breathing abnormalities; gas levels provide the basis for oxygen administration adjustment, need for position change; continuous monitoring by oximetry or transcutaneous electrode reduces need for arterial punctures to determine hypoxemia and hypercapnia.
Assess for changes in consciousness and activity, presence of irritability and restlessness.	Reveals hypoxic state as oxygen level in blood reduces, causing decrease of oxygen to brain.
Place child in semi- or high Fowler's position; orthopenic position for older child unless contraindicated (specify).	Promotes chest expansion and ease of breathing, gas distribution, and pulmonary blood flow, all of which enhance gas exchange.
Administer humidified oxygen via hood (infant), tent (young child), cannula, or face mask (older child) at rate prescribed, and adjust according to blood gas levels (specify).	Ensures adequate oxygen intake to maintain desired level; a PO_2 of less than 60 mm Hg and PCO_2 of more than 50 to 55 mm Hg may indicate need for repositioning, stimulation, suctioning, or ventilator support.
Provide sedation for restlessness, irritability as ordered unless respirations are depressed (specify drug, dose, route, and times).	Promotes rest and ease of respiratory effort to support ventilation, especially if anxiety present (action of drug).
Observe for early stages of hypoxemia and effects on nervous system (mood changes, anxiety, confusion), circulatory system (tachycardia, hypertension), respiratory system (altered depth and pattern,	Promotes careful evaluation of early signs and symptoms of insufficient alveolar ventilation and prevention of respiratory failure or arrest.

(continues)

(continued)

INTERVENTIONS	RATIONALES
dyspnea, retractions, grunting, prolonged expiration), gastrointestinal system (anorexia).	
Discuss disease process, causes, signs and symptoms with parents and child appropriate to age.	Provides information about reason for how to control symptoms and promote general health.
Explain all procedures and use of equipment to parents and child appropriate to age.	Reduces anxiety, which reduces oxygen requirements in the child.
Teach and demonstrate oxygen administration showing correct device to deliver O$_2$, amount to deliver, frequency, type of oxygen system, safety factors to parents; allow for return demonstration.	Maintains oxygen levels with amounts given, preventing hypoxia as well as oxygen, toxicity methods and amounts vary with age and condition of infant/child.
Instruct and demonstrate use of apnea monitor to parents; allow for return demonstration of application, setting, alarms, power source, inform of when and how to respond to changes in respiration and heart rate.	Alerts parents to presence of prolonged periods of apnea in infant in order to prevent hypoxia and possible death.

INTERVENTIONS	RATIONALES
Teach parents of respiratory signs and symptoms that must be reported indicating blood gas imbalance: fatigue, mental confusion, increasing dyspnea and tachypnea.	Assessing and reporting prevents potential for hypoxemia, hypercapnia, and more serious complications of respiratory failure.

NIC: *Respiratory Monitoring*

Evaluation

(Date/time of evaluation of goal)

(Has goal been met? Not met? Partially met?)

(What are ABG values?)

(Revisions to care plan? D/C care plan? Continue care plan?)

CHAPTER 3.1

APNEA

Apnea in the infant is the periodic absence of breathing for more than 15 seconds in the full-term or more than 20 seconds in the preterm infant. It may be associated with gastroesophageal reflux, seizures, sepsis or the impairment of breathing during sleep in the infant, although it is not uncommon to find no apparent causative factor. Apnea occurs during infancy and is usually resolved by one year of age without resulting in the death of the infant. The apparent life-threatening event (ALTE) that is indicative of apnea is not considered a cause of SIDS (sudden infant death syndrome), although the infant with apnea is at slightly higher risk. Both apnea and high-risk SIDS infants may be monitored by an apnea-monitoring device as a preventive measure.

MEDICAL CARE

Apnea Monitor: a device attached to the infant by electrodes placed on a belt that is wrapped around the infant's chest; alarms sound when respiratory or heart rate changes occur that are more or less than the rates set revealing apneic episodes.

Oxygen Therapy: treats hypoxia during apneic periods.

Chest X-ray: reveals respiratory infection if present.

Electrocardiogram: reveals presence of arrhythmias caused by bradycardia associated with apnea.

Electroencephalogram: reveals changes associated with seizures.

Pneumocardiogram: reveals cardiorespiratory patterns of heart and breathing rates, nasal airflow, and oxygen saturation.

Polysomnography: measures brain waves, eye movement, esophageal manometry, and end-tidal CO_2 levels during sleep.

pH Probe Study: 24-hour measurements of pH from a probe in the esophagus to reveal reflux.

Upper Gastrointestinal X-ray: reveals reflux associated with apnea.

Arterial Blood Gases: monitors respiratory function for pO_2 and pCO_2 changes resulting from abnormal ventilatory drive.

Methylxanthines: a drug used to stimulate respiration; theophyline or caffeine.

Metoclopramine (Cisapride): drug used to increase emptying a duodenum and tone of esophageal sphincter.

Nasal CPAP: continuous positive airway pressure may be used for preterm-birth apnea thought to be related to collapse of airway.

COMMON NURSING DIAGNOSES

See INEFFECTIVE BREATHING PATTERN

Related to: Impaired regulation.

Defining Characteristics: (Specify: respiratory depth changes, apnea during sleep, cyanosis, abnormal arterial blood gases.

See IMPAIRED GAS EXCHANGE

Related to: Ventilation perfusion imbalance.

Defining Characteristics: (Specify: preterm birth, hypoxia, apnea, bradycardia, hypercapnia, pallor.)

See IMBALANCED NUTRITION: LESS THAN BODY REQUIREMENTS

Related to: Inability to ingest food because of biologic factors.

Defining Characteristics: Choking and gasping during feeding, apneic or cyanotic episodes, reflux.

ADDITIONAL NURSING DIAGNOSES

RISK FOR ALTERED PARENTING

Related to: (Specify, e.g., adolescent parent.)

Defining Characteristics: Verbalization of role inadequacy, inappropriate caretaking behaviors (use of apnea monitoring device, cardiopulmonary resuscitation), request for information about care of infant and parenting skills (specify).

Goal: Parents will demonstrate necessary skills for caring for their child by (date/time to evaluate).

Outcome Criteria

✔ Verbalized readiness to deal with apneic episodes of infant.

✔ Demonstrates correct application and operation of apnea monitor.

✔ Becomes proficient at infant cardiopulmonary resuscitation (CPR).

NOC: *Role Performance*

INTERVENTIONS	RATIONALES
Assess history of apnea, life-threatening event of infant, SIDS of siblings or cousins.	Reveals risk factors associated with condition as basis for further evaluation.
Assess for presence of apneic or cyanotic episodes, bradycardia, upper respiratory infection, poor feeding with choking during feedings.	Identifies apneic episodes of more than 15 seconds in preterm or more than 20 seconds in full-term infant, associated factors, or potential for SIDS and need for monitoring.
Assess parents' ability to participate in apnea monitoring and/or CPR as an intervention in event of episode.	Fear and anxiety common to parents of apneic infant; feelings of guilt and inadequacy, fear of death of child presents obstacle to learning and interventions necessary for child's survival.
Encourage and allow parents to express feelings about unmet needs and ability to meet and develop self-expectations.	Identifies potential for isolation and social deprivation of mother, strategies to achieve realistic expectations.
Encourage touching and play activities between parents and infant.	Enhances bonding process and positive parental behaviors.
Provide calm, supportive and positive environment; encourage and praise positive parental behaviors.	Reduces anxiety for enhanced learning of infant care procedures.

INTERVENTIONS	RATIONALES
Provide written and/or pictorial instructions for parents of step-by-step procedures for apnea monitoring and resuscitation.	Provides reference as reinforcement of learning.
Demonstrate for parents, and allow for return demonstration, attaching electrodes to belt and monitor, applying belt to infant's chest, setting monitor, testing monitor alarms, turning monitor on, removal and care of monitor after use (add details).	Apnea monitor may be prescribed by physician for use in home for apneic and "near-miss" infants, although use is controversial; monitors cardiac and respiratory activity with an alarm system that wakes parents when rates are not within prescribed boundaries; electrodes, lead wires, and cable pick up on breathing and heart activity signals and limit apnea time by sounding alarm.
Teach parents safety issues of home apnea monitoring: remove leads from infant when not attached to monitor; unplug power cord when cord is not plugged into monitor; use safety covers on electrical outlets to discourage siblings from inserting other objects.	Prevent electrical accidents related to home monitor.
Demonstrate for parents and allow for return demonstration of CPR on infant model; instruct both parents and a family member in assessment of infant and need for CPR, correct mouth-to-mouth and cardiac compression techniques; supply written and pictorial instructions or booklet for review.	CPR done to resuscitate infant with cessation of breathing and presence of cyanosis.
Instruct parents to notify electric company and nearest 911 unit that monitor is being used; provide telephone numbers for emergency services and instruct to keep near phone.	Provides for emergency services if and when needed, including alternate electric sources.
Instruct other significant family members (grandparents) and support persons as to care for the child with a home monitor, including CPR (specify).	Promotes positive coping as parents can lessen continuous responsibility of home apnea monitoring.
Provide praise and support for parents as they learn to use the monitor and develop skill in CPR.	Positive reinforcement and support help the parents develop new parenting skills and feel confident in their abilities as parents.

INTERVENTIONS	RATIONALES
Explain the difference between apnea and SIDS.	Parental perception of the relationship between these conditions is often the basis for their fear of child's possible survival.
Instruct parents to place healthy infants on their back during sleep; avoid soft surfaces and soft objects (pillows) in the sleep environment.	Decreases the risk of SIDS, according to research; the American Academy of Pediatrics recommends that healthy infants be placed on their backs to sleep. Infants placed on their sides may roll to the prone position.
Suggest referral to home care agency, contact with family members and friends, other support services (specify).	Provides range of support and assistance, which helps to reduce anxiety and promote social activities.

NIC: *Role Enhancement*

Evaluation

(Date/time of evaluation of goal)

(Has goal been met? Not met? Partially met?)

(Did parents verbalize readiness to handle apnea? Provide quotes. Did parents demonstrate correct application of apnea monitor? Are parents proficient at infant CPR?)

(Revisions to care plan? D/C care plan? Continue care plan?)

COMPROMISED FAMILY COPING

Related to: Situational crisis.

Defining Characteristics: (Specify: family expresses concern and fear about infant's apnea episodes, displays protective behavior disproportionate to infant's need to grow and develop, describes a preoccupation with monitoring of infant apnea, chronic anxiety.)

Goal: Family will demonstrate adequate coping by (date/time to evaluate).

Outcome Criteria

✔ Family members are able to express feelings and needs to each other.

✔ Family members identify three healthy coping mechanisms.

NOC: *Family Coping*

INTERVENTIONS	RATIONALES
Assess family anxiety level, erratic behaviors (anger, tension, disorganization) perception of crisis situation.	Identifies information affecting ability of family to cope with infant apnea and monitoring.
Assess family coping methods used and perceived effectiveness.	Identifies need to develop new coping skills if existing methods are ineffective in changing exhibited behaviors.
Encourage expression of feelings and provide factual information about infant apnea.	Reduces anxiety and enhances family's understanding of condition.
Assist family to identify and use 3 techniques to cope with and solve problems and gain control over the situation (specify suggestions).	Provides support for problem solving and management of situation.
Reinforce appropriate coping behaviors.	Promote behavior change and adaptation to care of infant during apnea.
Suggest to parents that over-protective behaviors may hinder growth and development during infancy.	Enhances family understanding of condition and adverse effects of behaviors.
Reinforce need to maintain health of family members and social contacts.	Provides information about chronic anxiety, fatigue, and isolation as result of infant care and about their effects on health and care capabilities of family.

NIC: *Family Integrity Promotion*

Evaluation

(Date/time of evaluation of goal)

(Has goal been met? Not met? Partially met?)

(Did family members express feelings and needs to each other? Specify. Which three healthy coping mechanisms did family members identify?)

(Revisions to care plan? D/C care plan? Continue care plan?)

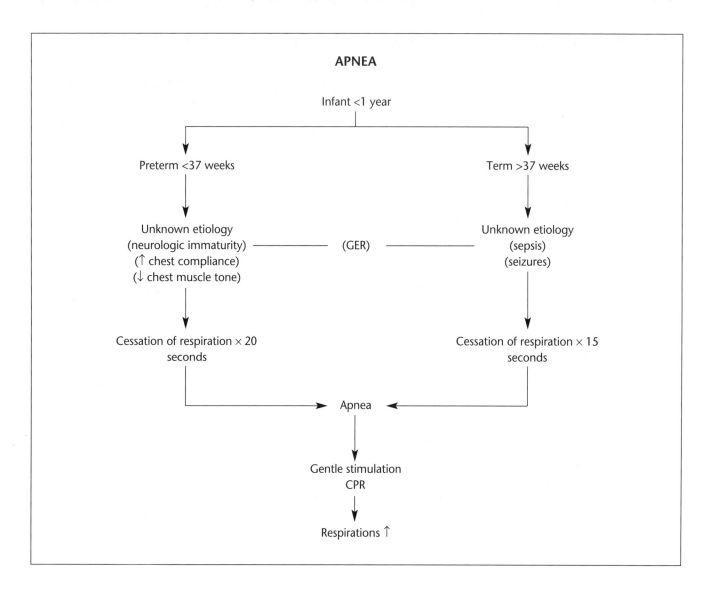

APNEA

Infant <1 year

Preterm <37 weeks

Term >37 weeks

Unknown etiology
(neurologic immaturity) —————— (GER) —————— Unknown etiology
($\uparrow$ chest compliance)   (sepsis)
($\downarrow$ chest muscle tone)   (seizures)

Cessation of respiration × 20
seconds

Cessation of respiration × 15
seconds

Apnea

Gentle stimulation
CPR

Respirations $\uparrow$

CHAPTER 3.2

ASTHMA

Asthma in children is a reversible airway-reactive disease characterized by bronchospasm, increased mucus production, and edema of the mucosa of the bronchioles. The result is obstruction, air trapping, and respiratory distress. Asthma is the leading chronic disorder in children. Most children experience their first attacks between 2 and 7 years of age with the onset of the most severe cases occurring after the age of 7. The onset of an attack may be gradual or immediate; continuous, with wheezing present at all times; or spasmodic, with intermittent attacks separated by intervals without symptoms. As an attack progresses, alveoli that are hyperinflated and poorly ventilated may lead to impaired gas exchange, hypoxemia, hypercapnia, and eventual respiratory acidosis and failure. The two types of asthma are extrinsic (immune mechanisms) and intrinsic (imbalance in the autonomic nervous system), both of which affect the bronchial tissue and mast cell function that produce the characteristics symptoms of the disease. Status asthmaticus is an acute condition characterized by an asthma attack that fails to respond to treatment and continues and increases in severity. It requires hospitalization of the child.

MEDICAL CARE

Preventive Medications: cromolyn sodium (Intel), PO or inhalation for children >5 years old: an NSAID that inhibits release of bronchoconstrictors from mast cells; beta-adrenergic agonists: PO, (albuterol, terbutaline) or inhaled (salmetrol) as prophylaxis for exercise-induced asthma.

Rescue Medications: corticosteroids: IV or possibly PO for short-term use to ↓ inflammation and ↓ airway obstruction; beta-adrenergic agonists: PO, IV (albuterol, terbutaline) or inhaled (salmetrol); methylxanthines (theophylline) PO, IV not usually used because of side effects and narrow margin of safety (toxicity at serum level >20 g/mL).

Antibiotics: given PO or IV specific to organism identified in culture and in sensitivity test of sputum.

Oxygen Therapy: treats hypoxemia as indicated by ABGs and is administered by tent, cannula, or face mask; use is usually reserved for status asthmaticus.

Chest X-ray: may reveal hyperinflation, infiltrates, or other pulmonary conditions such as atelectasis or pneumonia.

Pulmonary Function Testing; spirometry, peak expiratory flow rate (PEFR) compared with child's personal best flow rate. Measured in green (80–100% of personal best), yellow (50–80%), and red zones (<50% of personal best).

Sputum Culture: reveals large numbers of eosinophils and crystalloid fragments.

Arterial Blood Gases: reveals decreased pH, decreased pO_2, and increased pCO_2 as attack continues and ventilation perfusion imbalance occurs.

Complete Blood Count: reveals increased WBC if infection present, increased eosinophils in differential count of more than 5%, increased Hgb and Hct.

Skin Tests: done by scratch or intradermal to identify specific allergens for hypersensitization injection therapy for an older child.

Provocative Inhalation Test: reveals specific allergens and level that precipitates symptoms.

COMMON NURSING DIAGNOSES

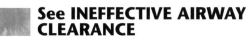 ### See INEFFECTIVE AIRWAY CLEARANCE

Related to: Tracheobronchial obstruction, secretions.

Defining Characteristics: (Specify: dyspnea; tachypnea; cough with or without sputum; uncontrollable cough that is hacking and paroxysmal, becomes rattling, and produces a clear, frothy sputum; abnormal breath sounds [wheezing on expiration and inspiration, fine and coarse crackles]; circumoral and nail bed cyanosis; fever; assuming orthopneic position.)

 ### See INEFFECTIVE BREATHING PATTERN

Related to: Inflammatory process, tracheobronchial obstruction, anxiety.

Defining Characteristics: (Specify: dyspnea, tachypnea, cough, nasal flaring, prolonged expiratory phase, intercostal and suprasternal retractions in infant, hyperresonance on percussion, shallow and irregular respirations, barrel chest configuration, abnormal ABGs, cyanosis, anxiety, restlessness, apprehension, speaks in short, broken phrases or unable to speak.)

See IMPAIRED GAS EXCHANGE

Related to: Ventilation perfusion imbalance.

Defining Characteristics: (Specify: restlessness, irritability, hypoxemia, hypercapnia, confusion, somnolence.)

 ### See RISK FOR DEFICIENT FLUID VOLUME

Related to: ↓ intake.

Defining Characteristics: (Specify: difficulty in drinking during panting, tachypnea, and dyspnea; thirst; dry skin and mucous membranes; diaphoresis; insensible loss.)

See SLEEP PATTERN DISTURBANCE

Related to: Interrupted sleep.

Defining Characteristics: (Specify: dyspnea, tachypnea, irritability, restlessness, inability to remain in prone or supine positions.)

 ### See IMBALANCED NUTRITION: LESS THAN BODY REQUIREMENTS

Related to: Chronic illness.

Defining Characteristics: (Specify: anorexia, nausea, vomiting, weight loss, dyspnea and tachypnea preventing intake of food.)

ADDITIONAL NURSING DIAGNOSES

ANXIETY

Related to: Threat of or change in health status (specify).

Defining Characteristics: (Specify: increased apprehension, fear with asthma attack, change in respiratory status, exposure to known or unknown allergens, tension and uncertainty about possible hospitalization for acute attack.)

Goal: Client will experience decreased anxiety by (date/time to evaluate).

Outcome Criteria

✔ Child verbalizes decreased anxiety.
✔ Child uses breathing exercises and relaxation techniques.

NOC: *Anxiety Control*

INTERVENTIONS	RATIONALES
Assess level of anxiety before, during, and after attack.	Provides information about anxiety level of child and parents as respirations become more difficult and fear of suffocation is present, and about fear of subsequent attacks.
Provide calm, supportive, and nonjudgmental environment, especially during an attack.	Reduces anxiety and calming effect allows and eases respirations for improved ventilation.
Allow parents and child to express fears and concerns and to ask questions about disease and what to expect.	Provides opportunity to vent feelings and secure information to reduce anxiety, especially if they know how to prevent or reduce frequency of attacks.
Prepare parents and child before all procedures and treatment.	Relieves anxiety caused by fear of unknown.
Stay with child during acute attack.	Provides comfort and support to the child.
Encourage quiet play and avoid any emotional stress.	Provides distractions from changes in breathing pattern and prevents emotional upsets, that increase respiratory difficulty or may initiate an acute attack.

INTERVENTIONS	RATIONALES
If hospitalized, allow open visitation, and telephoning; encourage parents to stay with child if possible, to bring toy or blanket from home, and to maintain home schedules for sleep, feeding, play as appropriate.	Relieves anxiety for parents and child when familiar people and routines are available.
Explain to parents and child the reason for and what to expect before and/or during attack; use drawings, pictures, models, and video tapes for child.	Promotes understanding of what is happening during attack and the possible causes in order to allay anxiety.
Inform parents and child of the reversibility of the disease, how the medications and treatment resolve the attack.	Reduces anxiety caused by fear of suffocation.
Clarify any misinformation and answer all questions honestly in simple understandable language for the parents and child.	Prevents unnecessary anxiety that results from inaccurate information or beliefs.
Instruct parents and child in environmental control and exercise limitations.	Provides anticipatory teaching that assists parents and child in preventing attacks.

NIC: *Anxiety Reduction*

Evaluation

(Date/time of evaluation of goal)

(Has goal been met? Not met? Partially met?)

(Did child verbalize decreased anxiety? Use quotes. Did child engage in breathing and relaxation exercises?)

(Revisions to care plan? D/C care plan? Continue care plan?)

ACTIVITY INTOLERANCE

Related to: (Specify: respiratory problem, fatigue.)

Defining Characteristics: (Specify: prolonged dyspnea from asthma attack; lethargy; exhausted appearance, inability to eat, speak, play.)

Goal: Child will experience increased tolerance for activity by (date and time to evaluate).

Outcome Criteria

✔ Child participates in usual activities (specify).

✔ Child verbalizes feeling less fatigued (specify).

NOC: *Activity Tolerance*

INTERVENTIONS	RATIONALES
Assess presence of weakness and fatigue caused by respiratory changes.	Provides information about energy reserves as dyspnea and work of breathing over period of time exhausts these reserves.
Schedule and provide rest periods in a quiet environment.	Promotes adequate rest and reduces stimuli.
Disturb only when necessary, perform all care at one time instead of spreading over a long period of time, avoid performing any care or procedures during an attack.	Conserves energy and prevents interruption in rest.
Provide for quiet play, reading, TV, games while at rest.	Prevents alteration in respiratory status and energy depletion caused by excessive activity.
Explain reason for need to conserve energy and avoid fatigue to parents and child.	Promotes understanding of effect of activity on breathing and need for rest to prevent fatigue.
Instruct in planning a schedule for bathing, feeding, rest that will conserve energy and prevent attack or promote resolution of an attack.	Provides care while promoting activities of daily care.
Inform of activity or exercise restrictions if these trigger attack; suggest medically approved activities (swimming, bicycling).	Provides preventive measures to offset possible attack.

NIC: *Energy Management*

Evaluation

(Date/time of evaluation of goal)

(Has goal been met? Not met? Partially met?)

(Describe activities in which child participated. Use quotes for child's verbalization of energy level)

(Revisions to care plan? D/C care plan? Continue care plan?)

HEALTH-SEEKING BEHAVIORS: PREVENTION OF ASTHMA ATTACK

Related to: Desire for information of preventive measures and behavior changes.

Defining Characteristics: (Specify: expressed desire for increased control of health practices and effect of current environmental conditions and behaviors on health status, increased frequency of attacks use quotes.)

Goal: Clients will obtain information about asthma.

Outcome Criteria

✔ Parents (and child if age-appropriate) verbalize understanding of triggering agents and prevention measures for asthma attacks.

NOC: *Knowledge: Health Promotion*

INTERVENTIONS	RATIONALES
Assess for knowledge of factors related to attacks, past history of respiratory infections and measures taken to maintain health of child.	Provides basis for information needed for health maintenance, as respiratory changes or infection can trigger an asthma attack.
Assess for use of over-the-counter medications, type used and effects.	Identifies whether products available for treatment of respiratory diseases should or should not be used, as they may interact with prescribed medications, causing attack to become more severe.
Assess health history of allergies in family members, what does or does not precipitate attack, and what behaviors result from the attack.	Identifies familial tendency to airway reactive disease or history of allergic rhinitis, eczema, urticaria.
Teach parents/child hand-washing technique, allow for demonstration.	Prevents transmission of micro-organisms from touching or handling supplies, touching face of child by parents or child without handwash.
Instruct child to avoid contact with those who have respiratory infections, how to cover mouth and nose when coughing or sneezing, and to dispose of tissues.	Prevents transmission of micro-organisms by airborne droplets.
Teach parents and child about physiology and signs and symptoms of the disease and possible precipitating factors influencing an attack (specify).	Provides information that will enhance performance of preventive measures and compliance to medical regimen.

INTERVENTIONS	RATIONALES
Discuss with parents and child the signs and symptoms indicating the onset of an attack (change in respirations, wheezing, dyspnea).	Teach actions to be taken to prevent a severe attack and when to notify physician.
Instruct child to avoid excessive activity, stressful situations.	Provides information on how to avoid situations that may provoke an attack.
Teach parents of effect of allergens and how to avoid exposure to offending environmental factors (cold air, humidity, air pollution, sprays, plants).	Reduces exposure to factors that precipitate an attack.
Suggest to parents actions to change home environment to reduce dust, exposure to pets and indoor plants, changing of filters, avoidance of foods (yellow dye), drugs (aspirin).	Reduces exposure to factors that precipitate an attack.
Teach child breathing exercises and controlled breathing and relaxation.	Prevents attack before it begins and increases ventilation.
Teach parents and child about medication administration as ordered (specify drug, dose, route, and times to be given) and how to manage method of administration; advise to avoid over-the-counter drugs without physician advice.	Promotes compliance in order to prevent attack and maintain wellness (action of drug).
Inform parents of skin testing for sensitivities to allergens.	Identifies allergies for hyper-sensitization regimen.
Suggest community agencies to contact for information and support.	Offers support to families with child suffering from asthma.

NIC: *Health Education*

Evaluation

(Date/time of evaluation of goal)

(Has goal been met? Not met? Partially met?)

(Did parents/child verbalize understanding of triggering agents and prevention measures for asthma attacks? Provide quotes.)

(Revisions to care plan? D/C care plan? Continue care plan?)

INTERRUPTED FAMILY PROCESSES

Related to: (Ill child.)

Defining Characteristics: (Specify: parental stress, which may result in parental dysfunction; stress may be manifested by excessive worry, withdrawal, denial, difficulty in making child-rearing decisions, overprotectiveness; alterations in the parent-child relationship which may hinder adjustment and decrease parent's ability to maximize child's growth and development potential.)

Goal: Family will resume supportive interaction by (date/time to evaluate).

Outcome Criteria

✔ Parents verbalize feelings and concerns related to the implications of the disease on the entire family.

✔ Family demonstrates acceptance, adjustment, and coping behaviors related to the symptoms and effects of asthma.

NOC: *Family Coping*

INTERVENTIONS	RATIONALES
Provide an opportunity for the family to adjust to the diagnosis; anticipate the normal grief reaction of "loss of the perfect child."	Reaction may occur in the early adjustment phase, after the diagnosis of a chronic disease, depending on the severity.
Explore the family's feelings regarding the child and the diagnosis.	Indicators of family-related psychologic stress often are obtained during open discussions as part of a history-taking; family stressors, if found early, can be the focus of preventive services to promote adaptation.
Assist the family to explore specific feelings regarding: guilt, anger, disappointment, irritation, and fear; discuss with parents their fears: dealing with the child's anxiety, fear of complications, fear of death, fear of tests and procedures, fear of treatments, and the child's potential inability to feel "normal" as compared to peers; help family to identify realistic and unrealistic fears.	Validates the normalcy of their feelings which promotes stress reduction and positive coping skills.

INTERVENTIONS	RATIONALES
Assess the family's coping skills and resources.	Promotes reinforcement of positive coping skills.
Foster positive family relationships; serve as a role model regarding attitudes and behaviors towards the child.	Promotes the family's ability to cope in a positive manner.
Assess interpersonal relationships within the family and support systems, with emphasis on the family's relationship with the child diagnosed with asthma; intervene appropriately with evidence of maladaptation; refer to counseling if appropriate (specify).	Promotes early identification of interpersonal problems, especially within the parent-child relationship.
Provide support to the family; assess family's support systems and encourage their appropriate use; refer to community agencies and support groups, as applicable (specify).	Promotes positive adaptation within the family.
Assess siblings and peers at intervals, as appropriate, providing time for questions and feelings.	Promotes positive relationships within siblings and peers, which can be altered by chronic illness that requires increased parental attention, and so forth.
Provide information to the family regarding the disorder, treatments, and implications; reinforce all information given; provide accurate information, paced at a rate appropriate for the family (specify).	Promotes a sense of control and alleviates stress; reinforcement and individualizing the approach promotes better understanding.
Encourage family in methods to promote the child's physical, psychological, and cognitive development, based on child's current developmental level (specify).	Provides parents accurate information on growth and development.
Assist family in the development and implementation of a home plan of care, utilizing age-appropriate goals consistent with activity tolerance.	Provides for an optimal level of care at home; parental input into that plan of care may serve to increase compliance and foster positive adaptation.
Explain to child/family the possible benefits of hyposensitization therapy where allergies cannot be avoided, as applicable.	Prevents potential asthma exacerbation when allergen induced.
Teach child and family correct use of metered dose inhaler, nebulizer, and peak flow meter;	Prevents and/or minimizes asthma exacerbation by early identification.

(continues)

(continued)

INTERVENTIONS	RATIONALES
emphasize understanding of equipment usage, cleaning, and strategies for compliance.	
Instruct child and family on preventive treatment when applicable (specify, i.e., prevention of exercise-induced asthma can be accomplished by use of certain medications prophylactically).	Prevents and/or minimizes asthma exacerbations.
Encourage child and family to engage in good health practices, such as balanced nutritional diet, adequate rest, good hygiene, and follow-up care.	Promotes the body's own natural defenses.
Reinforce methods to prevent infections: good handwashing, cleaning and care of equipment used, and avoidance of exposures.	Prevention of infection may minimize asthma exacerbations.

INTERVENTIONS	RATIONALES
Review with parents the signs of depression, especially in the adolescent; make appropriate referrals as needed (specify).	Promotes timely communication between parent and healthcare provider if concerns arise.

NIC: *Family Integrity Promotion*

Evaluation

(Date/time of evaluation of goal)

(Has goal been met? Not met? Partially met?)

(Did parents verbalize feelings and concerns? Provide quotes. Did family demonstrate acceptance, adjustment, and coping behaviors? Describe.)

(Revisions to care plan? D/C care plan? Continue care plan?)

ASTHMA

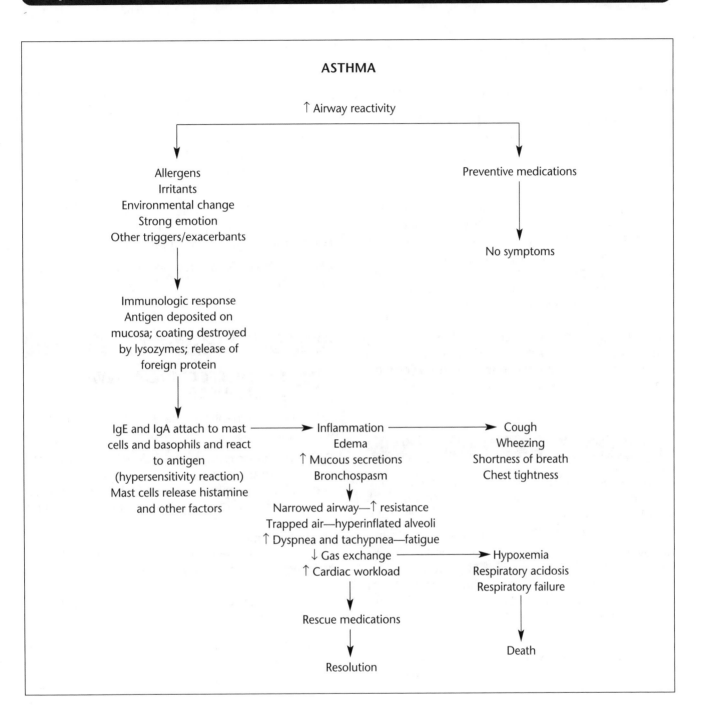

↑ Airway reactivity

Allergens
Irritants
Environmental change
Strong emotion
Other triggers/exacerbants

Preventive medications

No symptoms

Immunologic response
Antigen deposited on
mucosa; coating destroyed
by lysozymes; release of
foreign protein

IgE and IgA attach to mast → Inflammation ────────→ Cough
cells and basophils and react   Edema   Wheezing
to antigen   ↑ Mucous secretions   Shortness of breath
(hypersensitivity reaction)   Bronchospasm   Chest tightness
Mast cells release histamine
and other factors   Narrowed airway—↑ resistance
                      Trapped air—hyperinflated alveoli
                      ↑ Dyspnea and tachypnea—fatigue
                          ↓ Gas exchange ──────→ Hypoxemia
                          ↑ Cardiac workload   Respiratory acidosis
                                                    Respiratory failure

                          Rescue medications

                                                    Death

                          Resolution

CHAPTER 3.3

BRONCHIOLITIS

Bronchiolitis is an acute viral inflammation of the lower respiratory tract involving the bronchioles and alveoli. Accumulated thick mucus, exudate, and cellular debris and the mucosal edema from the inflammatory process obstruct the smaller airways (bronchioles). This causes a reduction in expiration, air trapping, and hyperinflation of the alveoli. The obstruction interferes with gas exchange, and in severe cases causes hypoxemia and hypercapnia, which can lead to respiratory acidosis. Children in a debilitated state who experience this disorder with other serious diseases are hospitalized.

MEDICAL CARE

Prevention: synagis IM monthly or RespiGam IV × 3 to 4 hours monthly. Drugs are reserved for high-risk infants (preterm, immune-compromised, <2 years old with chronic lung disease) during RSV season only.

Antipyretics: acetaminophen (Tylenol tablets, Pedric wafers or elixir, Liquiprin drops) PO to reduce fever. Ibuprofen (nonsteroidal anti-inflammatory) for children 6 months to 12 years; Motrin or Advil liquid suspension or tablets PO to reduce fever and inflammation.

Antivirals: ribavirin (Vilena, Viramid) via aerosol inhalation (hood, tent, or mask) during first 3 days of illness to prevent replication of the syncytial virus; controversial, usually reserved for use in those with or at risk for severe illnesses or complications.

Chest X-ray: reveals hyperinflation, atelectasis and areas of collapse, flattened diaphragm indicating air trapping; areas of consolidation may need differentiation from pneumonia.

Nasal/Nasopharyngeal Culture: reveals respiratory synctial virus by enzyme-linked immunosorbent assay method.

Arterial Blood Gases: reveals decreased pH, pO_2 under 60 mm Hg, pCO_2 over 45 mm Hg, indicating respiratory compromise and potential failure.

Complete Blood Count: reveals increased WBC, indicating infectious process.

COMMON NURSING DIAGNOSES

See INEFFECTIVE AIRWAY CLEARANCE

Related to: Tracheobronchial infection, obstruction, secretions.

Defining Characteristics: (Specify: abnormal breath sounds [diminished or absent, crackles, wheezes]; audible and palpable rhonchi; hyperresonance; change in rate and depth of respirations; tachypnea (50–80/min); paroxysmal, nonproductive, and harsh, hacking cough; dyspnea and shallow respiratory excursion; fever; increased mucus and nasal discharge.)

See INEFFECTIVE BREATHING PATTERN

Related to: Inflammatory process, tracheobronchial obstruction.

Defining Characteristics: (Specify: dyspnea, tachypnea, cough, nasal flaring, shallow respiratory excursion, suprasternal and subcostal retractions, abnormal ABGs.)

See IMPAIRED GAS EXCHANGE

Related to: Ventilation perfusion imbalance.

Defining Characteristics: (Specify: hypoxia, hypercapnia, irritability, restlessness, fatigue, inability to move secretions.)

See IMBALANCED NUTRITION: LESS THAN BODY REQUIREMENTS

Related to: Inability to ingest food because of fatigue.

Defining Characteristics: (Specify: dyspnea, fatigue, and weakness, causing difficulty in feeding, anorexia, weight loss.)

See RISK FOR DEFICIENT FLUID VOLUME

Related to: Excessive losses, altered fluid intake.

Defining Characteristics: (Specify: increased temperature, dry skin and mucous membranes, poor turgor.)

See HYPERTHERMIA

Related to: Respiratory infection.

Defining Characteristics (Specify: low-grade, moderate fever; give data, malaise.)

ADDITIONAL NURSING DIAGNOSES

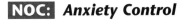

ANXIETY

Related to: (Specify: change in health status of infant or small child, threat of or actual hospitalization of infant/small child.)

Defining Characteristics: (Specify: increased apprehension that condition might worsen; expressed concern and worry about impending hospitalization, need for treatment such as mist tent, IV therapy while hospitalized.)

Goal: Clients will experience decreased anxiety by (date/time to evaluate).

Outcome Criteria

✔ Client verbalizes decreased anxiety.

✔ Client appears relaxed.

NOC: *Anxiety Control*

INTERVENTIONS	RATIONALES
Assess source and level of anxiety, how anxiety is manifested, and need for information that will relieve anxiety.	Provides information about anxiety level and the need for interventions to relieve it; sources of anxiety may include fear and uncertainty about treatment and recovery, guilt for presence of illness, possible loss of parental role, and loss of responsibility if hospitalized.
Allow expression of concerns and opportunity to ask questions about condition and recovery of ill infant/small child.	Provides opportunity to vent feelings, and to secure information needed to reduce anxiety.
Communicate openly with parents and answer questions calmly and honestly.	Promotes calm and supportive environment.
Encourage parents to remain calm and involved in care and decision-making regarding infant/small child noting any improvement that results.	Promotes constant monitoring of infant/small child for improvement or worsening of symptoms.
Encourage parents to stay with infant/small child or allow open visitation and telephoning, have parents assist in care (holding, feeding, diapering) and suggest routines and methods of treatment.	Allows parents to care for and support infant/small child; absence and wondering about condition of infant/small child may increase anxiety.
Teach parents about disease process and physical effects and symptoms of disease.	Provides information to relieve anxiety by informing parents of what to expect.
Explain reason for each procedure or type of therapy, effects of any diagnostic tests to parents (specify).	Prevents anxiety by reducing fear of unknown.
Clarify any misinformation and answer questions in lay terms when parents are able to listen, give same explanation other staff and/or physician gave regarding disease process and transmission.	Prevents unnecessary anxiety resulting from inaccurate knowledge or beliefs, or inconsistencies in information.

NIC: *Anxiety Reduction*

Evaluation

(Date/time of evaluation of goal)

(Has goal been met? Not met? Partially met?)

(Did parents verbalize decreased anxiety? Use quotes. Do parents appear more relaxed? Describe appearance contrasted to initial assessment of tension.)

(Revisions to care plan? D/C care plan? Continue care plan?)

FATIGUE

Related to: Respiratory effort.

Defining Characteristics: (Specify: lethargy or listlessness, emotional liability or irritability, exhausted appearance, inability to eat, limpness.)

Goal: Infant/child will experience increased energy level by (date/time to evaluate)

Outcome Criteria

✔ Infant/child is able to eat, drink, and play quietly.

NOC: *Activity Tolerance*

INTERVENTIONS	RATIONALES
Assess for extreme weakness and fatigue; ability to rest, sleep, and amount; movement in bed.	Provides information to determine effects of dyspnea and work of breathing over period of time, which becomes exhaustive and depletes infant/small child energy reserves and ability to rest, eat, drink.
Disturb infant/small child only when necessary, perform all care at one time instead of spreading over a long period of time.	Conserves energy and prevents interruptions in rest.
Schedule and provide rest periods in a quiet, comfortable environment (temperature and humidity).	Promotes adequate rest and reduces stimuli in order to decrease risk for fatigue.
Allow quiet play with familiar toy while maintaining bed rest.	Rest decreases fatigue and respiratory distress; quiet play prevents excessive activity, that depletes energy and increases respirations.
Encourage parents to use measures to prevent fatigue in infant/small child (holding and/or rocking, feeding in small amounts, playing with child, offering diversions such as TV, toys).	Provides support to infant/small child and conserves energy.

INTERVENTIONS	RATIONALES
Teach parents to pick up infant/small child if crying longer than 1 to 2 minutes.	Prevents fatigue, as prolonged crying is exhaustive.
Assist parents to develop a plan to provide feeding, bathing, changing diaper around rest periods.	Prevents interruption in rest and sleep.

NIC: *Energy Management*

Evaluation

(Date/time of evaluation of goal)

(Has goal been met? Not met? Partially met?)

(Provide data about child's eating and drinking including amounts taken. Describe child's play activity.)

(Revisions to care plan? D/C care plan? Continue care plan?)

DEFICIENT KNOWLEDGE: RSV

Related to: Lack of information about respiratory syncytial virus.

Defining Characteristics: Parents verbalize lack of understanding about RSV.

Goal: Parents will obtain knowledge about RSV.

Outcome Criteria

✔ Parents verbalize methods of prevention and treatment of RSV.

NOC: *Knowledge: Disease Process*

INTERVENTIONS	RATIONALES
Assess existing knowledge of disease prevention, transmission, and treatment.	Provides baseline for type of information needed to prevent infection transmission to child.
Teach that the virus is transmitted by direct and indirect contact via the nose and eyes, and that hands should be kept away from these areas.	Explains that kissing and cuddling infant/small child, and fomites that are on hard, smooth surfaces are sources of contact with the virus.

INTERVENTIONS	RATIONALES
Teach good handwashing technique for child and family members.	Prevents transmission by the hands, which are the main sources of contamination and carriers of organisms to the face area.
Suggest that plastic goggles may be worn when caring for infant/small child.	Prevents risk of contact with virus via the eyes.
Teach of potential for spread of virus to other family members and need for segregation of infant/small child from others.	Explains that virus is easily transmitted, with an incidence as high as half of family members acquiring viral infections.
If hospitalized, adhere to infection control policies for clients with RSV (specify).	Protects from exposure to secretions and transmission of virus to other patients.
Teach parents about the administration of medications prescribed (specify).	Improves consistency of medication administration and the recognition of adverse side effects.
Teach parents on the signs and symptoms of respiratory distress and infection, including fever, dyspnea, tachypnea, and expectoration of yellow/green sputum.	Encourages parents to seek prompt medical attention, as needed.
Encourage parents to provide good nutrition and hydration, emphasizing a high-calorie balanced diet and increased fluids (specify amounts).	Promotes liquification of secretions and replaces calories used to fight infection, thereby boosting the child's own natural body defense.
Encourage and teach parents to provide care for the hospitalized child at a level they are comfortable with and within the constraints of necessary treatments. Teach parents about the prophylactic drugs (if ordered) of RespiGam or Synagis (specify) • These drugs are given to high-risk infants only during the RSV season to prevent RSV infection of compromised infants. • RespiGam is RSV immune globulin that is administered once a month during RSV season by IV infusion lasting several hours. The drug interferes with vaccine effectiveness.	Promotes parental identity and control; may lessen anxiety and stress.

INTERVENTIONS	RATIONALES
• Synagis is a synthetic monoclonal antibody that is administered IM once a month during RSV season. The drug does not interfere with vaccines. It is very expensive.	
(Instruct parents regarding the drug Ribavirin if used during hospitalization: • Side effects • Type and purposes of isolation, including use of masks, gloves, and/or gowns as applicable (specify) • Precautions utilized for parents, staff, and visitors, including information regarding potential risks of environmental exposure; advise pregnant women not to directly care for child; decrease potential exposure by temporarily stopping the aerosols when tent/hood is opened and administer drug in well-ventilated rooms (at least 6 air exchanges per hour) • Strict handwashing before and after leaving the child's room)	Promotes understanding which may lessen anxiety; prevents accidental exposures to the drug.
Teach family members about the appropriate disposal of soiled tissues, and so forth.	Prevent the transmission of the disease.
Instruct parents on the importance of limiting the number of visitors and screening them for recent illness.	Prevent transmission of the disease to others; prevent further complications in the child with RSV.

NIC: *Parent Education*

Evaluation

(Date/time of evaluation of goal)

(Has goal been met? Not met? Partially met?)

(Did parents verbalize methods of prevention and treatment of RSV? Provide quotes.)

(Revisions to care plan? D/C care plan? Continue care plan?)

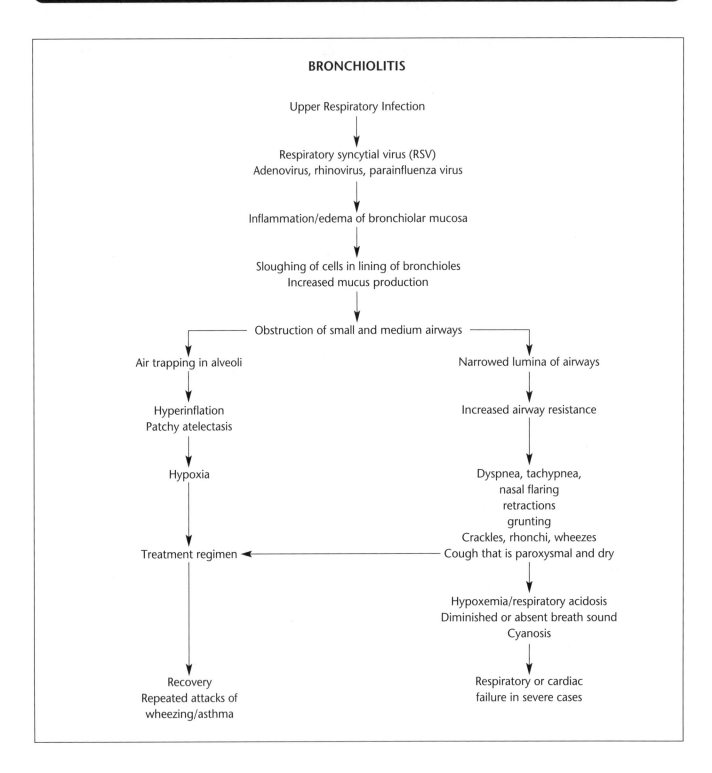

BRONCHIOLITIS

Upper Respiratory Infection

↓

Respiratory syncytial virus (RSV)
Adenovirus, rhinovirus, parainfluenza virus

↓

Inflammation/edema of bronchiolar mucosa

↓

Sloughing of cells in lining of bronchioles
Increased mucus production

↓

Obstruction of small and medium airways

Air trapping in alveoli

↓

Hyperinflation
Patchy atelectasis

↓

Hypoxia

↓

Treatment regimen

↓

Recovery
Repeated attacks of
wheezing/asthma

Narrowed lumina of airways

↓

Increased airway resistance

↓

Dyspnea, tachypnea,
nasal flaring
retractions
grunting
Crackles, rhonchi, wheezes
Cough that is paroxysmal and dry

↓

Hypoxemia/respiratory acidosis
Diminished or absent breath sound
Cyanosis

↓

Respiratory or cardiac
failure in severe cases

CHAPTER 3.4

BRONCHOPULMONARY DYSPLASIA

Bronchopulmonary dysplasia (BPD) is a chronic lung condition most common in infants that were preterm or small for gestational age (SGA) at birth. It is characterized by varying degrees of lung damage past the age of 1 month. BPD is caused by the use of assistive ventilation with the administration of high concentrations of oxygen to treat respiratory distress syndrome (RDS) or other serious disorders of the neonate. The lung and airway damage affects pulmonary function which leads to oxygen dependence, abnormal ABGs, and chest findings on X-ray examination, as well as susceptibility to pulmonary infections resulting in frequent and/or lengthy hospitalizations. BPD may resolve by the time the child is 3 to 4 years of age.

MEDICAL CARE

Prevention: prenatal glucocorticoid therapy given to mothers expected to deliver premature infants, and exogenous surfactant replacement therapy at birth.

Bronchodialators: albuterol, terbutaline, theophylline to relax bronchial smooth muscle.

Antimicrobials: cefaclor, amoxicillin, ampicillin sodium, carbenicillin disodium, vancomycin, third generation cephalosporins or other antibiotics to treat infection based on culture results and severity of infection.

Diuretics: furosemide, spironolactone to promote fluid removal and excretion which will reduce edema if heart failure present.

Cardiac Glycosides: digitalis to increase force and strength of heart contractions if heart failure or pulmonary hypertension present.

Corticosteroids: dexamethasone given to decrease the inflammation of the lung tissue.

Oxygen Therapy: treats hypoxemia as indicated by ABGs or transcutaneous O_2 monitoring or oximetry;

oxygen level delivered varies according to severity of disease, per nasal cannula or endotracheal tube.

Pulmonary Toilet: chest physiotherapy, postural drainage, and suction timed to allow maximum rest for the infant.

Chest X-ray: reveals bilateral infiltration, with areas of hyperaeration and cystic areas at base of lungs as disease progresses; "whiteout" and consolidation visible if condition worsens or increases in healing tissue visible if improving.

Serial Echocardiograms: reveal right ventricular hypertrophy and possible failure.

Pulmonary Function: reveals prolonged ratio between inspiratory and expiratory phases.

Throat/Tracheal Cultures: reveal and identify infectious agent and sensitivity to specific antimicrobial treatment if infection present.

Arterial Blood Gases: reveal hypoxemic state by decreases in pO_2 of less than 55 to 60 mm Hg and increases in pCO_2 of more than 45 to 65 mm Hg which determine oxygen administration adjustments based on chronic hypoxemia associated with this condition; increased HCO_3 in presence of respiratory failure (chronic or acute).

Electrolyte Panel: reveals hypokalemia if diuretics given, calcium and phosphorus deficits if nutrition inadequate.

Complete Blood Count: reveals increased WBC if infection is present.

COMMON NURSING DIAGNOSES

See INEFFECTIVE BREATHING PATTERN

Related to: Inflammatory process.

Defining Characteristics: (Specify: dyspnea, tachypnea, use of accessory muscles, increased anteroposterior diameter, abnormal ABGs, cyanosis, recurrent wheezing, crackles and presence of respiratory infections [bronchitis, bronchiolitis, pneumonia].)

See IMPAIRED GAS EXCHANGE

Related to: Tissue damage.

Defining Characteristics: (Specify: hypoxemia, hypercapnia, restlessness, confusion, irritability, somnolence.)

See IMBALANCED NUTRITION: LESS THAN BODY REQUIREMENTS

Related to: Inability to ingest food.

Defining Characteristics: (Specify: hypoxia during feeding, poor feeder, decreased weight gain, increased energy/metabolic need for work of breathing, altered physical growth.)

See EXCESS FLUID VOLUME

Related to: Compromised regulatory mechanisms (presence of right heart failure).

Defining Characteristics: (Specify: edema, pulmonary effusion, weight gain, dyspnea, crackles, change in respiratory pattern, pulmonary congestion.)

See DELAYED GROWTH AND DEVELOPMENT

Related to: Separation from significant others.

Defining Characteristics: (Specify: frequent or prolonged hospitalizations.)

Related to: Environmental and stimulation deficiencies.

Defining Characteristics: (Specify: isolation, listlessness, decreased responses.)

Related to: Effects of physical disability/chronic illness.

Defining Characteristics: (Specify: delay or difficulty in performing motor, mental, social skills typical of age group.)

ADDITIONAL NURSING DIAGNOSES

RISK FOR INFECTION

Related to: Chronic respiratory disease.

Defining Characteristics: (Specify: reduced ciliary activity, lung damage, decreased lung capacity and acces-

sory muscles' inability to move secretions, increased temperature, yellow or green sputum in increased amounts, diminished breath sounds; presence of respiratory and suction of family membranes.)

Goal: Infant will not experience a respiratory infection by (date/time to evaluate).

Outcome Criteria

✔ Temperature <101° F, clear respiratory secretions, breath sounds consistent for infant (specify).

✔ Behavior is consistent for infant.

NOC: *Risk Control*

INTERVENTIONS	RATIONALES
Assess for change in breathing pattern, color of mucus, rise in temperature, diminished breath sounds; presence of respiratory infection of family members.	Indicates presence or potential for infection, which may be life threatening in infants with this disease.
Avoid exposure to persons with respiratory infections; isolate from infectious patients.	Infants have a low respiratory reserve and are prone to infection transmission from others.
Utilize and teach good hand-washing technique before giving care to infant.	Prevents transmission of microorganisms to infant.
Remove secretions by CP and PD and suctioning via sterile technique as needed.	Stasis of secretions provide medium for infection.
Obtain sputum for culture as needed.	Identifies presence of pathogenic organisms.
Teach parents about infant's susceptibility to infection and to avoid contact with anyone with a respiratory infection.	Any illness, even a minor one will compromise the infant's respiratory status.
Reinforce to parents to maintain an environment free of smoke, sprays, or other irritating substances.	Avoids irritation of airways that might increase risk of infection.
Encourage parents to provide adequate fluid and nutritional intake.	Maintains fluid and nutritional requirements of infant to provide adequate defenses.
Refer parents for cardiopulmonary resuscitation (CPR) class.	Provides anticipatory knowledge to perform life-saving measure if needed.
Teach parents of need to have periodic X-rays and laboratory tests.	Monitors progress of disease.

INTERVENTIONS	RATIONALES
Instruct parents to report any changes in mucus or respiratory distress to physician.	Provides for immediate interventions, if needed, to control infection.

NIC: *Infection Control*

Evaluation

(Date/time of evaluation of goal)

(Has goal been met? Not met? Partially met?)

(What is temperature? Are respiratory secretions clear? Describe. Describe breath sounds and infant behavior and compare to usual parameters.)

(Revisions to care plan? D/C care plan? Continue care plan?)

COMPROMISED FAMILY COPING

Related to: (Specify, e.g., prolonged disease that exhausts supportive capacity of significant people; lack of coping skills.)

Defining Characteristics: (Specify: preoccupation of significant persons with anxiety, guilt, fear regardless of infant/child illness; display of protective behaviors by significant persons that are disproportionate to infant/child needs (too much or too little), frequent hospitalizations, prolonged hospitalization.)

Goal: Family will improve coping skills by (date/time to evaluate).

Outcome Criteria

✔ Family expresses major stressors accompanying infant's illness.

✔ Family identifies 3 coping mechanisms/support systems they can use.

NOC: *Family Coping*

INTERVENTIONS	RATIONALES
Assess anxiety, fear, erratic behavior, perception of crisis situation by family members.	Provides information affecting family ability to cope with infant/child prolonged illness.
Assist family to discuss coping methods used and effectiveness.	Identifies coping methods that work and need to develop new coping skills.

INTERVENTIONS	RATIONALES
Encourage expression of feelings and questions in accepting, nonjudgmental environment.	Reduces anxiety and enhances family's understanding of infant's condition.
Encourage family involvement in care during and after hospitalization.	Provides for reduction of anxiety and fear of equipment used in care.
Allow for open visitation, encourage telephone calls to hospital by family members.	Encourages bonding and assists in coping with infant/child hospitalization if family unable to stay.
Provide place for family members to rest, freshen up.	Promotes comfort of family.
Suggest social worker referral as needed (specify).	Provides support and resources for financial or infant/child care relief.
Give positive feedback and praise family efforts in developing coping and problem-solving techniques and caring for infant.	Encourages parents and family to participate in care and gain some control over the situation.
Suggest and reinforce appropriate coping behaviors (provide examples).	Promotes behavior change and adaptation to care of infant with oxygen dependence.
Reinforce need to maintain health of family members and emotional status of parents.	Chronic anxiety, fatigue will affect health and care capabilities of family.
Provide information regarding infant's condition and progress, oxygen dependence needs, and reason for care and medications.	Reduces anxiety of parents and family and anticipates need for knowledge about disease and care.
Suggest that assistance may be secured by telephoning hospital after discharge.	Provides family with resource in crisis situation.
Arrange education about cardiopulmonary resuscitation (CPR), oxygen administration, and safety measures to eliminate fire hazards.	Empowers family to manage emergency situation and maintain safe oxygen administration.

NIC: *Family Integrity Promotion*

Evaluation

(Date/time of evaluation of goal)

(Has goal been met? Not met? Partially met?)

(What stressors did the family identify? List at least three coping mechanisms or support systems the family plans to use.)

(Revisions to care plan? D/C care plan? Continue care plan?)

DISORGANIZED INFANT BEHAVIOR

Related to: Environmental stimulation.

Defining Characteristics: (Specify, e.g., alterations in heart rate, respirations, color changes, erratic body movements, difficulty with feedings or prolonged periods of wakefulness.

Goal: Infant will display increased organization of behavior by (date/time to evaluate).

Outcome Criteria

✔ Infant demonstrates quiet alert state and ability to habituate to environmental stimuli.

✔ Color changes with handling and movement are decreased.

✔ Demonstrates smoother transitions between sleeping and waking (specify how to measure).

NOC: *Child Development: Infant*

INTERVENTIONS	RATIONALES
Assess behavioral states of the infant including: periods of quiet and active sleep, habituation, orientation, and self-consoling ability.	Assessment provides information about the infant's unique abilities to cope with environmental stimulation. Allows planning of individualized supportive care.
Introduce one caregiving intervention at a time, observing responses; allow for "time out" if infant displays stress signals, such as finger splaying, grimacing, tongue extension, worried alertness, spitting up, back arching, gaze aversion, yawning, hiccuping, color changes, or changes in cardiac or respiratory functioning.	Prevents overstimulation and further maladaptation to the environment.
Cluster caregiving, while not overstimulating infant; continuously monitor infant for signs of stress during caregiving, providing rest periods as needed.	Promotes longer periods of alert and/or deep sleep which will enhance the body's own natural defenses; providing rest periods will allow infant to recover prior to initiation of additional caregiving; prevents sudden disruptions in sleep; promotes stability and adaptive behaviors.

INTERVENTIONS	RATIONALES
Remain at bedside after procedures/caregiving to assess infant's response; if maladaptive responses occur, use "time-out" to allow infant to adapt.	Prevents or minimizes maladaptive responses which often occurs up to 20 minutes after caregiving is completed.
Alter physical environment by decreasing light and sound.	Prevents or decreases maladaptive behaviors; both light and sound levels in the NICU have been implicated in interfering with sleep and stable physiological functioning.
Facilitate handling by providing containment: holding infant's arms and legs in a flexed position, close to their midline using the caregiver's hands and/or positioning aids such as rolled blankets; premature or ill infants should be positioned prone or side-lying, maintaining soft flexion.	Promotes flexion and stabilizes infant's motor and physiologic systems.
Place the infant in a flexed position with hands to midline, or swaddled with hands free; providing pacifier and/or fingers to suck on; providing objects to encourage hand grasping such as blankets, tubing, and fingers during caregiving.	Promotes self-consoling/soothing behaviors which facilitate organization and adaptive behaviors.
Provide a primary care team to work collaboratively with the parents in developing an individualized plan of care reviewed daily and discussed at intervals with the parents.	Promotes element of trust for both the infant and family, improving parent-infant relationships; allows caregivers to identify infant's behavioral cues.
Provide individualized feeding support determined by the infant's own needs and strengths; feeding focus should be positive and pleasurable, with attention to infant's cues or signals.	Promotes positive feeding experiences, that facilitate weight gain and feeding competency.
Provide optimal level of family support through utilization of family centered caregiving principles: enhanced parental involvement in all aspects of caregiving and decision-making; promote family comfort with homelike environment.	Promotes feelings of belonging and control which enhances parent-infant relationship.

INTERVENTIONS	RATIONALES
Assist parents in learning their infant's signals or cues and interpreting them appropriately.	Promotes positive parenting role and minimizes infant's maladaptive behaviors, promoting improved long-term growth and development.
Instruct and encourage parents in caregiving activities throughout the NICU stay, at a level parents are comfortable with (specify).	Promotes improved parental confidence, enhances parenting skills, and improves parent-infant relationship/interactions.
Teach and assist parents in promoting infant adaptive behaviors through use of containment, swaddling, promotion and maintenance of flexion, non-nutritive sucking, and finger grasping.	Promotes positive adaptive behaviors in the infant and increases parental participation and feelings of control.
Encourage parents to personalize infant bed space by bringing in clothes, blankets to be used over isolettes/cribs, and pictures from home.	Promotes positive parental identity and feelings of control. Decreases NICU stimulation.
Teach and encourage parental participation in Kangaroo care or skin-to-skin holding when infant is medically stable; this method is accomplished by placing infant on parent's chest under their clothing.	Promotes stable physiologic functioning, maintains thermoregulation, improves quiet/alert sleep periods, improves weight gain, promotes positive parent/infant relationship and improves parental confidence.
Support parents in making the difficult transition from hospital	Promotes feelings of control and mastery through education and

INTERVENTIONS	RATIONALES
to home; allow ample time for teaching and communication of needs and feelings; validate feelings of anxiety as normal; give brief and accurate information, with time for clarification and provide supplemental written materials; allow parents permission to be in control of decisions and maintain structure in their own lives; discuss feelings of anger and guilt openly; adapt teaching and communication techniques to different family styles, customs, and cultures.	open communication; this will enhance the parent-infant relationship and foster the child's growth and development.

NIC: *Developmental Enhancement*

Evaluation

(Date/time of evaluation of goal)

(Has goal been met? Not met? Partially met?)

(Did infant demonstrate quiet alert state and ability to habituate to environmental stimuli? Describe. Were color changes with handling and movement decreased? How was this measured? Did infant demonstrate smoother transitions between sleeping and waking? How was the change measured?)

(Revisions to care plan? D/C care plan? Continue care plan?)

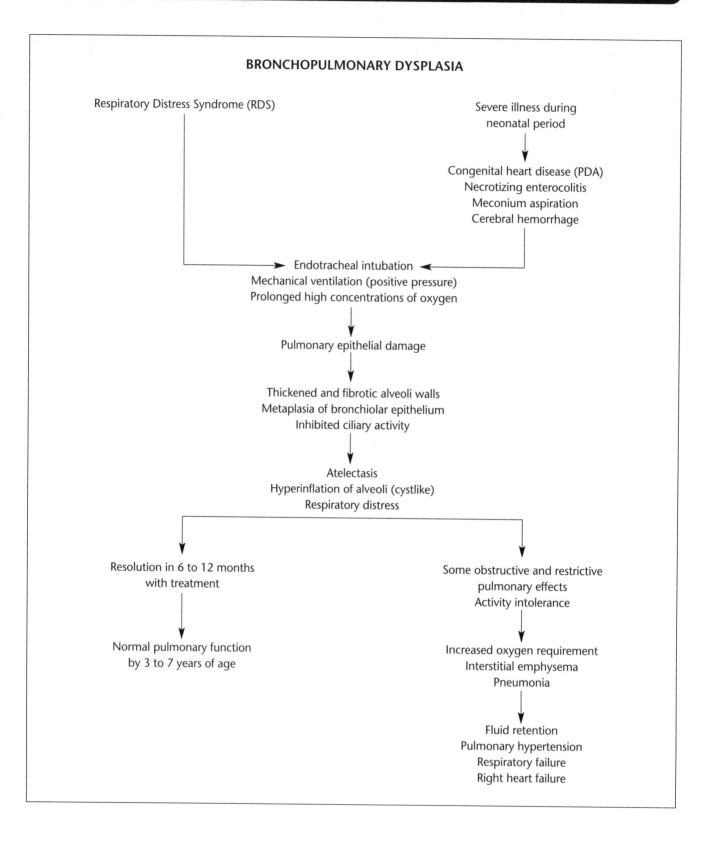

BRONCHOPULMONARY DYSPLASIA

Respiratory Distress Syndrome (RDS)

Severe illness during
neonatal period

Congenital heart disease (PDA)
Necrotizing enterocolitis
Meconium aspiration
Cerebral hemorrhage

Endotracheal intubation
Mechanical ventilation (positive pressure)
Prolonged high concentrations of oxygen

Pulmonary epithelial damage

Thickened and fibrotic alveoli walls
Metaplasia of bronchiolar epithelium
Inhibited ciliary activity

Atelectasis
Hyperinflation of alveoli (cystlike)
Respiratory distress

Resolution in 6 to 12 months
with treatment

Some obstructive and restrictive
pulmonary effects
Activity intolerance

Normal pulmonary function
by 3 to 7 years of age

Increased oxygen requirement
Interstitial emphysema
Pneumonia

Fluid retention
Pulmonary hypertension
Respiratory failure
Right heart failure

CHAPTER 3.5

CYSTIC FIBROSIS

Cystic fibrosis (mucoviscidosis) is the most common life-shortening hereditary illness in children. It is an autosomal-recessive trait disorder affecting the exocrine glands. The disease produces abnormal ion transport in epithelial tissues, which results in dehydration of secretions causing mucus to become thick and tenacious and causing mechanical obstruction in ducts and glands. Organs affected are the pancreas, small intestine, liver, lungs, and reproductive organs. Severity of the disease varies. Although an increased survival rate has been evident in recent years, death is the final result as progressive pulmonary complications occur and create a serious threat to the child's life. Children with cystic fibrosis and their families are continuously faced with the daily implementation of a medical regimen that may deplete their physical, emotional, and financial resources. As the disease is chronic, hospitalization may be frequent.

MEDICAL CARE

Bronchodilators/Adrenergic Agonists: via nebulizer, or hand-held inhalator to relieve bronchospasms and facilitate removal of pulmonary secretions by bronchial dilatation and smooth muscle relaxation.

Mucolytics: acetylcysteine (Mucomyst) used in the nebulizing solution for mist tent, face mask to liquefy mucus; recombinant human deoxyribonuclease (Pulmozyme) used as an aerosolized medication to decrease the viscosity of mucus.

Vitamins: if liver involved, vitamin A, D, E, and K given as replacement in water-miscible preparations.

Pancreatic Enzymes: given to replace enzyme deficiency in powder, granules, packet, or tablet form to assist in digestion and bowel elimination.

Antibiotics: selection dependent on identification and sensitivity to organism revealed by culture, whether therapy is prophylactic, and term of treatment.

Oxygen Therapy: continuous, low-volume oxygen administered with caution for acute respiratory distress.

Pulmonary Toilet: chest PT and postural drainage and aerobic exercise enhances movement of secretions.

Chest X-ray: reveals patchy areas of atelectasis and generalized obstructive emphysema, with later infiltratives and dissemination of bronchopneumonia evident.

Pulmonary Function: reveals severity of lung involvement and general condition.

Iontophoresis of Pilocarpine Sweat Test: reveals sweat chloride content greater than 60 mEq/L, obtained by electrode stimulation of the sweat glands and measurement of the chloride content in the laboratory, is the most definitive test for cystic fibrosis.

Stool Test: reveals fecal fat (steatorrhea) in a 5-day stool collection specimen and calculated to determine impaired fat absorption.

Alanine Aminotransferase (ALT)/Aspartate Aminotransferase (AST): reveals elevation of these enzymes in liver damage.

COMMON NURSING DIAGNOSES

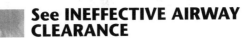

See INEFFECTIVE AIRWAY CLEARANCE

Related to: Tracheobronchial secretions and obstruction.

Defining Characteristics: (Specify: dyspnea; tachypnea; increasing amount of thick, tenacious sputum; nonproductive cough; wheezy respirations with expiratory obstruction.)

See INEFFECTIVE BREATHING PATTERN

Related to: Tracheobronchial obstruction; decreased energy and fatigue.

Defining Characteristics: (Specify: dyspnea, tachypnea, cough, increased anteroposterior diameter (barrel chest), cyanosis, prolonged expiratory phase, finger and toe clubbing with continued ventilatory impairment.)

See IMBALANCED NUTRITION: LESS THAN BODY REQUIREMENTS

Related to: Inability to digest food or absorb nutrients.

Defining Characteristics: (Specify: reduced weight gain; failure to thrive; weight loss with adequate food intake and increased appetite; vomiting; thin and wasted appearance of extremities and buttocks; absence of pancreatic enzymes, causing increased amount of stool; foul-smelling loosely formed bulky stools; steatorrhea, prolapse of the rectum.)

See RISK FOR DEFICIENT FLUID VOLUME

Related to: Excessive losses through normal routes.

Defining Characteristics: Tachypnea, vomiting, diarrhea, profuse sweating, loss of sodium and chloride.

See DECREASED CARDIAC OUTPUT

Related to: Electrical factors.

Defining Characteristics: (Specify: dysrhythmias; ECG changes; variations in hemodynamic readings [VS and BP]; dyspnea; pale, cold, clammy skin; cyanosis; edema; complication of heart failure.)

See DISTURBED SLEEP PATTERN

Related to: Interrupted sleep.

Defining Characteristics: (Specify: cough, dyspnea, fatigue, increasing irritability, restlessness, lethargy, listlessness, average number of hours.)

See RISK FOR IMPAIRED SKIN INTEGRITY

Related to: Bed rest.

Defining Characteristics: (Specify: disruption of skin surface, redness or rash on genitalia and buttocks, redness and irritation at bony prominences; describe.)

See DELAYED GROWTH AND DEVELOPMENT

Related to: Effects of physical illness and disability.

Defining Characteristics: (Specify: altered physical growth, delay or difficulty in performing motor, social skills typical of age group; describe.)

ADDITIONAL NURSING DIAGNOSES

RISK FOR ACTIVITY INTOLERANCE

Related to: Deconditioned status.

Defining Characteristics: (Specify: weakness, fatigue, inability to participate in self-care, physical and social activities.)

Related to: Respiratory problems.

Defining Characteristics: (Specify: dyspnea, tachypnea, exertional discomfort.)

Goal: Infant/child will maintain usual activity levels by (date/time to evaluate).

Outcome Criteria

✔ Infant/child engages in activities (specify) without fatigue or respiratory distress.

NOC: *Energy Conservation*

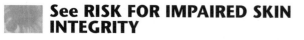

INTERVENTIONS	RATIONALES
Assess level of fatigue and activity in relation to respiratory status (specify frequency).	Provides information about energy reserves as dyspnea and work of breathing over period of time exhausts these reserves.
Schedule care and provide rest periods in a quiet environment.	Promotes adequate rest and reduces stimuli.
Disturb only when necessary for care and procedures; provide quiet play appropriate for age (specify), interests, and energy level.	Conserves energy and prevents interruption in rest; prevents alteration in respiratory status and energy depletion caused by excessive activity.

INTERVENTIONS	RATIONALES
Perform respiratory physiotherapy (specify when); avoid treatment before or after meals.	Reduces work while promoting effectiveness of breathing.
Assist to perform breathing exercises.	Improves ventilation and strengthens chest muscles.
Explain to parents and child the reasons for need to conserve energy and to rest to avoid fatigue.	Promotes understanding of effect of activity on breathing and importance of rest to prevent fatigue.
Discuss with parents and child any activity or exercise restrictions, how to engage in activities without tiring or affecting respiratory status; discuss types of activities child enjoys.	Measures to prevent fatigue while engaging in as near normal participation as possible.
Instruct child to ask for assistance if needed for daily activities; assist to plan a schedule for ADL that will conserve energy.	Prevents overtiring and fatigue.

NIC: *Energy Management*

Evaluation

(Date/time of evaluation of goal)

(Has goal been met? Not met? Partially met?)

(Did infant/child engage in the activity specified without fatigue or respiratory difficulty? Describe behavior.)

(Revisions to care plan? D/C care plan? Continue care plan?)

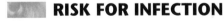

RISK FOR INFECTION

Related to: Chronic pulmonary disease.

Defining Characteristics: Presence of and stasis of mucus in respiratory tract, increased environmental exposure, change in respiratory pattern and mucus color, temperature, steroid administration (specify).

Goal: Client will not experience any infection by (date/time to evaluate).

Outcome Criteria

✔ Absence of infection.

✔ (Specify individual parameters to monitor for infection, e.g., behavioral, VS, lab values, changes in secretions and breathing.)

NOC: *Risk Control*

INTERVENTIONS	RATIONALES
Assess for change in breathing pattern, color of mucus, diminished breath sounds, ability to cough and raise secretions (specify frequency).	Indicates presence of respiratory infection.
Teach to avoid exposure to persons with respiratory infections; isolate from infectious patients.	Prevents transmission of microorganisms as disease increases susceptibility to infection.
Teach and use good hand-washing technique before giving care.	Prevents transmission of microorganisms to child.
Assist to cough or remove secretions by suctioning.	Stasis of secretions provide medium for infection.
Use medical asepsis techniques or sterile techniques when administering respiratory care (specify).	Prevents exposure to infectious agents.
Administer antibiotics as ordered (specify drug, dose, route, and times).	Provides prophylactic antibiotics, that are often prescribed as a preventive measure. Specify drug action.
Instruct parents of child's high susceptibility to infection and to avoid contact of child with persons or family members with respiratory infections.	Prevents any infection that will compromise respiratory status and that could be life-threatening.
Teach parents about antibiotic regimen (specify) and inform of need to have influenza immunization and to avoid cough suppressants.	Promotes use of preventive measures to control possible infection, cough suppressants prevent cough needed to bring up secretions.
Teach parents to report any changes in mucus or respiratory status to physician.	Provides for immediate interventions to control infection.

NIC: *Infection Control*

Evaluation

(Date/time of evaluation of goal)

(Has goal been met? Not met? Partially met?)

(Provide evaluative data on parameters specified in outcome criteria, e.g., VS, behavior, etc.)

(Revisions to care plan? D/C care plan? Continue care plan?)

ANTICIPATORY GRIEVING

Related to: Potential loss of significant other by parents, perceived potential loss of physiopsychosocial well-being by child.

Defining Characteristics: (Specify: expression of distress at potential loss, poor prognosis for child [premature death], anger, guilt, sadness, fear, long-term chronic illness of child; use quotes.)

Goal: Clients will express their grief by (date/time to evaluate).

Outcome Criteria

✔ Clients express concerns about the future.

✔ Clients verbalize the stages of grieving.

✔ Clients identify support systems available to them.

NOC: *Family Coping*

INTERVENTIONS	RATIONALES
Assess stage of grief process, problems encountered, feelings regarding potential loss.	Allows for information regarding stage of grieving, as time to work through grieving varies with individuals and the longer the illness, the better able the parents and family will be able to move through the stages towards acceptance.
Provide emotional and spiritual comfort in an accepting environment.	Provides for emotional needs of parents; assists them in coping with ill child.
Answer all questions honestly, clarify any misconceptions.	Promotes trust and reduces parental anxiety.
Accept parental and child's responses and allow for their expression of feelings.	Allows for reactions necessary to work through grieving.
Assist in identifying and using effective coping mechanisms and in accepting situations over which they have no control.	Promotes use of defense mechanisms to progress through grief.
Encourage parents to assist child with normal development and discipline.	Promotes sense of normalcy and well-being for child.

INTERVENTIONS	RATIONALES
Allow child to talk about any concerns regarding death and respond to questions honestly.	Promotes expression of feelings and concerns for understanding grieving process and behaviors.
Provide information to child based on age and developmental level (specify).	Ensures that child receives information he or she can understand. Promotes trust.
Inform parents and child of stages of grieving and of behaviors that are common in resolving grief.	Promotes understanding of feelings and behaviors that are manifested by grief.
Suggest to parents coping skills and approaches that may be used (give examples).	Promotes coping ability over prolonged period of illness.
Refer to (specify) counseling services, clergy, local support agencies for cystic fibrosis, Cystic Fibrosis Foundation.	Provides support and assistance in adapting to chronic illness and potential early death of child.
Discuss with parents and child the disease process and what can be expected from chronic nature and systems involved with the illness.	Provides a realistic view of the child's illness.

NIC: *Grief-Work Facilitation*

Evaluation

(Date/time of evaluation of goal)

(Has goal been met? Not met? Partially met?)

(Did clients express concerns about the future? Did clients verbalize the stages of grieving? What support systems did clients identify as available to them? Provide quotes.)

(Revisions to care plan? D/C care plan? Continue care plan?)

ANXIETY

Related to: (Specify: threat of or change in health status; threat of or change in environment (hospitalization), threat of death, threat of illness occurring in healthy children or future children.

Defining Characteristics: (Specify, e.g., parent—increased apprehension that condition might worsen or infection develop, expressed concern and worry about possible hospitalization, fear of consequences of disease, increased tension and uncertainty; child—unhappy and sad attitude, withdrawal or aggressive behavior, somatic and fatigue complaints, poor school attendance and performance.)

Goal: Clients will experience decreased anxiety by (date/time to evaluate).

Outcome Criteria

✔ Clients identify cause of anxiety and 3 coping mechanisms.

✔ Clients verbalize decreased feelings of anxiety.

NOC: *Anxiety Control*

INTERVENTIONS	RATIONALES
Assess source and level of anxiety, how anxiety is manifested, and need for information that will relieve anxiety of client.	Provides information about anxiety level and the need for interventions to relieve it, sources may include fear and uncertainty about treatment and recovery, guilt for presence of illness, possible loss of parental role, and loss of responsibility if hospitalized.
Allow parents and child to express fears and concerns and to ask questions about disease and what to expect.	Provides opportunity to vent feelings and secure information to reduce anxiety.
Assist clients to identify effective coping mechanisms they may use for anxiety (suggest possibilities as needed, e.g., relaxation techniques, listening to music, playing with clay).	Promotes clients' active participation in decreasing anxiety.
Communicate with parents and answer questions calmly and honestly.	Promotes calm and supportive environment.
Provide supportive and nonjudgmental environment.	Promotes trust and reduces anxiety.
Inform parents and child of all procedures and treatments.	Relieves anxiety caused by fear of the unknown.
Allow parents to stay with child, allow open visitation and telephone communications; encourage to participate in care that is planned around usual home routines.	Reduces anxiety for child by allowing presence and involvement in care, and familiar routines and persons.
If hospitalization is frequent, assign same personnel to care for child if appropriate.	Promotes trust and comfort and reduces anxiety when cared for by familiar persons.
Explain changes in condition and need for hospitalization.	Promotes understanding of disease complications and nature of chronic disease.

INTERVENTIONS	RATIONALES
Explain to parents and child as appropriate for age, reason for each procedure or type of therapy, effects of any diagnostic tests.	Prevents anxiety by reducing fear of unknown.
Clarify any misinformation with honesty and in simple, understandable language.	Prevents unnecessary anxiety resulting from inaccurate information or beliefs.
Refer to counseling, community groups for cystic fibrosis (as needed; specify).	Provides support to parents and child, and information from those with similar problems, which reduces anxiety.

NIC: *Anxiety Reduction*

Evaluation

(Date/time of evaluation of goal)

(Has goal been met? Not met? Partially met?)

(Which causes of anxiety did clients identify? Did clients verbalize decreased anxiety? Provide quotes. Specify 3 coping mechanisms identified by clients.)

(Revisions to care plan? D/C care plan? Continue care plan?)

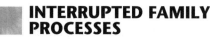

INTERRUPTED FAMILY PROCESSES

Related to: Chronic illness.

Defining Characteristics: (Specify: family system unable to meet physical, emotional needs of its members; inability to express or accept wide range of feelings; family unable to deal with or adapt to chronic illness of child in a constructive manner; excessive involvement with ill child by parents/siblings; evidence of marital and social discord exhibited by parents; guilt expressed by parents/siblings; irritability as a response to the ill child; lack of support from family/friends.)

Goal: Family will regain a functional family system by (date/time to evaluate).

Outcome Criteria

✔ Family members display supportive behaviors to one another.

✔ Family members report open discussions to solve problems.

✔ Family members identify how ill child will be cared for.

NOC: *Family Functioning*

INTERVENTIONS	RATIONALES
Assess family ability to cope with ill child, strain on family relationships, developmental level of family, response of siblings, knowledge of health practices, family rule behavior and attitude toward long-term care, economic pressures and resources to care for long-term illness.	Provides information about family attitudes and coping abilities, that directly affect the child's health and feeling of well-being; chronic illness of a child in a family may strengthen a family or strain family relationships; members may develop emotional problems when family is under stress.
Assist individual family members to identify stressors and behaviors and to define them in positive terms.	Individual problems that are defined and explored have meaning for the entire family.
Assist family members in expressing problems and exploring solutions, responsibilities.	Provides opportunity to express feelings, problems, and problem-solving strategies by whole family.
Assist in establishing short- and long-term goals in maintaining child care and family integration of child into home routine.	Promotes inclusion of ill child in family routines and activities.
Support and encourage parental caretaking efforts.	Reinforces roles and reduces stress in family members.
Discuss family dynamics and need to tolerate conflict and individual behaviors.	Provides knowledge and assists in understanding family behaviors leading to problem resolution.
Discuss needs of all family members and inform of methods to provide care and attention to all members.	Allows for ongoing responsibility for care of all family members.
Inform parents of local agencies, respite care, support groups for family assistance, Cystic Fibrosis Foundation (specify).	Provides information, economic and emotional support for family as a group or individual.
Suggest to family methods to maintain child's independence and role in the family and that discipline of child and well children should be the same.	Ensures acceptance of child into family routines.
Encourage that family health must be maintained and social contacts encouraged.	Health and attitude of family promotes ill child's coping ability.

INTERVENTIONS	RATIONALES
Provide referrals to parents about where health care may be secured (dentist, physical therapy, pulmonary physiotherapy (specify).	Ensures ongoing health care for child with chronic illness.

NIC: *Family Mobilization*

Evaluation

(Date/time of evaluation of goal)

(Has goal been met? Not met? Partially met?)

(Describe family members' behavior toward each other. Did family members report open discussions? Use quotes. Specify the plan family members identified to care for ill child.)

(Revisions to care plan? D/C care plan? Continue care plan?)

IMPAIRED HOME MAINTENANCE

Related to: Complexity of home care management of cystic fibrosis patient.

Defining Characteristics: (Specify: frequent exacerbations of respiratory infections; inadequate understanding of illness and home care components; child not functioning up to full potential in terms of growth and development, independence issues; stressors within family relationships.)

Goal: Family will provide a safe, hygienic home for ill child by (date/time to evaluate).

Outcome Criteria

✔ Parents obtain and learn to operate equipment needed to care for child (specify).

✔ Family provides appropriate care for ill child (specify parameters to evaluate).

NOC: *Family Functioning*

INTERVENTIONS	RATIONALES
Assess home environment and families' ability to maintain a safe, clean home for the ill child.	Provides baseline data on which to plan interventions.

INTERVENTIONS	RATIONALES
Develop a flexible home plan of care, with input from all family members.	Promotes less disruption to family routines.
Assist parents in locating the appropriate equipment and supplies necessary for home care; provide opportunities to learn and practice use prior to discharge; anticipate problems.	Promotes feelings of control; may decrease anxiety and stressors.
Instruct parents in all aspects of home care; reinforce teaching with written materials; return demonstrations, as applicable: oral hygiene chest physiotherapy (CPT)—parents adjust frequency based on individual child's needs; use of games and childhood activities can be incorporated into the therapy (somersaults, wheelbarrow); antibiotic therapy for respiratory exacerbations; facilitate arrangements with home health nursing (as applicable), nutrition management including pancreatic enzyme replacement, health practices—adequate rest, good hygiene, importance of follow-up care, exercise, prevention of illness.	Promotes understanding of care needed for child at home to provide optimal health and promote normal growth and development; promotes body's own natural defenses. Use of play will increase the likelihood of success.
Instruct parents on the signs of depression, especially in adolescents; make appropriate referral as needed (specify).	Promotes good communication between parent and health professional if a concern arises.

INTERVENTIONS	RATIONALES
Organize and coordinate services from health professionals involved in the home care of the child, including home health nursing, respiratory therapy, physicians, social services (as applicable).	Promotes family support which is crucial for a positive adaptation to care at home; may lessen anxiety and stressors.
Discuss impact of caregiving at home with family members to assess potential problems; include siblings.	Promotes improved communication between family members and health professionals; promotes positive relationships between parent-child and child-sibling.
Provide support and praise for family members as they take over the care of their child.	Positive reinforcement empowers the family to provide optimum care.

NIC: *Family Mobilization*

Evaluation

(Date/time of evaluation of goal)

(Has goal been met? Not met? Partially met?)

(Did family obtain and demonstrate use of equipment? Did family care for child as indicated in specified outcome parameters?)

(Revisions to care plan? D/C care plan? Continue care plan?)

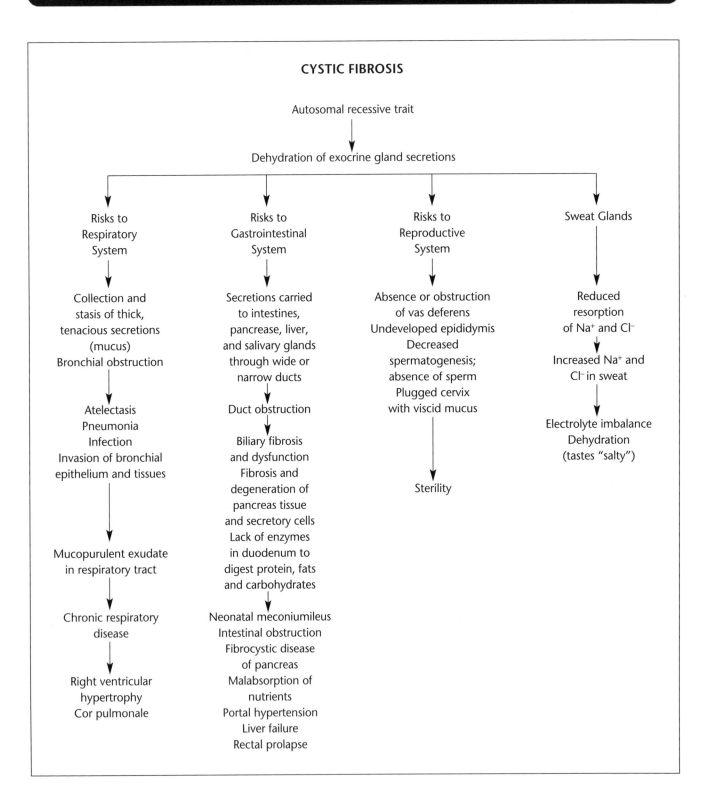

CYSTIC FIBROSIS

Autosomal recessive trait

Dehydration of exocrine gland secretions

Risks to Respiratory System

Collection and stasis of thick, tenacious secretions (mucus)
Bronchial obstruction

Atelectasis
Pneumonia
Infection
Invasion of bronchial epithelium and tissues

Mucopurulent exudate in respiratory tract

Chronic respiratory disease

Right ventricular hypertrophy
Cor pulmonale

Risks to Gastrointestinal System

Secretions carried to intestines, pancrease, liver, and salivary glands through wide or narrow ducts

Duct obstruction

Biliary fibrosis and dysfunction
Fibrosis and degeneration of pancreas tissue and secretory cells
Lack of enzymes in duodenum to digest protein, fats and carbohydrates

Neonatal meconiumileus
Intestinal obstruction
Fibrocystic disease of pancreas
Malabsorption of nutrients
Portal hypertension
Liver failure
Rectal prolapse

Risks to Reproductive System

Absence or obstruction of vas deferens
Undeveloped epididymis
Decreased spermatogenesis; absence of sperm
Plugged cervix with viscid mucus

Sterility

Sweat Glands

Reduced resorption of Na^+ and Cl^-

Increased Na^+ and Cl^- in sweat

Electrolyte imbalance
Dehydration (tastes "salty")

CHAPTER 3.6

EPIGLOTTITIS

Epiglottitis is the acute inflammation of the epiglottis and surrounding laryngeal area with the associated edema that constitutes an emergency situation as the supraglottic area becomes obstructed. The child characteristically appears very ill with a fever, severe sore throat, muffled voice, and insists on sitting upright with the chin extended and mouth open. Drooling is common because of inability to swallow, and respiratory distress is progressive as the obstruction advances. No examination of the oropharynx is performed until emergency equipment and personnel are readily available. Respiratory distress must be relieved by endotracheal intubation or tracheostomy in severe cases. Onset is rapid (over 4–12 hours) and breathing pattern usually re-established within 72 hours following intubation and antimicrobial therapy. Children most commonly affected are between 2 and 7 years of age.

MEDICAL CARE

Immunization: hemophilus, type B vaccination, to protect against the *Hemophilus influenzae*, type B, the most common cause of epiglottitis.

Antipyretics/Analgesics: acetaminophen to reduce fever and relieve throat pain. Ibuprofen (nonsteroidal anti-inflammatory) for children 6 months to 12 years; to reduce fever and inflammation.

Antibiotics: ampicillin; chloramphenicol (Chloromycetin Palmitate suspension); cefuroxime sodium.

Corticosteroids: reduces inflammation of the epiglottis, improving oxygenation; dexamethasone.

Oxygen Therapy: treats potential hypoxia; administered by tent, mask, cannula or via endotrachial tube.

Neck X-ray: may be done to view lateral neck to diagnose condition.

Throat Culture: reveals and identifies causative agent and sensitivity to specific antimicrobial therapy. Done only under direct supervision of a physician, emergency equipment for intubation should be readily available.

Blood Culture: reveals and identifies causative agent or presence of other infectious agent.

Arterial Blood Gases: reveals decreased pH, pO_2; increased pCO_2 as respiratory distress becomes more acute and ventilation perfusion disturbance occurs.

COMMON NURSING DIAGNOSES

See INEFFECTIVE AIRWAY CLEARANCE

Related to: Obstruction.

Defining Characteristics: (Specify: sudden increase in temperature, dyspnea, tachypnea, drooling, difficulty in swallowing, bright red epiglottis with edema, decreased breath sounds, muffled voice, sore throat, neck X-ray results.)

See INEFFECTIVE BREATHING PATTERN

Related to: Inflammatory process, obstruction.

Defining Characteristics: (Specify: air hunger, dyspnea, tachypnea, use of accessory muscles [intercostal, sub or suprasternal retractions], assumption of three-point position, sitting up with mouth open and chin forward, stridor or croaking sound on inspiration.)

See RISK FOR DEFICIENT FLUID VOLUME

Related to: Loss of fluid through respirations and temperature, altered intake.

Defining Characteristics: (Specify: increased body temperature, dry skin and mucous membranes, decreased skin turgor, increased pulse and respirations, sore throat and difficulty in swallowing, refusal to drink fluids.)

See HYPERTHERMIA

Related to: Inflammation/infection of epiglottis.

Defining Characteristics: (Specify: sudden increase in body temperature above normal range, specify, warm to touch, increased pulse and respirations, positive culture.)

ADDITIONAL NURSING DIAGNOSES

ANXIETY

Related to: Specify: change in health status of child; change in environment (hospitalization); change in role functioning (parenting).

Defining Characteristics: (Specify: verbalization of extreme fear and apprehension by parents; agitation, crying, irritability, air hunger and extreme expression of fear [child].)

Goal: Clients will experience decreased levels of anxiety by (date/time to evaluate).

Outcome Criteria

✔ Clients verbalize decreased anxiety.

✔ Child appears calm without crying or irritability.

NOC: *Anxiety Control*

INTERVENTIONS	RATIONALES
Assess severity of fear and anxiety of parents and child.	Provides information about presence of extreme anxiety as symptoms of disease become more acute and breathing more difficult.
Provide calm and supportive environment and reassure parents that best care is being given to child.	Provides reassurance and reduces anxiety of parents.
Allow child to assume position of comfort, provide familiar object (toy, blanket); tripod position may offer the most comfort.	Promotes comfort and security for child.

INTERVENTIONS	RATIONALES
Remain with child at all times during acute stages.	Provides constant assessment for emergency interventions and reassurance for parents.
Encourage parents to stay with child, provide a place for rest.	Promotes security needs for child and assists in reducing parental anxiety.
Teach parents about all procedures, care, and changes in the child's condition.	Reduces anxiety caused by fear of the unknown.
Avoid any care or procedures that are not necessary during acute stage.	Prevents increase of anxiety which increases respiratory distress.
Allow child to remain seated on parent's lap during all care, including lateral neck X-ray if ordered.	Reduces child's anxiety and avoids precipitating a complete obstruction.
Allow for expression of fears and feelings of parents and child and for behaviors caused by severe anxiety.	Reduces anxiety and embarrassment.
Orient parents and child to room, equipment, supplies and policies.	Familiarizes them to hospital environment.
Teach parents that swelling subsides 24 hours after antibiotic therapy is initiated and epiglottis usually returns to normal in about 3 days.	Provides confirmation of positive outcome and reduces anxiety.

NIC: *Anxiety Reduction*

Evaluation

(Date/time of evaluation of goal)

(Has goal been met? Not met? Partially met?)

(Did client verbalize decreased anxiety? Use quotes. Describe child's behavior.)

(Revisions to care plan? D/C care plan? Continue care plan?)

RISK FOR SUFFOCATION

Related to: Disease process.

Defining Characteristics: (Specify: supraglottic edema; obstruction; dysphasia; hypoxia; cyanosis; extreme anxiety, with struggle to breathe.)

Goal: Child will not experience suffocation by (date/time to evaluate).

Outcome Criteria

✔ Preventive measures taken to ensure patent airway.

✔ Child's airway remains open either naturally or by means of ET tube or tracheostomy.

NOC: *Risk Control*

INTERVENTIONS	RATIONALES
Assess for changes in skin color from pallor to cyanosis, severe dyspnea and sternal and intercostal retractions, lethargy, increased pulse (specify when).	Provides information about increasing airway obstruction.
Allow to sit up and avoid forcing child to lie down.	Lying down may cause epiglottis to fall backward, causing airway obstruction.
Avoid inspecting throat with tongue blade or obtaining throat culture unless immediate emergency equipment and personnel at hand.	Leads to airway spasms and obstruction.
Administer O$_2$ and monitor via pulse oximeter.	Promotes oxygenation of tissues and prevents hypoxemia.
Have emergency intubation equipment at hand and assist with endotracheal intubation or tracheostomy if necessary, or prepare for procedure in surgery.	Establishes airway if obstruction present and respiratory failure and asphyxia imminent.
Provide parents with explanation of care and all procedures and reason and procedure for emergency intubation or tracheostomy if needed while hospitalized.	Explanations provide information and support for parents who are not familiar with procedures.
Inform parents of reason for restraints if emergency procedure done, that swelling is reduced after 24 hours of therapy and tube will probably be removed after 3 days.	Prepares parents with information of what to expect.

NIC: *Airway Management*

Evaluation

(Date/time of evaluation of goal)

(Has goal been met? Not met? Partially met?)

(Describe status of child's airway.)

(Revisions to care plan? D/C care plan? Continue care plan?)

DEFICIENT KNOWLEDGE (PREVENTIVE CARE)

Related to: The promotion of health-seeking behaviors within the hospital and/or home to prevent complications and speed recovery (specify).

Defining Characteristics: (Specify: parents request information about caregiving and preventive measures; child readmitted to hospital with complications.)

Goal: Parents will gain understanding of preventive care by (date/time to evaluate).

Outcome Criteria

✔ Parents verbalize signs and symptoms to report to the physician.

✔ Parents demonstrate correct medication administration for the child.

NOC: *Knowledge: Treatment Regimen*

INTERVENTIONS	RATIONALES
Teach parents on the administration of prescribed medications (specify).	Promotes understanding that may improve consistency of medication administration and recognition of adverse effects.
Teach parents the signs and symptoms of respiratory distress (specify).	Encourages parents to seek prompt medical treatment as necessary.
Instruct parents on the importance of rest and good nutrition, to prevent illness.	Prevents secondary infections; promotes body's own natural defenses.
Encourage and teach parents to provide care for the hospitalized child at a level they are comfortable with and within the constraints of necessary treatments.	Promotes parental identity and control; may lessen anxiety and stress.
Teach parents, child, and family members, as applicable, on good handwashing techniques and the proper disposal of soiled tissues, and so forth.	Prevents transmission of illness.
Evaluate parents' understanding of teaching and reinforce as needed. Offer praise for efforts.	Provides information about additional teaching needs. Positive reinforcement promotes self-esteem and pride in caring for the child properly.

NIC: *Teaching: Prescribed Medication*

Evaluation

(Date/time of evaluation of goal)

(Has goal been met? Not met? Partially met?)

(Did parents verbalize understanding of signs to report? Provide quotes. Did parents demonstrate medication administration?)

(Revisions to care plan? D/C care plan? Continue care plan?)

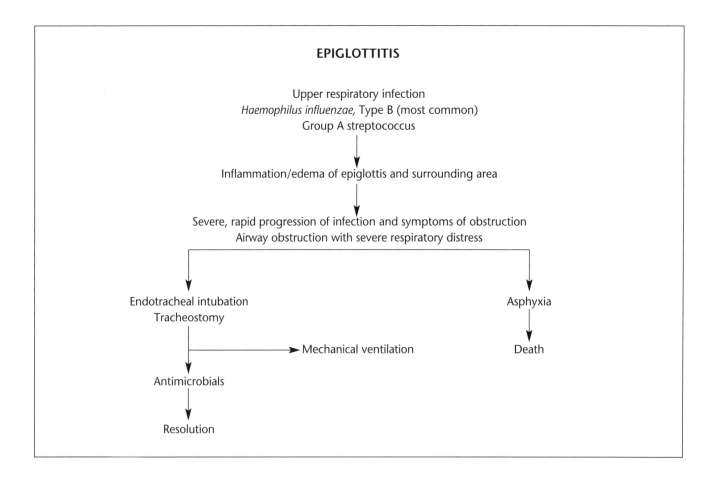

EPIGLOTTITIS

Upper respiratory infection
Haemophilus influenzae, Type B (most common)
Group A streptococcus

Inflammation/edema of epiglottis and surrounding area

Severe, rapid progression of infection and symptoms of obstruction
Airway obstruction with severe respiratory distress

Endotracheal intubation
Tracheostomy

Asphyxia

Mechanical ventilation

Death

Antimicrobials

Resolution

CHAPTER 3.7

CROUP

Laryngotracheobronchitis (LTB) is the most common form of croup. It is characterized by an acute viral infection of the larynx, trachea, and bronchi which causes obstruction below the level of the vocal cords. Spasmodic croup is croup of sudden onset, occurring mainly at night and characterized by laryngeal obstruction at the level of the vocal cords caused by viral infections or allergens. Both occur as a result of upper respiratory infection, edema, and spasms that cause respiratory distress in varying degrees depending on the amount of obstruction. The disease most commonly affects infants and small children between 3 months and 3 years of age and occurs in the winter months. Hospitalization is reserved for those with severe symptoms and compromised respiratory function caused by the obstruction.

MEDICAL CARE

Antipyretics: acetaminophen to reduce fever; Ibuprofen (nonsteroidal anti-inflammatory) for children 6 months to 12 years; to decrease fever and inflammation.

Bronchodilators: racemic epinephrine inhalant given by nebulizer or intermittent positive pressure breathing device (IPPB) to relax respiratory smooth muscle and relieve stridor respirations.

Corticosteroids: to reduce inflammation and edema around the vocal cords.

Antibiotics: antibiotic selection dependent on culture sensitivity results.

Oxygen Therapy: treats hypoxemia based on reduced pO_2 levels of ABGs, administered by tent or hood.

Chest/Neck X-rays: differentiate between croup disorders and epiglottitis.

Throat Culture: reveals and identifies infectious agent and sensitivity to specific antimicrobial therapy.

Arterial Blood Gases: reveal hypoxemic states that require oxygen therapy; decreased pH, and changes in oxygen and carbon dioxide levels, indicating respiratory acidosis or failure in severe cases.

Complete Blood Count: reveals increased WBC if infection present.

COMMON NURSING DIAGNOSES

See INEFFECTIVE AIRWAY CLEARANCE

Related to: Tracheobronchial obstruction.

Defining Characteristics: (Specify: dyspnea; thick secretions; tachypnea; hoarseness; persistent barking cough; diminished breath sounds, with scattered crackles and rhonchi; cyanosis; restlessness; tachycardia; hypoxemia; hypercapnia.)

See INEFFECTIVE BREATHING PATTERN

Related to: Inflammatory process, laryngotracheobronchial obstruction.

Defining Characteristics: (Specify: dyspnea, tachypnea, abnormal ABGs, barking, metallic sounding cough, nasal flaring, inspiratory stridor, subclavicular and substernal retractions, cyanosis or pallor, restlessness, irritability.)

See RISK FOR DEFICIENT FLUID VOLUME

Related to: Loss of fluid through normal routes (respirations and temperature), altered intake.

Defining Characteristics: (Specify: low grade temperature, dry skin and mucous membranes, increased pulse and respiration, difficult swallowing, poor skin turgor, sunken fontanels, and absence of tears.)

See DISTURBED SLEEP PATTERN

Related to: Difficult breathing.

Defining Characteristics: Interrupted sleep caused by cough, restlessness, irritability (describe).

ADDITIONAL NURSING DIAGNOSES

ANXIETY

Related to: Change in health status of infant/small child; threat to or change in environment (hospitalization).

Defining Characteristics: (Specify: increased apprehension that condition might worsen and hospitalization might be necessary [parental]; crying and clinging behaviors, refusal to eat or play [infant or small child]; persistent cough and breathing difficulty [infant/small child].)

Goal: Client will experience decreased anxiety by (date/time to evaluate).

Outcome Criteria

✔ Parent verbalizes decreased anxiety.

✔ Child is calm, not crying.

NOC: *Anxiety Control*

INTERVENTIONS	RATIONALES
Assess level and sources of anxiety of parents and child and identify behaviors caused by anxiety.	Provides information about need for interventions to relieve anxiety and concern.
Allow parents to express concerns and to ask questions about course of disease and what to expect.	Provides opportunity to vent feelings, secure information needed to reduce anxiety.
Encourage parents and child to remain calm and provide a quiet environment.	Anxiety affects respirations and calm environment reduces anxiety.
Inform parents and child of all procedures, especially use of croup tent, care and any changes in condition.	Relieves anxiety resulting from fear of the unknown.
Encourage parents to stay with infant/small child if hospitalized, bring toy, blanket from home; allow visits from siblings.	Allows parents to care for and support child and provide familiar objects and people to reduce child's anxiety.

INTERVENTIONS	RATIONALES
If hospitalized, carry out home routines for feeding, sleep.	Prevents anxiety associated with changes in daily rituals.
Explain course of disease to parents and child, that recovery is fairly prompt with proper therapy, and that cough may persist for a week or more after recovery.	Reduces anxiety caused by the sound of the breathing and appearance of the infant/small child.
Clarify any misinformation and answer all questions regarding the disease process and manifestations.	Prevents unnecessary anxiety resulting from inaccurate information or beliefs.
If tent is used, instruct and assist parents in interacting with child.	Promotes support to child and relieves anxiety.
Inform and discuss signs and symptoms indicating increasing severity of disease and actions to take.	Reduces anxiety caused by increasing acuteness of condition by knowledge of what to do and when to report to physician.

NIC: *Anxiety Reduction*

Evaluation

(Date/time of evaluation of goal)

(Has goal been met? Not met? Partially met?)

(What did parent say about anxiety level? Describe child's behavior)

(Revisions to care plan? D/C care plan? Continue care plan?)

FATIGUE

Related to: Dyspnea.

Defining Characteristics: (Specify: lethargy or listlessness, emotional lability or irritability, exhausted appearance, inability to eat.)

Goal: Child will experience increased energy by (date/time to evaluate).

Outcome Criteria

✔ Child sleeps (specify number of hours) without interruption.

✔ Child eats and drinks (specify amount or percentage).

NOC: *Energy Conservation*

INTERVENTIONS	RATIONALES
Assess for weakness and fatigue, ability to rest, sleep, and eat.	Dyspnea and work of breathing over period of time exhausts the infant/child's energy reserves affecting ability to rest, eat, drink.
Disturb only when necessary, perform all care at one time instead of spreading over a long period of time.	Conserves energy and prevents interruptions in rest.
Schedule and provide rest periods in a quiet, comfortable environment (temperature and humidity).	Promotes adequate rest and reduces stimuli to decrease fatigue.
Allow quiet play while maintaining bed rest.	Rest decreases fatigue and respiratory distress; quiet play prevents excessive activity, which depletes energy and increases respirations.
Explain need to conserve energy and avoid fatigue to parents and child.	Promotes understanding of infant/young child's response to respiratory distress and importance of rest and support to prevent fatigue.
Suggest measures to take to prevent fatigue (holding and/or rocking infant/young child, feeding slowly in small amounts, playing with child, offer TV and other diversions).	Provides support to infant/small child and conserves energy.
Teach parents to decrease crying and not allow infant to cry longer than 1 to 2 minutes.	Prevents fatigue, as prolonged crying exhausts infant.
Assist parents to make a plan for providing bathing, feeding, changing diaper around rest periods.	Prevents interruption in rest or sleep.

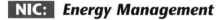 **Energy Management**

Evaluation

(Date/time of evaluation of goal)

(Has goal been met? Not met? Partially met?)

(Specify how long child sleeps and describe how much child is eating.)

(Revisions to care plan? D/C care plan? Continue care plan?)

DEFICIENT KNOWLEDGE OF PARENTS: CARETAKER

Related to: Caregiving to prevent complications and speed recovery.

Defining Characteristics: (Specify, use quotes: parents request information about the home care of the child and/or preventive measures.)

Goal: Parents will understand how to care for ill child by (date/time to evaluate).

Outcome Criteria

✔ Parents verbalize how to provide warm mist for spasmodic croup.

✔ Parents identify when to seek medical care for their child.

NOC: *Knowledge: Treatment Regimen*

INTERVENTIONS	RATIONALES
Assess parent's understanding of child's illness.	Provides baseline data for teaching.
Teach parents to seek medical care if their child has a high fever (>101° F) or any signs of respiratory distress.	Provides parents with guidelines to obtain health care when needed.
Instruct parents on the administration of prescribed medications (specify).	Improves consistency of medication administration and recognition of adverse side effects.
Teach parents the importance of rest (specify quantity).	Prevents secondary infections and/or relapses.
Teach parents to provide good nutrition and hydration, emphasizing a high calorie balanced diet and increased fluids (specify).	Promotes liquification of secretions, and replaces calories used to fight infections, boosting the child's own natural defenses.
Teach parents how to provide humidity by sitting in the bathroom with the door closed and a hot shower running, while holding the child. Protect the child from burns. Also, teach that taking the child out into the cool night air when taking child to the hospital, may decrease the symptoms.	Decreases bronchial spasms and inflammation.

(continues)

(continued)

INTERVENTIONS	RATIONALES
Encourage and teach parents to provide care for the hospitalized child at a level they are comfortable with, and within the constraints of necessary treatments (specify).	Promotes parental identity and control; may lessen anxiety and stress.
Teach good handwashing techniques, and the appropriate disposal of soiled tissues.	Prevents transmission of illness.
Encourage parents to limit visitors and screen them for recent illness.	Prevents transmission of illness; prevents or minimizes risk of complications for the infected child.
Teach parents that spasmodic croup may reoccur for 1 or 2 nights.	Provides anticipatory guidance to parents.

NIC: *Teaching: Individual*

Evaluation

(Date/time of evaluation of goal)

(Has goal been met? Not met? Partially met?)

(Using quotes, what did parents say about how to provide warm mist for spasmodic croup? When did they say they would seek medical care for their child?)

(Revisions to care plan? D/C care plan? Continue care plan?)

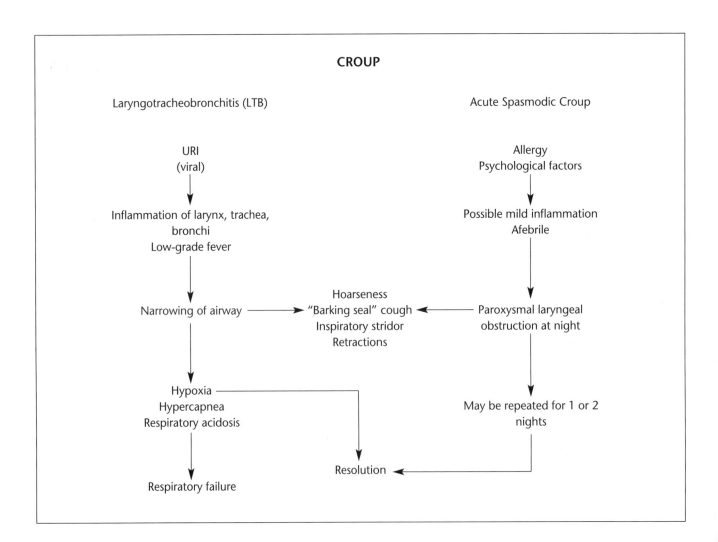

CHAPTER 3.8

OTITIS MEDIA

Otitis Media (OM) is an infection of the middle ear most common in infants and toddlers during the winter months. It may be either viral or bacterial. Inflammatory obstruction of the eustachian tube causes accumulation of secretions in the middle ear and negative pressure from lack of ventilation. The negative pressure pulls fluid and microorganisms into the middle ear through the eustachian tube resulting in otitis media with effusion. The illness usually follows a URI or cold. The older child runs a fever, is irritable, and complains of severe earache, while a neonate may be afebrile and appear lethargic. The child may or may not have a purulent discharge from the affected ear. Myringotomy is a surgical procedure performed to equalize the pressure by inserting tubes through the tympanic membrane. The tympanostomy tubes remain in place until they spontaneously fall out. Most children outgrow the tendency for OM by the age of 6. There is a higher incidence in children exposed to passive tobacco smoke and decreased incidence in breast-fed infants.

MEDICAL CARE

Antipyretics and Analgesics: to decrease fever and pain.

Antibiotics: when indicated for bacterial infection, a full 10 day course of an appropriate antibiotic: amoxicillin-clavulanate, trimethorprim-sulfamethoxazole, erythromycin, sulfonamides, cephalosporins, and so forth.

Tympanometry: provides information about pressure on the tympanic membrane.

Otoscopy: reveals a red, bulging tympanic membrane.

COMMON NURSING DIAGNOSES

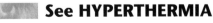 ### See HYPERTHERMIA

Related to: Acute illness.

Defining Characteristics: (Specify infant/child's temperature.)

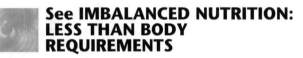 ### See RISK FOR DEFICIENT FLUID VOLUME

Related to: Inadequate intake.

Defining Characteristics: (Specify client's intake and output; describe feeding behavior of infant, e.g., begins to suck and pulls away crying; poor skin turgor, dark urine, etc.)

See IMBALANCED NUTRITION: LESS THAN BODY REQUIREMENTS

Related to: Inadequate intake for age and size.

Defining Characteristics: (Specify: e.g., refusal to eat; picks at food; cries that ear hurts when swallowing; low percentage of meals eaten [specify]; weight loss.)

See DISTURBED SLEEP PATTERN

Related to: Ear discomfort.

Defining Characteristics: (Specify: child wakes crying; sleeps fitfully.)

ADDITIONAL NURSING DIAGNOSES

PAIN

Related to: Increased pressure in the middle ear.

Defining Characteristics: (Specify: e.g., infant is pulling at ear and crying, child states "my ear hurts"; rate pain on an appropriate pain scale for age and development.)

Goal: Client will experience relief from pain by (date/time to evaluate).

Outcome Criteria

✔ Child rates pain < (specify for scale used).

✔ Infant does not pull at ear, is calm and not crying, pain rating is < (use a pain scale designed for infants).

NOC: *Comfort Level*

INTERVENTIONS	RATIONALES
Assess client's pain (specify how frequently) using the (specify) pain scale. Note if infant is irritable or pulling or rubbing an ear.	Use of a pain scale allows measurement of changes in level of pain by different providers. Preverbal infants frequently pull or rub the affected ear and appear irritable.
Assess vital signs (specify which, e.g., TPR or TPR or BO) q 4h and as indicated by client's condition.	Pain may cause tachycardia and tachypnea; fever may increase discomfort.
Administer pain medication (specify drug, dose, route, and times) as ordered.	Specify the action of the medication to decrease pain.
Monitor child for relief of pain (specify appropriate time frame for drug) and any side effects of medication (specify).	Provides information about the effectiveness of the medication and prevents complications.
Encourage and assist the parent to hold and comfort the client. (Specify: e.g., holding, rocking, or kangaroo care for an infant.)	Provides tactile comfort and distraction for the ill child.
Suggest that a warm heating pad or an ice pack might provide comfort. (Specify if the child is old enough to choose.) Ensure safety by turning the heating pad only to low and covering it with a towel. Teach parents to check for overheating and to never turn the control higher than low.	Heat may facilitate vasodilation and drainage if the child lies on the affected side. Cold may reduce edema and pain.
Reassure parents that the discomfort usually subsides within a day on antibiotics but reinforce that the whole prescription should be taken.	Parents may be concerned about their child's pain but may not know to continue the antibiotic after symptoms subside.

NIC: *Kangaroo Care*

Evaluation

(Date/time of evaluation of goal)

(Has goal been met? Not met? Partially met?)

(Using quotes when possible, what is pain rating after implementation of care plan? Describe infant's behavior.)

(Revisions to care plan? D/C care plan? Continue care plan?)

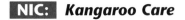

DISTURBED SENSORY PERCEPTION: AUDITORY

Related to: Inflammation and edema of middle ear.

Defining Characteristics: (Specify: child complains of not being able to hear; does not respond when spoken to; infant does not respond to sounds as usual.)

Goal: Client will regain usual hearing level by (date/time to evaluate).

Outcome Criteria

✔ Specify, e.g., child states that hearing has returned to "normal."

✔ Infant responds to sounds made behind him or her.

NOC: *Anxiety Control*

INTERVENTIONS	RATIONALES
Observe the client's response to sound. Ask an older child to describe hearing loss (e.g., do things sound muffled, or is there no sound in the affected ear?).	Provides baseline assessment data about degree of hearing loss.
Reassure parents and child that hearing loss is temporary and will resolve with treatment. Provide information about OM and answer any questions.	Decreases anxiety over sensory loss.
Speak in a loud and clear voice and face child when talking. Encourage parents also to do this.	Assists the client to hear what is being said.
Administer medications as ordered (specify drugs, doses, routes, times).	Describe action of drug that will resolve OM and restore hearing.
Decrease unnecessary environmental noise (specify, e.g., TV, alarms, staff noise, etc.)	The child may be confused and frightened by sounds he or she cannot hear properly.
Notify caregiver of changes in hearing ability or drainage from affected ear.	Complications of OM may include conductive hearing loss or a perforated tympanic membrane.

NIC: *Communication Enhancement: Hearing Deficit*

Evaluation

(Date/time of evaluation of goal)

(Has goal been met? Not met? Partially met?)

(Did child report that hearing was improved? Use quotes. Describe infant's behavior related to sounds—compare to before interventions.)

(Revisions to care plan? D/C care plan? Continue care plan?)

 DEFICIENT KNOWLEDGE: PARENTS, PREVENTION OF OM

Related to: (Specify, e.g., lack of information; lack of recall of information; misinterpreted information.)

Defining Characteristics: (Specify, e.g., parents allow smoking in the home so child is exposed to passive smoke; infant is bottle-fed and sometimes the infant lies flat with the bottle propped.)

Goal: Parents will gain knowledge about prevention of OM by (date/time to evaluate).

Outcome Criteria

✔ Parents verbalize understanding of OM.

✔ Parents verbalize understanding of 3 factors that may contribute to OM.

NOC: *Knowledge: Disease Process*

INTERVENTIONS	RATIONALES
Provide privacy for discussion, promote trust, remain nonjudgmental, and support parents.	Shows respect for the parents and opens communication.
Assess parent's current understanding of OM, the risks of exposing the infant/child to passive smoking, feeding activities with infant, and exposure to illness.	Provides baseline information about current knowledge.

INTERVENTIONS	RATIONALES
Teach parents (and child if age-appropriate) about OM using an ear model for demonstration. Ask parents to verbalize their understanding of teaching.	Provides information by auditory and visual means and assesses understanding.
Discuss possible causes of OM: exposure to illness of others, irritation from environmental smoke, and/or formula entering the eustachian tube when the infant is fed in a supine position.	Provides information about health promotion.
Assist parents to plan ways to decrease the chances of recurrent OM. Make suggestions as needed: take entire course of antibiotic; avoid sick people; maintain a smoke-free home; feed the infant while being held in a sitting position.	Empower parents to make good parenting decisions for their child to help prevent OM.
Provide praise for decisions that will promote wellness for the child and family.	Positive reinforcement supports decision to improve lifestyle.
Refer parents to (specify, e.g., caregiver, smoking cessation, or parenting skills class) as needed.	Encourages follow-up and gaining additional knowledge and skills.

NIC: *Health Education*

Evaluation

(Date/time of evaluation of goal)

(Has goal been met? Not met? Partially met?)

(Did parents verbalize understanding of OM? What 3 factors did parents identify that may contribute to OM? Use quotes.)

(Revisions to care plan? D/C care plan? Continue care plan?)

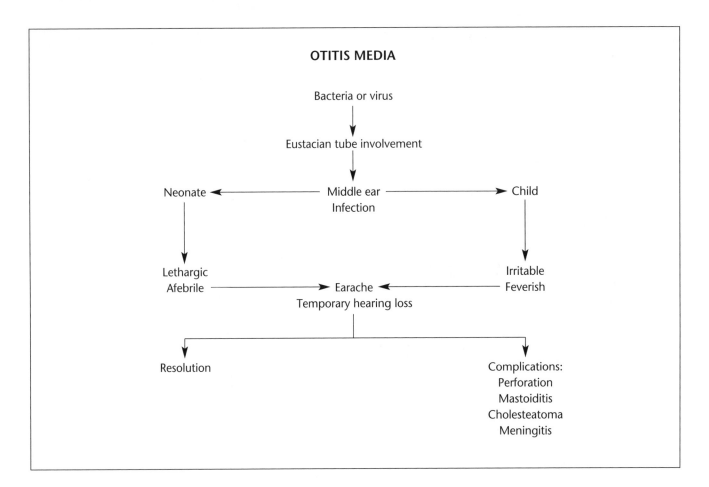

OTITIS MEDIA

Bacteria or virus

Eustacian tube involvement

Middle ear
Infection

Neonate

Child

Lethargic
Afebrile

Irritable
Feverish

Earache
Temporary hearing loss

Resolution

Complications:
Perforation
Mastoiditis
Cholesteatoma
Meningitis

CHAPTER 3.9

PNEUMONIA

Pneumonia is a lower respiratory condition characterized by the inflammation or infection of the pulmonary parenchyma. It is caused by bacteria, viruses, or fungi, or by the aspiration of a foreign substance. It may occur as a primary infection or secondary to another illness or infection. Pneumonia is most common in infants and small children, but it can occur throughout childhood. Signs and symptoms of the disease depend on the age, causative agent, extent of the disease, and the degree of obstruction it causes and the systemic reaction to the infection. The treatment and care is similar for all types of pneumonia.

MEDICAL CARE

Antipyretics: acetaminophen to reduce fever; Ibuprofen (nonsteroidal anti-inflammatory) for children 6 months to 12 years; to reduce fever and inflammation.

Antibiotics: penicillin G to treat pneumococcal, streptococcal, or staphylococcal pneumonia; Erythromycin, Trimethoprimsulfamethoxazole, Climadycin, Chloramphenicol, or cephalosporins for penicillin-allergic children.

Oxygen Therapy: treats hypoxemia, administered by oxygen tent or hood.

Chest X-ray: reveals patchy areas of consolidation in one lobe or throughout lung, varying sizes of pneumatoceles or disseminated infiltration dependent on causative agent.

Sputum Culture: reveals and identifies infectious agent and sensitivity to specific antimicrobial therapy.

Blood Culture: reveals positive reaction for causative agent.

Complete Blood Count: increased WBC of 15,000 or over 20,000/cu mm.

Antistreptolysin-O Titer: elevation indicates recent streptococcal infection if above 333 Todd units.

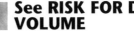

COMMON NURSING DIAGNOSES

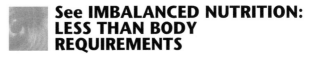 See INEFFECTIVE BREATHING PATTERN

Related to: Inflammatory process.

Defining Characteristics: (Specify: dyspnea, tachypnea, grunting and nonproductive cough in small child, nasal flaring, decreased dull breath sounds, crackles, productive cough in older child, use of accessory muscles with retractions, circumoral cyanosis, shallow respirations, increased fremitus.)

See RISK FOR DEFICIENT FLUID VOLUME

Related to: Excessive losses through normal routes, ↓ fluid intake.

Defining Characteristics: (Specify: increased temperature and pulse rate tachypnea, vomiting and diarrhea in young child, reduced fluids in proportion to output, provide I&O.).

See IMBALANCED NUTRITION: LESS THAN BODY REQUIREMENTS

Related to: Inability to ingest food or digest food.

Defining Characteristics: (Specify: lack of interest in food, anorexia, cough, abdominal pain, vomiting and diarrhea in younger child.)

115

ADDITIONAL DIAGNOSES

▨▨ HYPERTHERMIA

Related to: Illness of lower respiratory tract infection.

Defining Characteristics: (Specify: abrupt onset of high body temperature, tachycardia, tachypnea, chills, myalgia, warm to touch, flushed cheeks, convulsions in infant/young child.)

Goal: Client will be normothermic by (date/time to evaluate).

Outcome Criteria

✔ Temperature between 97 and 100° F.

NOC: *Thermoregulation*

INTERVENTIONS	RATIONALES
Assess temperature (specify route and frequency).	Provides information about the effectiveness of care.
Administer antipyretic medications as ordered (specify drug, dose, route, and times) and reassess temperature (state when).	Specify action of drug in lowering temperature. Specify timing until peak action of specific medication.
Remove any extra clothing or covers the child may have on after the antipyretic has taken effect.	Helps reduce skin temperature by convection after the set point has been lowered.
Encourage fluids (specify if IV running or PO amounts—at least 30 cc/hr) that child likes (specify).	Additional fluids help prevent elevated temperature associated with dehydration.
Teach parents how to take the child's temperature (specify).	Teaching empowers parents to care for their child.
Teach parents about possible side effects of antipyretic medications (specify).	Information helps prevent adverse effects from medications.
Provide parents with instructions about management of childhood fever per caregiver preference (specify, e.g., when to use antipyretics, when to call the caregiver, etc.).	Empowers parents to care for their child.

NIC: *Fever Treatment*

Evaluation

(Date/time of evaluation of goal)

(Has goal been met? Not met? Partially met?)

(What is client's temperature?)

(Revisions to care plan? D/C care plan? Continue care plan?')

▨▨ RISK FOR INJURY

Related to: Pulmonary complications.

Defining Characteristics: (Specify: fluid accumulation in the pleural cavity, dyspnea, pneumothorax, empyema, decreased breath sounds with crackles, seizure activity with high temperature, staphylococcal-type pneumonia in infant, pneumococcal-type pneumonia in child.)

Goal: Client will not experience injury by (date/time to evaluate).

Outcome Criteria

✔ Breath sounds clear.

✔ Temperature <100° F.

NOC: *Risk Control*

INTERVENTIONS	RATIONALES
Assess vital signs and breath sounds, cough and ability to cough up secretions (specify when).	Changes revealed in early stages of complications and reveals airway patency and dyspnea caused by fluid accumulation in pleural cavity and secretion accumulation in airways.
Prepare (infant/child) for procedure and assist with thoracentesis; use therapeutic play to prepare child.	Performed to drain fluid to be cultured or to instill antibiotics if infection present.
Monitor temperature for sudden rise (specify frequency).	Reveals a sudden, rapid rise in temperature which may trigger a febrile seizure.
Report detection of possible respiratory complications (chest pain, dyspnea, cyanosis, abdominal distention), to physician.	Allows for immediate preventive measures to be taken during course of disease.
Reassure parents that complications are uncommon because of effectiveness of antibiotic therapy.	Promotes a positive feeling in parents for recovery of child.

INTERVENTIONS	RATIONALES
Inform parents that recovery from the disease is usually rapid and uneventful if symptoms are reported early for proper treatment.	Promotes awareness and compliance of parents to note respiratory changes and report them immediately to prevent complications.
Teach parents and child to report changes in respirations, sputum, temperature elevation.	Indicates possible pulmonary infection.

NIC: *Infection Control*

Evaluation

(Date/time of evaluation of goal)

(Has goal been met? Not met? Partially met?)

(Describe breath sounds; what is client's temperature?)

(Revisions to care plan? D/C care plan? Continue care plan?)

 DEFICIENT KNOWLEDGE: PNEUMONIA

Related to: Unfamiliarity with disease and complications, measures to control and prevent transmission of respiratory disease.

Defining Characteristics: (Specify: use quotes, verbalization of need for information about medications, activity and rest, nutritional and fluid requirements and medical asepsis techniques to prevent spread of infection.)

Goal: Parents will obtain knowledge about pneumonia by (date/time to evaluate).

Outcome Criteria

✔ Parents verbalize understanding about disease and treatment methods.

✔ Parents verbalize signs of respiratory distress to report (specify).

✔ Parents demonstrate correct handwashing and disposal of used tissues.

NOC: *Knowledge: Treatment Regimen*

INTERVENTIONS	RATIONALES
Assess parents' knowledge of disease and methods to control and resolve disease.	Promotes plan of instruction that is realistic and prevents repetition of information.
Provide information and explanations in clear, understandable language; use pictures, pamphlets, video tapes, model in teaching about disease (specify).	Ensures understanding based on readiness and ability to learn; visual aids reinforce learning.
Instruct in administration of medications including action of drugs, dosages, times, frequency, side effects, expected results, methods to give medications; provide written instructions and schedule to follow and inform to administer full course of antibiotic to child (provide specifics).	Provides information about drug therapy, which is the most important treatment for the cure of pneumonia, and about prevention of lung complications resulting from the disease; bacterial pneumonia is treated with antibiotic therapy.
Instruct and assist to plan feedings and/or develop menus for appropriate inclusion of nourishing fluids, daily caloric and basic four requirements for age group (specify).	Promotes proper diet, which enhances health status, and adequate fluid intake, which prevents dehydration.
Teach about any activity restrictions and of adequate rest during illness and convalescence.	Promotes more rest and possible restriction of activity needed during more acute stages of disease.
Teach about care of used tissues and to cover mouth and nose when coughing or blowing nose; proper handwashing technique for parents and child.	Prevents transmission of microorganisms by droplets dispersed into the air or by hands.
Instruct parents on the signs and symptoms of impending respiratory distress (specify).	Encourages parents to seek prompt medical treatment as necessary.

NIC: *Teaching: Disease Process*

Evaluation

(Date/time of evaluation of goal)

(Has goal been met? Not met? Partially met?)

(Did parents verbalize understanding about the disease and treatment and signs of respiratory distress to report? Provide quotes. Did parents wash hands and dispose of used tissues correctly or indicate that they would?)

(Revisions to care plan? D/C care plan? Continue care plan?)

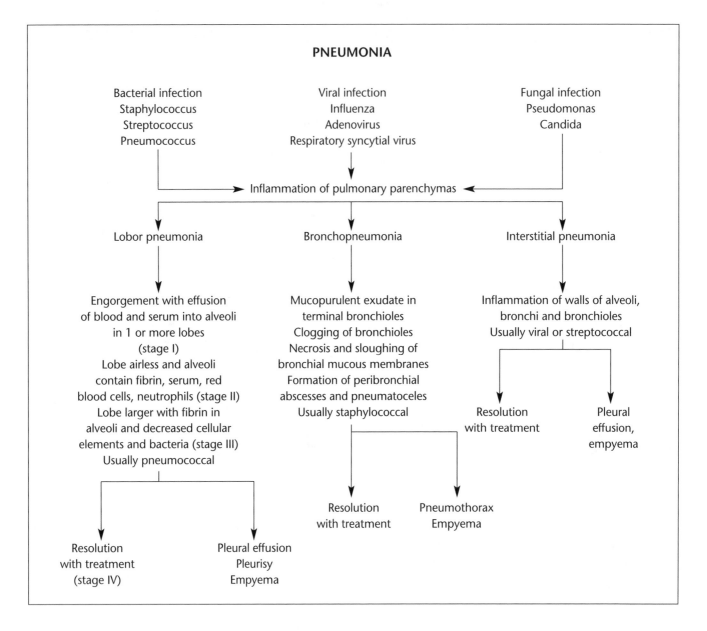

PNEUMONIA

Bacterial infection
Staphylococcus
Streptococcus
Pneumococcus

Viral infection
Influenza
Adenovirus
Respiratory syncytial virus

Fungal infection
Pseudomonas
Candida

Inflammation of pulmonary parenchymas

Lobor pneumonia

Bronchopneumonia

Interstitial pneumonia

Engorgement with effusion
of blood and serum into alveoli
in 1 or more lobes
(stage I)
Lobe airless and alveoli
contain fibrin, serum, red
blood cells, neutrophils (stage II)
Lobe larger with fibrin in
alveoli and decreased cellular
elements and bacteria (stage III)
Usually pneumococcal

Mucopurulent exudate in
terminal bronchioles
Clogging of bronchioles
Necrosis and sloughing of
bronchial mucous membranes
Formation of peribronchial
abscesses and pneumatoceles
Usually staphylococcal

Inflammation of walls of alveoli,
bronchi and bronchioles
Usually viral or streptococcal

Resolution
with treatment

Pleural
effusion,
empyema

Resolution
with treatment
(stage IV)

Pleural effusion
Pleurisy
Empyema

Resolution
with treatment

Pneumothorax
Empyema

CHAPTER 3.10

TONSILLITIS

Tonsillitis is an infection of the tonsils, which consist of pairs of lymph tissue in the nasal and oropharyngeal passages. Bacterial or viral pharyngitis usually precedes infection of the tonsils. Inflammation and edema of the tonsillar tissue creates difficulty swallowing and talking, and forces the child to breathe through the mouth. Advanced infection can lead to cellulitis in adjacent tissue or formation of an abscess which may require drainage. The tonsils removed during a tonsillectomy are the palatine tonsils located in the oropharynx. The adenoids are tonsils located in the nasopharynx and also sometimes removed by adenoidectomy.

MEDICAL CARE

Rapid Strep Test/Throat Culture: to identify streptococcal tonsillitis requiring antibiotic treatment.

Antibiotics: for streptococcal tonsillitis: penicillin, erythromycin, amoxicillin, azithromycin, cephalosporins.

Antipyretics/Analgesics: acetaminophen to reduce fever and discomfort; throat lozenges.

Tonsillectomy, Possibly with Adenoidectomy (T & A): may be done for recurrent bouts of tonsillitis or severe inflammation leading to obstruction. Surgery is delayed for 6 weeks after an acute infection.

COMMON NURSING DIAGNOSES

See INEFFECTIVE AIRWAY CLEARANCE

Related to: Obstruction by inflamed lymphoid tissue.

Defining Characteristics: (Specify, e.g., child complains of difficulty swallowing; breathes through mouth only.)

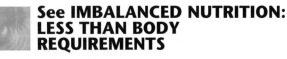 See IMBALANCED NUTRITION: LESS THAN BODY REQUIREMENTS

Related to: Discomfort associated with swallowing.

Defining Characteristics: (Specify: e.g., child refuses to eat, states "throat hurts"; give percentages of meals eaten.)

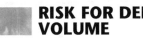 See ANXIETY

Related to: Perceived threat to biologic integrity of child secondary to invasive procedures.

Defining Characteristics: (Specify, e.g., parents state they are anxious, confused about indications for surgery; parent is crying or irritable; describe behaviors.)

ADDITIONAL NURSING DIAGNOSES

RISK FOR DEFICIENT FLUID VOLUME

Related to: Inadequate oral intake, excessive losses through abnormal route.

Defining Characteristics: (Specify, e.g., child states it hurts to drink, decreased intake [specify amount]; post-tonsillectomy risk for hemorrhage.)

Goal: Child will not experience deficient fluid volume by (date/time to evaluate).

Outcome Criteria

✔ Intake equals output.
✔ No signs of bleeding from operative site.

NOC: *Fluid Balance*

INTERVENTIONS	RATIONALES
Assess hourly intake and output. Monitor skin turgor and moisture of mucous membranes.	Provides information about physiologic fluid balance and signs of dehydration.
Observe post-tonsillectomy client for signs of bleeding: assess operative site using a flashlight (specify frequency), monitor child for excessive swallowing, even during sleep.	Provides information about the integrity of the surgical site. Bleeding from the operative site may cause the child to swallow frequently.
Monitor vital signs per protocol (specify which parameters and frequency).	Tachycardia and hypotension are physiologic responses to deficient fluid volume.
Monitor and maintain IV fluids via pump as ordered (specify fluid and rate). Evaluate IV site hourly.	Replaces losses from surgery and maintains hydration if child is unable to drink.
Encourage child to drink small amounts of favorite clear liquids (specify, e.g., 30 cc per hour of apple juice). Avoid red or brown-colored liquids or citrus. Do not allow use of a straw.	Small amounts may be more easily tolerated. Red or brown may be confused with bleeding if child vomits. Suction created by sucking could disrupt operative site, avoids risk for injury.
Use creative, developmentally appropriate techniques to make a game of drinking (specify, e.g., placing stars or coloring in blocks on a chart or earning stickers.	Child's desire to play or to gain approval can help promote increased intake.
Teach child to avoid excessive coughing or clearing of throat. Administer antiemetics as ordered (specify) to prevent vomiting.	Excessive coughing, clearing the throat, or vomiting may disrupt the operative site.
Provide parents with discharge teaching regarding fluid intake, activity, and when to seek medical care (specify caregiver's orders).	Teaching ensures that parents will continue to monitor fluid balance.

NIC: *Fluid Management*

Evaluation

(Date/time of evaluation of goal)

(Has goal been met? Not met? Partially met?)

(Provide intake and output specifying time frame. Is there any bleeding from operative site?)

(Revisions to care plan? D/C care plan? Continue care plan?)

PAIN

Related to: Invasive procedure.

Defining Characteristics: (Specify date/type of surgery; client statements about pain [use quotes], pain rating on a scale [specify which scale is used]; nonverbal indications of discomfort such as grimacing, crying, clinging to parent.)

Goal: Child will experience decreased pain by (date/time to evaluate).

Outcome Criteria

✔ (Specify, e.g., child states pain is less; rates pain lower on same scale; child not grimacing, crying, or clinging to parent.)

NOC: *Pain Level*

INTERVENTIONS	RATIONALES
Assess pain using appropriate pain scale for child's age and development (specify).	Use of a pain scale allows objective measurement of subjective pain perception.
Observe child for nonverbal indications of pain such as crying, grimacing, irritability.	Provides additional information about pain. Child may find speaking causes discomfort.
Administer pain medications as ordered (specify drug, dose, route, and time). Monitor for effectiveness and side effects (specify when).	Specify action of medication in relieving pain.
Encourage child to try placing an ice collar on the neck or to eat frozen pops.	Cold causes vasoconstriction and reduces edema that contributes to pain.
Suggest quiet activity such as listening to music, watching TV (specify).	Provides distraction from discomfort.

NIC: *Pain Management*

Evaluation

(Date/time of evaluation of goal)

(Has goal been met? Not met? Partially met?)

(Did child report decreased pain? How did child rate pain? Describe nonverbal behavior.)

(Revisions to care plan? D/C care plan? Continue care plan?)

DEFICIENT KNOWLEDGE: POSTOPERATIVE HOME CARE

Related to: Lack of information about tonsillectomy and postoperative care.

Defining Characteristics: (Specify, e.g., parents state or demonstrate lack of understanding of how to care for child after surgery.)

Goal: Parents will gain the knowledge to care for the postoperative child safely at home by (date/time to evaluate).

Outcome Criteria

✔ Parents verbalize understanding of postoperative care information.

✔ Parents demonstrate appropriate postoperative care of child (specify, e.g., encouraging child to drink 30 cc/hr).

NOC: *Knowledge: Treatment Regimen*

INTERVENTIONS	RATIONALE
Assess parents' understanding of the illness and treatment.	Provides baseline information about parents' comprehension of illness.
Allow time for teaching, use a variety of methods (specify, e.g., written instructions, pictures, verbal instruction), encourage questions and reassure parents about child's condition.	Facilitates learning by ensuring parents' comfort. A variety of methods ensures that even illiterate parents will receive appropriate teaching.
Provide information about the surgery as needed. Teach parents that an important risk after a tonsillectomy is excessive bleeding from the operative site. Teach to observe for excessive swallowing and to encourage the child to avoid putting anything in the mouth, and to avoid excess coughing and clearing the throat. Provide physician's instructions regarding any bleeding (specify).	Provides necessary information for parents to recognize and prevent complications.

INTERVENTIONS	RATIONALE
Instruct parents to keep the child quiet for the first few days (specify physician's orders) and inform when the child may return to school (specify).	Provides information to prevent complications.
Teach parents to encourage child to drink clear liquids the first day, advance to soft foods as per physician's preference (specify). Show parents how to evaluate for dehydration; how to monitor intake and output and test skin turgor.	Provides information to prevent dehydration.
Provide medication teaching as needed (specify drug, dose, route, and times ordered) and instruct parents to avoid giving the child aspirin.	Specify action of medications. Aspirin may interfere with blood clotting.
Provide phone numbers in case parents have additional questions after discharge.	Provides additional information as needed.

NIC: *Teaching: Disease Process*

Evaluation

(Date/time of evaluation of goal)

(Has goal been met? Not met? Partially met?)

(Did parents verbalize understanding of care? Provide quotes. Describe parental behavior which indicates understanding of teaching.)

(Revisions to care plan? D/C care plan? Continue care plan?)

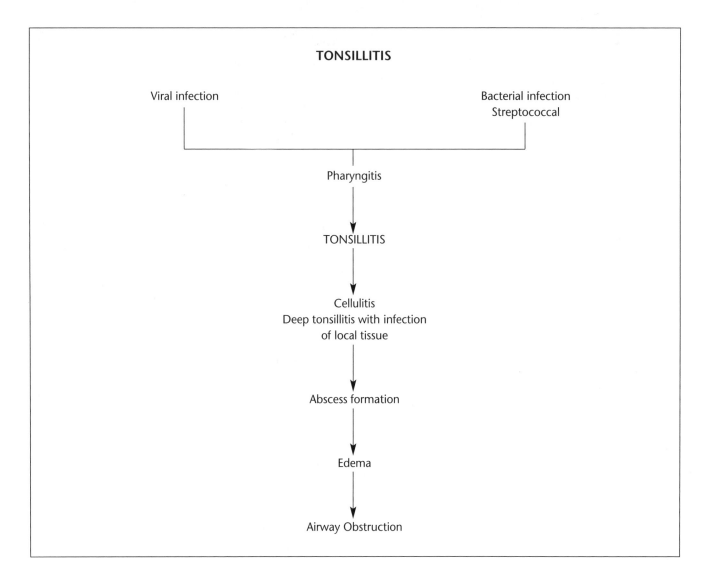

CHAPTER 3.11

TRACHEOSTOMY

The surgical creation of an opening in the trachea between the second and fourth rings is known as a tracheostomy. In children, it may be done to provide an airway to by-pass an acute upper airway obstruction (subglottic stenosis, vocal cord paralysis, epiglottitis, croup) or for long-term mechanical ventilation administration. A plastic tube that softens at body temperature, usually without an inner cannula, is inserted in place and anchored with long sutures taped to the chest during surgery. These sutures remain in place for five days to hold the stoma open until a tract is formed in the trachea and skin. Routine care includes suctioning, cleaning and changing the tracheostomy tube, changing the ties that hold the tube in place, and dressing changes. Temporary tubes are removed when the condition permits and they are no longer needed. Long-term tubes are removed by weaning to the smallest tube with subsequent occlusion of the tube for a day and then final removal.

MEDICAL CARE

Cleansing Agents: hydrogen peroxide at half strength to cleanse around the stoma.

Oxygen Therapy: supplements oxygen when ventilator removed for procedures to prevent hypoxemia, administered with humidication.

Emergency Endotracheal Intubation: procedure done to provide airway in an emergency situation until crisis is resolved or tracheostomy is performed.

COMMON NURSING DIAGNOSES

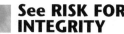 See INEFFECTIVE AIRWAY CLEARANCE

Related to: Tracheobronchial secretion, obstruction.

Defining Characteristics: (Specify: abnormal breath sounds [crackles, wheezes], change in rate or depth of respirations, dyspnea, cyanosis, tube dislodgement or decannulation, tube occlusion, viscous secretion.)

See IMPAIRED GAS EXCHANGE

Related to: Altered oxygen supply.

Defining Characteristics: (Specify: hypoxia, hypercapnia, inability to move secretions, improper suctioning procedure.)

See RISK FOR IMPAIRED SKIN INTEGRITY

Related to: Presence of tracheostomy.

Defining Characteristics: (Specify: secretions around tracheostomy tube; rash or redness around site; low environmental humidity; dry, crusting secretions around site; mechanical factor of pressure and irritation of tube movement.)

See INEFFECTIVE BREATHING PATTERN

Related to: Tracheobronchial obstruction, anxiety.

Defining Characteristics: (Specify: tube occlusion or accidental decannulation, dyspnea, tachypnea, respiratory depth changes, viscous secretions, nasal flaring, accessory muscle retractions.)

See IMBALANCED NUTRITION: LESS THAN BODY REQUIREMENT

Related to: Inability to ingest food.

Defining Characteristics: (Specify: poor feeding with tube in place, difficulty swallowing, choking.)

ADDITIONAL NURSING DIAGNOSES

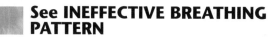 ANXIETY

Related to: Threat to self-concept (tracheostomy); change in health status.

Defining Characteristics: (Specify: increased apprehension, fear of procedures to care for tracheostomy, uncertainty about possible respiratory status changes, expressed feelings of distress over presence of tracheostomy.)

Goal: Clients will experience decreased anxiety by (date/time to evaluate).

Outcome Criteria

✔ Reduced parental and child anxiety verbalized.

NOC: *Coping*

INTERVENTIONS	RATIONALES
Assess level and manifestations of anxiety in parents and child.	Provides information needed for interventions and clues to severity of anxiety.
Allow parents and child to express fears and concerns and to ask questions about disease and what to expect.	Provides opportunity to vent feelings and secure information to reduce anxiety.
Provide supportive and nonjudgmental environment.	Promotes trust and reduces anxiety.
Encourage parents to stay with child, allow open visitation and telephone communications; encourage to participate in care that is planned around usual home routines.	Reduces anxiety by allowing presence and involvement in care, familiar routines and persons for child.
Inform of all procedures and care and any changes in the child's condition.	Reduces anxiety caused by fear of the unknown.
Provide child with pencil and paper, pictures, slate as age allows (specify).	Provides means of communication and interaction with the child.
Provide child with medical play objects such as a doll with a tracheostomy, suction catheters, tracheostomy tubes and ties, as applicable (specify).	Provides child the opportunity to have hands on experience with supplies; improves their understanding of procedures; gives health care professionals some insight into the child's understanding of the procedure.
Allow child to assume position of comfort, provide familiar object (toy or blanket).	Promotes comfort and security.
Provide child/parents tours of the PICU and the floor prior to the surgical procedures as applicable.	Promotes understanding of what to expect which may help to decrease anxiety.

INTERVENTIONS	RATIONALES
Inform of disease process and behaviors and physical effects and symptoms of tracheostomy; assure parents that tracheostomy will facilitate breathing.	Relieves anxiety by knowing what to expect, especially if tracheostomy is long-term.
Explain to parents and child in age-related fashion reason for tracheostomy procedure or therapy, effects of presence of tracheostomy, how procedures are performed (specify).	Reduces anxiety caused by fear of unknown.
Clarify any misinformation with honesty and in simple understandable language.	Prevents any unnecessary anxiety resulting from inaccurate information or beliefs.
Refer to counseling, community groups or agencies (specify).	Reduces anxiety by providing to parents and child support and information from those with similar problems.

NIC: *Anxiety Reduction*

Evaluation

(Date/time of evaluation of goal)

(Has goal been met? Not met? Partially met?)

(Did clients verbalize decreased anxiety? Provide quotes.)

(Revisions to care plan? D/C care plan? Continue care plan?)

▓▓ RISK FOR INFECTION

Related to: Invasive procedures (tracheostomy and care).

Defining Characteristics: (Specify: stasis of secretions, suctioning tracheostomy, redness, excoriation, swelling and drainage at tracheostomy site, change in breath sounds and sputum, increased temperature, presence of infection of family members.)

Goal: Client will not experience infection by (date/ time to evaluate).

Outcome Criteria

✔ Client's temperature remains <100° F.

✔ Breath sounds and secretions remain clear.

NOC: *Risk Control*

INTERVENTIONS	RATIONALES
Assess for change in breathing pattern, color of mucus, diminished breath sounds, ability to cough and raise secretions (specify when).	Indicates presence of respiratory infection.
Avoid exposure to persons with respiratory infection, isolate from infectious patients or family members.	Prevents increased susceptibility and risk for infection.
Utilize good handwashing technique before giving care or performing procedures.	Prevents transmission of microorganisms to child.
Demonstrate handwashing technique to parents and child and allow for return demonstration.	Prevents cross-contamination by hands.
Assist to cough or remove secretions by suctioning via sterile technique.	Stasis of secretions provide medium for infection.
Use medical asepsis techniques or sterile technique when administering tracheostomy and site care (specify).	Prevents exposure to infectious agents.
Change tracheostomy dressing, tube, and ties when soiled, wet, or encrusted with secretions as needed.	Maintains cleanliness of wound and removes risk of contact with infectious agents.
Administer antibiotic therapy if ordered. (Specify drug, dose, route, and times ordered.)	Provides protection from or treatment of infection by destroying or inhibiting growth of microorganisms (specify).
Obtain sputum or wound drainage culture, send to lab.	Identifies presence of pathogenic organisms.
Teach parents of child's susceptibility to infection and to avoid contact of child with persons or family members with respiratory infections.	Provides information that any infection will compromise respiratory status and could be life-threatening.
Encourage parents to provide humidity to environment by vaporizer.	Provides humidity normally obtained through mouth and pharynx.
Inform parents to provide adequate fluid and nutritional intake based on age (specify).	Maintains fluid and nutritional requirements of infant/child.
Teach parents to report any changes in sputum, respiratory status, skin at tracheostomy site to physician.	Provides for immediate interventions to control infection.
Instruct parents and allow for demonstration of sterile or clean technique.	Promotes sterility or cleanliness of procedures based on healing of tracheostomy site.

NIC: *Infection Protection*

Evaluation

(Date/time of evaluation of goal)

(Has goal been met? Not met? Partially met?)

(What is temperature? Describe breath sounds and secretions.)

(Revisions to care plan? D/C care plan? Continue care plan?)

RISK FOR ASPIRATION

Related to: Presence of tracheostomy or endotracheal tube.

Defining Characteristics: (Specify: impaired swallowing, vomiting, choking.)

Goal: Client will not aspirate by (date/time to evaluate).

Outcome Criteria

✔ Client swallows meals without choking, coughing, or changing color.

NOC: *Risk Control*

INTERVENTIONS	RATIONALES
Assess ability to swallow, type of food consistency (solid or formula), age of child.	Provides information about potential for choking or aspiration.
Offer small amounts of liquids initially and follow with increases as tolerated; add cereal to infant formula or offer thick milkshakes to child (specify).	Provides fluids and nutrients of a consistency that is best managed and swallowed to prevent choking.
Place in upright or sitting position for feedings (or place on lap or in infant seat); allow to remain in position for 30 minutes afterwards.	Promotes flow of fluids and foods by gravity.
If choking occurs, suction fluids from mouth and airway; avoid suctioning procedure after feedings.	Removes fluid or food from airway to prevent aspiration; suctioning after feedings may cause nausea or vomiting.
Instruct parents in types of foods and liquids to offer infant/child.	Promotes nutrition requirements that are easier to tolerate and swallow with tube in place.

(continues)

(continued)

INTERVENTIONS	RATIONALES
Teach parents actions to take when choking occurs; positions that are most effective, procedure for feeding (specify).	Prevents aspiration of fluid or food into airway.
Teach parents to suction airway if choking, perform after other measures have failed.	Removes fluid or feedings from airway.
Inform parents to notify physician in presence of respiratory distress.	Prevents life-threatening situation caused by suffocation.

NIC: *Aspiration Precautions*

Evaluation

(Date/time of evaluation of goal)

(Has goal been met? Not met? Partially met?)

(Did client swallow meal without choking, coughing, or changing color?)

(Revisions to care plan? D/C care plan? Continue care plan?)

RISK FOR INJURY

Related to: Tracheostomy complications.

Defining Characteristics: (Specify: damage to tracheal mucosa by inappropriate suctioning, excessive movement or dislodgement of tube, accidental decannulation.)

Goal: Client will not experience injury related to tracheostomy by (date/time to evaluate).

Outcome Criteria

✔ Absence of respiratory distress (define).

✔ Tracheostomy tube remains in place and patent.

NOC: *Risk Control*

INTERVENTIONS	RATIONALES
Assess for proper tube placement, presence of an air leak around tube, patency of tube (specify when/how).	Ensures effective tube function to provide airway for ventilation.
Assess security of tapes and knots, tightness of tapes by inserting small finger between tape and neck (when?).	Promotes safe use of ties to stabilize tube, which should not be frayed and should fit snugly without compromising circulation.

INTERVENTIONS	RATIONALES
Assess need for suctioning by noting change in breath sounds and respiratory rate, depth, and ease.	Allows for removal of secretions to prevent obstruction and respiratory distress.
Assess stay sutures if new tracheostomy by noting security of tapes on side of neck, any movement or dislodgement of tube.	Ensures safe placement of tracheostomy tube and prevents dislodgement.
Hold tube in place when dressing changed, ointment applied under wings of tube, changing tapes, or suctioning tube.	Prevents manipulation of tube that causes mechanical irritation and may dislodge tube.
Restrain if appropriate developmentally and if needed; inform parents and child of reason. Monitor skin under restraints per protocol (specify).	Prevents child from pulling tube out accidentally; prevents injury.
Suction carefully and intermittently, use proper catheter size and technique (specify).	Clears airway and tube of secretions without damage to trachea, prolonged suctioning causes vagal stimulation and bradycardia and high pressure may damage mucosa of trachea.
Provide spare tracheostomy tube, scissors, bag, and proper sized mask and adaptor, oxygen source, and suctioning equipment at bedside.	Provides for emergency interventions for airway obstruction or decannulation.
Change tapes 3 days after surgery and tube 2 weeks after surgery per physician order, with 2 nurses present or respiratory therapist.	Ensures safety of procedures with help at hand if needed.
Change tube if obstructed, reinsert new tube if dislodged; have 2 people present.	Maintains effective tube functioning and airway patency.
Teach, demonstrate, and allow parents to return demonstration of the tube change (insertion and removal) to be done every month or as needed, tube ties change, suctioning and cleansing of tube if long-term care needed.	Promotes continuity of care by parents if able to perform skills and approved by physician; promotes independence and control of family in child's care.
Teach parents of positive effects of tracheostomy, such as ease of breathing, improved rest and feeding, progress in developmental tasks.	Provides emotional support to parents and family.

INTERVENTIONS	RATIONALES
Teach parents of equipment and supplies to have on hand. Assist family to obtain needed equipment.	Provides support for any emergency.
Inform parents to clothe child in loose-fitting clothing around neck with no loose threads or frayed material, remove crumbs, beads or dangerous toys, careful bathing with elimination of water near tube; cover tube with bib when drinking or eating meals.	Prevents obstruction of tube or entry of foreign materials.
Instruct parents to report any swelling or bleeding around tube, increased respiratory effort, change in skin color, absence of air moving in and out of tube, inability to insert suction tube, excessive choking during feeding.	Prevents complications that may compromise respiratory status.

NIC: *Airway Management*

Evaluation

(Date/time of evaluation of goal)

(Has goal been met? Not met? Partially met?)

(Provide data about respiratory status. Is tracheostomy tube in place and patent?)

(Revisions to care plan? D/C care plan? Continue care plan?)

DEFICIENT KNOWLEDGE

Related to: Lack of understanding of the care necessary for a child at home with a tracheostomy; impending discharge of child to home.

Defining Characteristics: (Specify: parents request information regarding care of the child at home; child returns to the hospital because of problems encountered during/with caregiving at home.

Goal: Parents will gain knowledge about caring for the child with a tracheostomy by (date/time to evaluate).

Outcome Criteria

✔ Parents verbalize and demonstrate proper care of tracheostomy: site assessment, suctioning techniques, site care, tube changes, and emergency protocols (specify).

NOC: *Knowledge: Treatment Regimen*

INTERVENTIONS	RATIONALES
Instructions should be in short sessions, tailored to parents' specific learning styles and needs; written materials should be given after each session if literate.	Understanding will be improved when sessions are short and individualized; written materials reinforce learning and improve comprehension.
Notify local utilities and EMS regarding the child's condition.	Response time may be heightened if the appropriate personnel are notified in advance.
Facilitate the acquisition of necessary supplies and equipment needed at home, including suction apparatus, oxygen, pulse oximetry, and so forth; coordinate the necessary teaching regarding the equipment as applicable.	Ensures appropriate supplies and equipment are available at discharge; promotes understanding of how equipment works.
Contact local home health nursing agencies, as applicable; facilitate arrangements.	Promotes feelings of control and decreases anxiety within parents; discharge is often a time of higher stress for parents, and they can become easily overwhelmed.
Demonstrate all aspects of tracheostomy care for the child (if applicable), family, and other significant caregivers; observe return demonstrations; teaching should include: tracheostomy site assessment, suctioning techniques, tracheostomy site care, tracheostomy changes, and emergency protocols.	Including all family members and significant others may help expand the level of support felt by the immediate family; stress will be decreased if they have a sense that they can have some time away, while still leaving the child in good hands.
Instruct all caregivers on CPR, with return demonstrations encouraged; reinforce with written materials or video.	Promotes increased understanding of emergency resuscitation needs of patient; prior knowledge of CPR may reduce stress felt by the family.
Teach and encourage the family to treat the child as normally as possible, including information on growth and development, discipline, school, sibling reactions, the importance of play, and trips outside the home.	Promotes normalcy within the family which facilitates positive adaptation; lessens anxiety and stress.
Teach child and parents vocalization techniques as applicable.	Promotes communication which enhances self-esteem and facilitates normal growth and development.

NIC: *Teaching: Procedure/Treatment*

Evaluation

(Date/time of evaluation of goal)

(Has goal been met? Not met? Partially met?)

(Did parents verbalize and demonstrate proper care of tracheostomy: site assessment, suctioning techniques, site care, tube changes, and emergency protocols?)

(Revisions to care plan? D/C care plan? Continue care plan?)

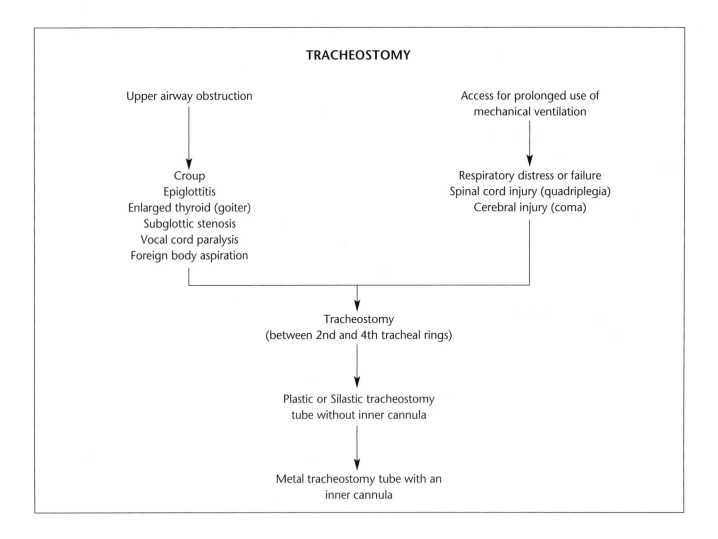

TRACHEOSTOMY

Upper airway obstruction

Access for prolonged use of mechanical ventilation

Croup
Epiglottitis
Enlarged thyroid (goiter)
Subglottic stenosis
Vocal cord paralysis
Foreign body aspiration

Respiratory distress or failure
Spinal cord injury (quadriplegia)
Cerebral injury (coma)

Tracheostomy
(between 2nd and 4th tracheal rings)

Plastic or Silastic tracheostomy
tube without inner cannula

Metal tracheostomy tube with an
inner cannula

CHAPTER 3.12

TUBERCULOSIS

Tuberculosis (TB) in children is usually contracted from an infected adult by droplets expelled from the respiratory tract and dispersed into the air. Although the incidence and death rate from TB are greater in other parts of the world, there has been an increase of cases in the United States. Rates are high among migrant workers, the homeless, and those who are HIV-positive. Most cases are managed at home with drug therapy. Only patients with more serious forms of the disease or who need special diagnostic tests are hospitalized.

MEDICAL CARE

Anti-infectives/Antituberculosis: isoniazid (INH) in combination with rifampin or pyrazinamide to inhibit bacterial growth (bacteriostatic action).

Skin Tests: intradermal Mantoux test (purified protein derivative (PPD)) to screen for sensitivity to the bacillus as a result of past exposure, or to test for suspected tuberculosis. The American Academy of Pediatrics (2000) does not recommend tuberculin skin testing of children with no TB risk factors who live in communities with a low prevalence of TB.

Sputum or Gastric Washing Culture: identifies causative agent in sputum coughed up from lower respiratory tract in children or fasting gastric contents in infants or young children who swallow sputum.

Chest X-ray: reveals tuberculosis lesion if disease is suspected, but radiography results are difficult to differentiate from other diseases.

COMMON NURSING DIAGNOSES

 ### See IMBALANCED NUTRITION: LESS THAN BODY REQUIREMENTS

Related to: Inability to ingest food because of biologic, economic factors.

Defining Characteristics: Inadequate food intake, lack of food availability, pyridoxine deficiency as result of drug therapy.

ADDITIONAL NURSING DIAGNOSES

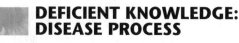 ### DEFICIENT KNOWLEDGE: DISEASE PROCESS

Related to: Unfamiliarity with disease and treatment.

Defining Characteristics: (Specify: verbalization of need for information about medications, activity and rest, nutritional requirements, and infection transmission prevention.)

Goal: Parents will obtain knowledge about tuberculosis by (date/time to evaluate).

Outcome Criteria

✔ Parents verbalize understanding about tuberculosis and planned treatment.

✔ Parents demonstrate correct medication administration (specify drugs, dose, routes, and times).

NOC: *Knowledge: Disease Process*

INTERVENTIONS	RATIONALES
Assess knowledge of disease and methods to control and resolve disease.	Promotes plan of instruction that is realistic; prevents repetition of information.
Provide information and explanations in clear, understandable language; use pictures, pamphlets, video tapes, model in teaching about disease.	Ensures understanding based on readiness and ability to learn; visual aids reinforce learning.
Teach about administration of medications, including action of drugs, dosages, times, frequency, side effects, expected results,	Provides information about drug therapy which is the most important treatment for the cure of tuberculosis and is

INTERVENTIONS	RATIONALES
methods to give medications; provide written instructions and schedule to follow (specify).	administered for at least 9 months during the course of the disease and for 6 months after negative cultures secured; isoniazid alone or in combination with other antituberculosis drugs administered for active tuberculosis and conversion from negative to positive skin testing.
Instruct and assist in planning feedings and/or developing menus for appropriate inclusions of meat and milk and daily caloric and basic four requirements for age group.	Ensures proper diet that enhances health status, and adequate amounts of meat and milk supply vitamin B_6 (pyridoxine) in those receiving isoniazid to prevent peripheral neuritis.
Teach about activity or activity restrictions and adequate rest during convalescence (specify).	More rest and possible restrictions of activity needed during active stage of disease, but school or nursery school attendance is encouraged if asymptomatic.
Provide information about limiting competitive and contact sport activities when the disease is active.	Promotion of optimal health without injury will enhance complete recovery.
Teach about care of used tissues and to cover mouth and nose when coughing or blowing nose, proper handwashing technique.	Prevents transmission of microorganisms by droplets dispersed into the air.
Teach parents about prevention of unnecessary exposure to other infectious diseases, including maintaining the appropriate immunizations as applicable (specify).	Promotes the body's own defenses; prevents secondary infection and/or complications.
Provide information about testing family members and follow-up skin tests for exposed contacts.	Provides early detection of disease and possible source of disease, and prevents potential spread of disease.

INTERVENTIONS	RATIONALES
Provide parents information on isolation procedures, as needed, during the active stage of the illness (specify).	Prevents transmission of the disease.
Reinforce to parents the importance of maintaining the treatment regimen over long period of time; offer information and support for continued care.	Recovery requires extended period of time and support helps to ensure compliance with regimen.
Teach parents about protecting the child from stressors, including parental anxieties.	Promotes body's own use of natural defenses; stress may further weaken those defenses.
Encourage parents to verbalize and demonstrate understanding of teaching. Provide praise and support to family.	Reinforces teaching and promotes optimal caregiving.

NIC: *Teaching: Disease Process*

Evaluation

(Date/time of evaluation of goal)

(Has goal been met? Not met? Partially met?)

(Did parents verbalize understanding about tuberculosis and planned treatment? Provide quotes. Did parents demonstrate correct medication administration?)

(Revisions to care plan? D/C care plan? Continue care plan?)

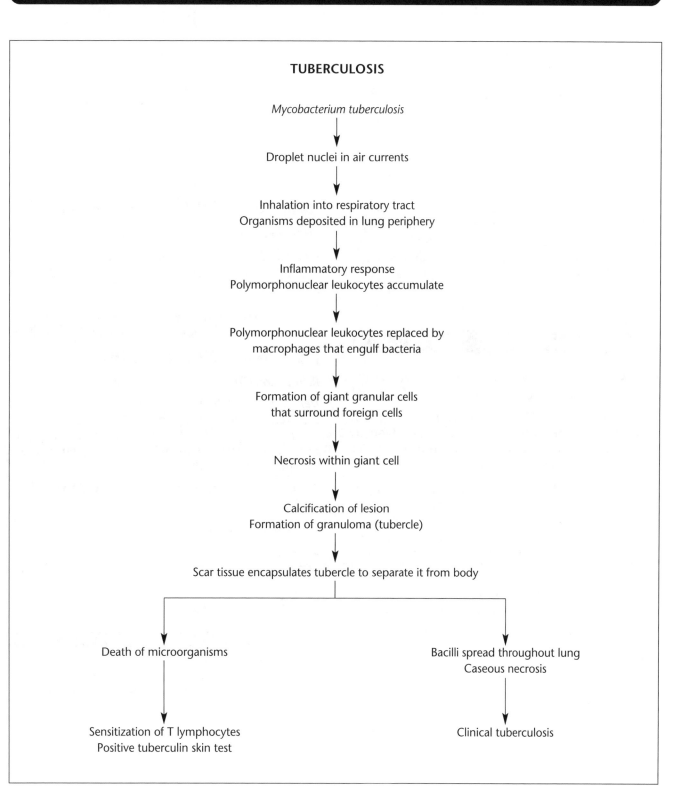

TUBERCULOSIS

Mycobacterium tuberculosis

↓

Droplet nuclei in air currents

↓

Inhalation into respiratory tract
Organisms deposited in lung periphery

↓

Inflammatory response
Polymorphonuclear leukocytes accumulate

↓

Polymorphonuclear leukocytes replaced by
macrophages that engulf bacteria

↓

Formation of giant granular cells
that surround foreign cells

↓

Necrosis within giant cell

↓

Calcification of lesion
Formation of granuloma (tubercle)

↓

Scar tissue encapsulates tubercle to separate it from body

Death of microorganisms   Bacilli spread throughout lung
                                                            Caseous necrosis

↓   ↓

Sensitization of T lymphocytes   Clinical tuberculosis
Positive tuberculin skin test

CHAPTER 3.13

ALLERGIC RHINITIS

Allergic rhinitis is an episodic or perennial upper respiratory tract condition characterized by sneezing, itching nose and eyes, and discharge from the nose and throat. Chronic nasal stuffiness and obstruction to airflow cause mouth breathing, otitis media, and eustachian tube abnormalities. Allergic rhinitis may manifest itself at any age in childhood.

MEDICAL CARE

Antihistamines (H1 receptor antagonist): given alone or in combination with a decongestant for nasal congestion and cough.

Antihistamines (phenothiazine derivatives): given to prevent action of histamine, which provides relief from allergic conditions.

Decongestants: nose drops or spray for older infants (over 6 months) and children; pseudoephedrine given for children over 2 years of age to relieve nasal congestion and clear passages; nose drops reduce swelling by vasoconstriction resulting from topical application.

Skin Tests: identify allergic responses and sensitivities to antigens as a basis for desensitization therapy.

Nasal Culture: reveals presence of eosinophils.

Biopsy of Nasal Mucous Membrane: reveals eosinophils and abnormal mucosa.

RAST Test: reveals and measures the immunoglobulin.

COMMON NURSING DIAGNOSES

See INEFFECTIVE BREATHING PATTERN

Related to: Inflammatory process, obstruction.

Defining Characteristics: Nasal stuffiness and obstruction, mouth breathing, mucus secretion and drainage, respiratory changes, breathing difficulty.

See DISTURBED SLEEP PATTERN

Related to: Internal factors of illness.

Defining Characteristics: (Specify: interrupted sleep, irritability, restlessness, inability to breathe through nose).

ADDITIONAL NURSING DIAGNOSES

RISK FOR INFECTION

Related to: Chronic disease (allergy).

Defining Characteristics: (Specify: nasal discharge; red, itchy conjunctiva; purulent discharge from nose or eyes; allergic shiners [dark areas under eyes], frequent colds, otitis media with pain and temperature elevation; pharyngitis.)

Goal: Client will not experience an infection by (date/time to evaluate).

Outcome Criteria

✔ Temperature <100° F.
✔ Secretions remain clear.

NOC: *Risk Control*

INTERVENTIONS	RATIONALES
Assess for rubbing of nose, nasal discharge and its characteristics (clear, amount, purulent), dark areas around eye, nose itching and pushing hand up and back of nose, frequent sneezing, red and itchy eyes and drainage or watering (specify when).	Provides information about physical and behavioral effects of allergic rhinitis; chronic nasal obstruction causes edema and discoloration of the eyes and mouth breathing, wrinkling of face is caused by attempt to avoid rubbing or scratching of nose.
Inspect nasal passages and throat with penlight for redness, swelling, and presence of mucus and/or exudate; check skin around nares for redness, irritation (when).	Reveals inflammation and risk of infection spread.

INTERVENTIONS	RATIONALES
Assess for knowledge and use of preventive measures needed to avoid spread of microorganisms.	Provides basis for information needed for health maintenance.
Assess for frequency of upper respiratory infections among family members; attendance at school, daycare, nursery school.	Persistent reinfection usually the result of repeated exposures to microorganisms.
Assess use of over-the-counter medications and type used.	Combination products are not particularly useful; symptomatic treatment more effective in controlling upper respiratory responses; overuse of some medications may cause undesirable side effects (drowsiness) or rebound effects (return of symptoms).
Provide vaporizer or humidifier if nasal and oral mucous membranes are dry.	Maintains moist mucous membranes to prevent breaks and soreness.
Administer antihistamines and immunotherapy if ordered alone or in combination with decongestants (specify).	Provides control of the symptoms when exposed to allergens.
Teach handwashing technique after exposure to nasopharyngeal secretions (sneezing, blowing nose).	Hands found to be most common carrier of microorganisms.
Instruct in disposal of tissues used for cough or nose wiping.	Prevents transmission of microorganisms.
Inform to avoid contact with infected people or family members, although transmission commonly occurs in families, schools, nursery schools, recreational gatherings.	Prevents exposure to the infectious agent, although isolation is not realistic within a family.

INTERVENTIONS	RATIONALES
Instruct parents in administration of medications via oral and inhalation routes (specify).	Ensures compliance with medication regimen to control symptoms and prevent infection.
Instruct to administer all of the antibiotic prescribed for infection (if present).	Ensures effective treatment of bacterial infection for prompt response within 24 hours after antibiotic administration.
Teach about desensitization injection schedule.	Allays child's anxiety and fear caused by injections.
Teach parents measures to control environment (air conditioning; removal of dust, pets, smoke).	Supports environment free of allergens or irritants that cause attacks.
Inform to notify physician if the temperature increases, ear hurts, throat is sore or nose has purulent drainage.	Allows for immediate interventions to treat at complications.

NIC: *Infection Prevention*

Evaluation

(Date/time of evaluation of goal)

(Has goal been met? Not met? Partially met?)

(What is temperature? Describe secretions.)

(Revisions to care plan? D/C care plan? Continue care plan?)

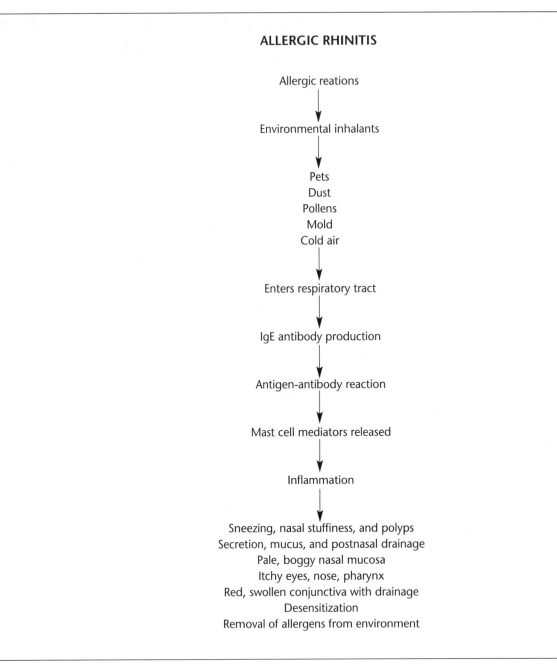

ALLERGIC RHINITIS

Allergic reations

↓

Environmental inhalants

↓

Pets
Dust
Pollens
Mold
Cold air

↓

Enters respiratory tract

↓

IgE antibody production

↓

Antigen-antibody reaction

↓

Mast cell mediators released

↓

Inflammation

↓

Sneezing, nasal stuffiness, and polyps
Secretion, mucus, and postnasal drainage
Pale, boggy nasal mucosa
Itchy eyes, nose, pharynx
Red, swollen conjunctiva with drainage
Desensitization
Removal of allergens from environment

UNIT 4

GASTROINTESTINAL SYSTEM

CHAPTER 4.0

GASTROINTESTINAL SYSTEM: BASIC CARE PLAN

The gastrointestinal (GI) tract is a long passageway that functions to allow ingestion, digestion, and absorption of nutrients and fluids, and elimination of solid wastes from the body. The components of the GI tract are the mouth, teeth, salivary glands, esophagus, stomach, small intestine, pancreas, liver, gallbladder, large intestine, and anus. Inherited defects in structure or function, or infection, physiologic and psychological factors may affect ingestion, digestion, or elimination. The system is a common site of minor disorders in infants and children.

GASTROINTESTINAL GROWTH AND DEVELOPMENT

- Tooth eruption in infancy at 6 to 8 months with the primary set of teeth completed by approximately 2 years of age.

- Striated muscles in the throat develop by 6 weeks of age and cerebral connections are developed at 6 months of age to assist in swallowing, which is a reflex activity up to 3 months of age and is stimulated by the flow of milk into the mouth. A coordinated muscular action of swallowing and sucking is necessary.

- Sucking pads present in cheeks to assist sucking and remain until sucking not needed to obtain nutrition.

- Stomach is round in shape until 2 years of age, elongates until 7 years of age when it assumes shape and position of an adult.

- Stomach capacity increases:

Newborn:	10 to 20 ml
1 to 3 weeks:	30 to 100 ml
1 to 3 months:	90 to 200 ml
1 to 2 years:	200 to 500 ml
10 years:	750 to 900 ml

- Cardiac sphincter is immature and relaxed in infant causing regurgitation; as digestive system matures, this "spitting up" is outgrown by 6 to 7 months of age.

- The intestinal tract in the infant and young child is longer than in the older child and the musculature and sphincters are underdeveloped with a deficiency of elastin fibers in the very young child.

- Growth of the intestines increases between 1 to 3 years of age.

- Digestive and absorptive surfaces are completely developed at birth.

- The liver may sometimes be palpated 1 to 2 cm below the right costal margin in infants and young children. Palpation of the liver 3 cm or more below the costal margin indicates abnormal enlargement.

- Sucking and swallowing are reflex activities without voluntary control until 3 months of age. Infants are capable of swallowing, holding food in the mouth and spitting food out of mouth by 6 months of age; swallowing becomes more coordinated and solid foods more acceptable with growth.

- Chewing begins with eruption of primary teeth at about 6 months; a sense of taste with response to sweet and sour solutions is present at birth; sweet taste increases sucking and other tastes decrease sucking.

- Stomach empties in 3 to 4 hours (breast milk faster than formula) in infant and 3 to 6 hours in older infant and child; begins to enter small intestine in 1 to 2 minutes after ingestion.

- Immature system allows food to be propelled through system rapidly resulting in bowel elimination frequency and watery stools as water not absorbed as well as in older child; stool less frequent and more regular and becoming firmer as system becomes more efficient during the first year.

- Intestinal flora introduced through the mouth and established by 2 days of life.
- Stool changes from meconium to greenish black, greenish brown, greenish yellow (transitional stools) and then become yellowish and pasty in breast-fed infants and paler yellow in infants fed formula.
- Salivary glands increase in size and mature in function by 3 years of age.
- Gastric secretions increase in acidity with composition the same as an adult by 10 years of age.
- Pancreatic amylase and lipase are deficient in infant and affect utilization of complex carbohydrates, and absorption of fats.
- Liver function increases as growth takes place and liver matures; limited ability to conjugate bilirubin which may result in jaundice, but able to conjugate bilirubin and secrete bile by 2 weeks of age with bile composition mature at 6 months of age.
- Gluconeogenesis, formation of plasma proteins and ketones, storage of vitamins and the breakdown of amino acids by the liver achieved by 1 year of age.
- Basal metabolism rate is highest in infant and decreases as body increases in size; usually higher in boys than girls.
- Appetite decreases by 2 years of age as growth and metabolic rate slows and food requirements are reduced.
- Caloric requirements of child:

Infant:	110 to 120 cal/kg/day
Toddler:	1300 cal/day
Preschool:	1800 cal/day
School-age:	2400 cal/day

- Approximate weights (varies with sex, age frame, height):

Birth: 5½ to 10 lb (2500–4600 gm) at full term
Birth weight doubled by 5 months, tripled by 1 year
Gains approximately 30 gm/day

- Length at birth for full-term infant: 18 to 22 in (45–55 cm)

Growth rate/year:

2nd year:	11 cm
3rd year:	8 cm
4th year:	7 cm
up to 10 years:	5 to 6 cm

NURSING DIAGNOSES

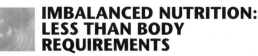

IMBALANCED NUTRITION: LESS THAN BODY REQUIREMENTS

Related to: (Specify: inability to ingest or digest food or absorb nutrients because of biologic or psychological factors.)

Defining Characteristics: (Specify: loss of weight with adequate intake, lack of interest in food, anorexia, nausea, vomiting, diarrhea, congenital defect of gastrointestinal system, regurgitation, abdominal pain, dysphagia, inability in infant to suck and swallow, failure to thrive, malabsorption syndromes, growth and developmental changes [food jags, fads, ritualisms, rejection of solid foods], vitamin deficiency, increased metabolic demand, chronic illness, poor nutrient quality of food.)

Goal: Client will experience balanced nutrition by (date/time to evaluate).

Outcome Criteria

✔ Adequate intake of appropriate nutrients for normal growth and development (specify).

✔ Height and weight parameters met and maintained based on individual determinations (specify).

NOC: *Nutritional Status: Nutrient Intake*

INTERVENTIONS	RATIONALES
Assess history of food intake (24-hour recall, amounts of food and formula or breast milk; financial and cultural influences; vitamin/mineral supplement; food allergies.	Provides information needed to evaluate nutritional pattern, habits and adequacy (deficiency or excess).
Assess appetite changes (poor or excessive), presence of illness and diagnosis, effect of nutrition on skin, hair, eyes, mouth, head, muscles, behavior.	Indicates health status and effect of illness which requires an increase in nutritional needs and appetite that is affected by illness and may result in malnutrition.
Assess height and weight, head circumference, skinfold thickness and arm circumference and compare with previous values and standard charts.	Provides anthropometric information about body's fat and protein content and general nutritional status.

(continues)

(continued)

INTERVENTIONS	RATIONALES
Assess difficulty in sucking, swallowing, chewing, gag reflex, teeth, oral mucous membrane, lips, and palate for abnormalities, presence of oral pain or infection.	Provides information about ability to ingest foods or formula necessary for normal growth and development; inadequate dental care, oral inflammatory disorders, congenital defects (cleft lip/palate) interferes with feeding.
Assess presence of nausea, vomiting and if spitting up, projectile; related to activity or intake or tension/stress; characteristics of vomits (bloody, bile, digested or undigested food), frequency and persistence, amount, associated conditions (diarrhea, fever, headache, motion sickness, anger, conflict with parent).	Provides information about emesis which affects nutrition and is controlled by the vomiting center in the medulla; causes include: blockage of the pylorus, reflex from incompetent esophageal sphincter, gastroenteritis, duodenal and gastric spasm, increased ICP, bowel obstruction, drugs and allergens; persistent losses may lead to fluid and electrolyte imbalance.
Assess abdominal girth, stool characteristics (odor, appearance), presence of diarrhea, bowel sounds for increased motility.	Provides information about ability to absorb foods; stool may be bulky and fatty in cystic fibrosis if bile flow obstructed and fats are not digested; diarrhea may cause carbohydrate malabsorption as motility increases and moves nutrients through the bowel before absorption takes place.
Place infant/child in position of comfort for feeding/meals: hold infant in arms or upright as condition indicates (cleft defect); child in sitting position at table within easy reach of food and with appropriate sized utensils (specify).	Provides most appropriate position to enhance movement of formula/solid food by gravity and peristalsis and to prevent vomiting and/or aspiration.
Offer feedings/meals as near usual to normal routine as possible; provide amounts (small when indicated) and frequency (infant feedings q 4h and progress to 3 meals/day with introduction of solid foods at proper age); if ill, spread over 6 meals/day (specify).	Promotes feedings/meals that are similar to established pattern and adjusted to special needs caused by specific illness or increased metabolic demand (fever, infection, chronic illness, malnutrition).
Request parent to bring foods from home if desired and serve in age appropriate quantities; allow child to eat in a community setting with other children.	Promotes appetite and increased independence and familiar types and preparation of foods.

INTERVENTIONS	RATIONALES
Offer age appropriate food consistency and foods that are not irritating to oral, stomach, bowel mucosa; thicken formula with cereal when necessary; modify other foods specific to disorder (specify).	Promotes ingestion and retention of foods and prevents exacerbation or increased severity of gastrointestinal disorders.
Maintain NPO status (if prescribed), provide infant with non-nutritional sucking.	Provides rest for gastrointestinal tract needed because of vomiting, diarrhea, preoperative preparation.
Initiate and monitor IV administration of nutrients as prescribed (specify fluid, rate and site and use of pump).	Provides short-term fluid and nutritional support via peripheral vein in those who are unable to ingest or retain nourishment (vomiting, diarrhea postoperative care).
Initiate and monitor IV total parenteral nutrition as prescribed (specify).	Provides long-term fluid and nutritional support via a right atrial catheter in a large vein in those who are nutritionally deficient as a result of a chronic disease (Crohn's disease) or negative nitrogen balance.
Insert nasogastric tube and initiate and monitor tube feedings as prescribed; initiate and monitor feedings and insertion site of gastrostomy if present (provide specifics).	Provides nutritional support for those with persistent weight loss; unable to chew, swallow, suck; who need an increase in nutrients while ill, but with intact digestive and absorption activity.
Avoid excessive handling of an infant after feeding.	Prevents possible vomiting from increased stimuli.
Administer vitamin/mineral supplements, digestive enzymes, antispasmodics, antibiotics (specify).	Provides or replaces necessary substances that may be deficient if absorption impaired, or be the cause of impaired digestion absorption; reduces peristalsis and infectious process affective nutritional status.
Consult or refer with nutritionist as needed.	Provides support for the infant/child's special dietary needs.
Instruct parents in the different food intake at different ages, the amount and types of foods appropriate to age using the food guide pyramid, how food intake relates to growth and development.	Promotes knowledge of needs that will ensure nutritional adequacy of child.
Teach parents to avoid including sugar and salt in diet; offer nutritious between-meal snacks.	Maintains and promotes health status.

INTERVENTIONS	RATIONALES
Teach parents about caloric needs for age of child and in weight and height measurement techniques (specify).	Promotes knowledge to ensure stable weight and gains proportionate to growth.
Teach about proper preparation and storage of foods; handwash before preparing or handling food.	Prevents spoiling and contamination of foods that may cause gastrointestinal symptoms.
Instruct parents in use of special devices or utensils for feeding or for self-feeding by child (specify).	Promotes food intake.
Inform parents of need for food supplements and that the quality of food is more important than the quantity of food ingested.	Ensures nutritional status and provides parents with realistic information about food intake.
Explain method of providing nutrition via IV or NG or gastrostomy tube (if used).	Reduces anxiety by understanding of alternate method of supplying nutrients to infant/child.
Discuss with parents how to wean child from breast or bottle, when to add solid foods to diet (specify).	Provides information if needed about infant's diet changes.
Instruct parents in menu planning that is age appropriate, acknowledging food preferences, consistency and texture, finger and raw foods, and allow child to participate in planning.	Encourages inclusion of necessary foods and acceptance of foods offered.

NIC: *Nutrition Management*

Evaluation

(Date/time of evaluation of goal)

(Has goal been met? Not met? Partially met?)

(Describe intake based on outcome criteria. What is height and weight?)

(Revisions to care plan? D/C care plan? Continue care plan?)

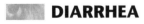 **DIARRHEA**

Related to: Dietary intake.

Defining Characteristics: (Specify: abdominal pain, cramping, increased frequency of bowel elimination and bowel sounds, loose, liquid stools, urgency, intake of high fiber, spicy foods.)

Related to: Inflammation, irritation or malabsorption of bowel.

Defining Characteristics: (Specify: abdominal pain and cramping, increased frequency of bowel elimination and bowel sounds, loose, liquid, unformed stools, urgency, blood, mucus or pus in stools.

Related to: Toxins, contaminants.

Defining Characteristics: (Specify: abdominal pain, increased frequency of bowel elimination and bowel sounds, loose, liquid stools, urgency, fever and malaise.)

Related to: Medications, radiation.

Defining Characteristics: (Specify: abdominal pain, increased frequency of bowel elimination and bowel sounds, loose, liquid stools, urgency, chemotherapeutic agents, external radiation treatments.)

Goal: Client will be relieved of diarrhea by (date and time to evaluate).

Outcome Criteria

✔ Resolution of diarrhea with establishment of pattern of soft formed stool elimination (specify).

✔ Absence of precipitating factors causing diarrheal episodes (specify).

NOC: *Bowel Elimination*

INTERVENTIONS	RATIONALES
Assess normal pattern of bowel elimination and characteristics of stool (frequency, amount, consistency, presence of blood, pus, mucus, color change), presence of diseases or contact with contaminants, infective organisms, medications being taken.	Provides information about baseline parameters for comparison, reason for changes; diarrhea may be acute caused by an inflammation, toxin or a systemic disease and last about 72 hours, or chronic caused by inflammation, allergy, malabsorption, bowel motility changes or disease and last longer than 72 hours; antibiotic therapy may cause diarrhea as it destroys the normal flora in the bowel.
Assess abdomen for distention palpation and bowel sounds for increases in auscultation (specify when).	Indicates a distended bowel with fluid and hypermotility of bowel which reduces the amount of material that is absorbed by the bowel mucosa.

(continues)

(continued)

INTERVENTIONS	RATIONALES
Assess for temperature elevation, irritability, flaccidity, lack of expression, whiny cry, lethargy, anorexia, vomiting, eyes lackluster.	Provides information about signs and symptoms associated with diarrhea.
Assess for fluid loss with a light weight loss, dry skin and mucous membranes, poor skin turgor, serum potassium, sodium for decreases (specify when).	Indicates possible dehydration associated with fluid/electrolyte loss from frequent watery stools and vomiting and insensible fluid loss from fever that leads to metabolic acidosis.
Obtain stool specimen for laboratory examination for toxins, ova and parasites, number of calories of infective organisms present; fecal analysis for occult blood, fat content; repeat specimen examination as needed to confirm presence of organism.	Indicates possible cause of diarrhea.
Place on enteric isolation and explain reasons why this is necessary until diagnosis is confirmed; maintain precautions if cause is identified as an infective organism.	Prevents undue anxiety and transmission of disease to others since bacterial and viral infections are the most common causes of diarrhea in children.
Place on NPO, administer and monitor IV fluids and electrolytes (specify).	Allows bowel to rest and IV replaces lost fluids and electrolytes.
Administer oral rehydration fluids q 4 to 6 hours and increase or decrease depending on hydration status; volume should equal stool losses and as prescribed, and maintenance therapy includes the addition of breast milk or plain water for every 2 bottles of rehydration fluid (specify).	Provides therapy of choice for milk or moderate dehydration in infants.
Encourage continuation or reintroduction of the child's regular diet as soon as possible.	A regular diet provides the nutrients the child needs and has been shown to have no adverse effects according to the American Academy of Pediatrics.
Administer anti-infective therapy and antidiarrheals as ordered (specify drug, dose, route, and times; include therapeutic and side effects to monitor for.	Specify drug action.
Change diaper frequently as needed (in infant), expose buttocks to air and apply skin protective ointment to buttocks	Protects skin from excretions and secretions that are irritating and cause excoriation and skin breakdown.

INTERVENTIONS	RATIONALES
and perianal area in infants and anal area in children if irritated and sore; wash area with warm water after each diarrhea episode (commercial wipes may be used if skin not irritated).	
Teach parents and child about enteric precautions including handwashing technique after bowel movement and before meals, disposal of and laundering of linens and articles contaminated by excrement, demonstrate and allow for return demonstration of handwashing.	Prevents transmission or spread of microorganisms causing diarrhea to others.
Teach parents signs and symptoms of dehydration or changes in characteristics of diarrhea and to report them to physician; diarrhea that becomes chronic or returns or diet that is not tolerated should be reported.	Provides for immediate treatment and prevention of severe complication of acidosis; diarrhea that persists longer than 12 to 24 hours in infant or longer than 48 hours in child should be reported.
Discuss proper refrigeration and handling of foods.	Preserves foods properly to prevent spoiling and possible source of diarrhea.
Instruct parents on procedure to collect stool specimen and take to laboratory labeled properly.	Provides specimen examination to identify cause of diarrhea.
Instruct parents to stop milk and solid foods if diarrhea starts again and begin with sips of fluid and advance diet as before.	Prevents recurrence of severe diarrhea or chronic type caused by intolerance to foods or effect of foods on diseased bowel.
Instruct parents in medication administration if prescribed and avoidance of medications in children under 12 years of age (absorbents, antidiarrheals).	Promotes correct administration of antibiotics for some types of diarrhea and avoidance of medications that may cause toxicity or mask fluid losses and prolong diarrhea caused by infectious agents by decreasing motility.

NIC: *Fluid and Electrolyte Management*

Evaluation

(Date/time of evaluation of goal)

(Has goal been met? Not met? Partially met?)

(Describe pattern and consistency of bowel movements. Have precipitating factors been eliminated? Describe.)

(Revisions to care plan? D/C care plan? Continue care plan?)

CONSTIPATION

Related to: Less than adequate dietary intake and bulk.

Defining Characteristics: (Specify: frequency less than usual pattern, hard, dry formed stool, decreased bowel sounds, straining at stool, decreased amount of stool, change from human to cow's milk in infancy.)

Related to: Personal habits.

Defining Characteristics: (Specify: environmental changes [school], stool withholding in young children, lack of privacy, inability of leisurely use of bathroom, not using bathroom when urge is felt by school-age children.)

Related to: Less than adequate physical activity or immobility.

Defining Characteristics: (Specify: frequency less than usual pattern, hard, dry formed stool, decreased bowel sounds, absence of stool, abdominal distention or rigidity or cramping, postoperative bed rest and immobility, bed rest status.)

Related to: Medications.

Defining Characteristics: (Specify: administration of diuretics, antacids, anticonvulsives, iron preparation to treat other conditions, diagnostic procedure using barium, hard, dry, less frequent stools.)

Related to: Neuromuscular or musculoskeletal impairment.

Defining Characteristics: (Specify: inability to feel urge to defecate, fecal impaction, hard, dry formed stool, locomotion impairment, inability to exert force necessary to defecate, painful defecation, mental retardation, poor and sphincter tone, paralysis, autonomic dysreflexia.)

Related to: Gastrointestinal obstructive lesions.

Defining Characteristics: (Specify: ribbon-like stools, less frequent or absence of stools, abdominal distention and pain, diminished or absence of bowel sounds.)

Goal: Client will obtain relief from constipation by (date and time to evaluate).

Outcome Criteria

✔ Resolution of constipation with establishment of pattern of soft formed stool elimination depending on age (specify).

✔ Bowel elimination alteration (constipation) relieved and return of preoperative or prehospitalization pattern (describe).

NOC: *Bowel Elimination*

INTERVENTIONS	RATIONALES
Assess normal pattern of bowel elimination and characteristics of stool (frequency, amount, shape and consistency), presence of diseases, abnormalities of the bowel caused by congenital defects.	Provides information that indicates baseline parameters for comparison; frequency varies among children depending on age and foods ingested, but may be as few as 3 to 5/day in infant, as few as 6/week in child less than 3 years of age, and few as 4/week in older child; presence of constipation may be associated with disorders in children that lead to obstruction.
Assess abdomen for hard mass or distention, measure abdominal girth, auscultate for bowel sounds that are diminished or absent (specify frequency).	Indicates accumulation of stool in bowel or reduction in peristalsis.
Assess for toilet training techniques, change in diet, change in environment.	Provides information that may lead to reasons for constipation.
Assess for intentional stool withholding, discomfort in defecation, word the child uses to indicate need to defecate.	Provides information about reason child might have for suppressing the urge to defecate.
Assess parents' feelings about bowel habits and toilet training.	Provides information about child's reaction to parental attitudes and may cause bowel elimination suppression.
Provide privacy during bowel elimination.	Promotes elimination by preserving privacy that a child considers important for a very private and intimate activity.
Allow child to sit up during bowel elimination on a bedpan if necessary or on a commode or toilet if possible.	Provides a normal position for easier bowel elimination; a bedpan may eliminate possibility of elimination.

(continues)

(continued)

INTERVENTIONS	RATIONALES
Encourage fluid intake and activity within limitations imposed by illness; add fruit, fiber, prune juice to diet (specify amounts).	Provides fluid and exercise for bowel motility and prevents hard, dry stool if water is reabsorbed because of lack of fluids, bulk in stool provided by fiber in the diet promotes motility.
Administer stool softeners, suppositories or isotonic enema as ordered for child (specify), explain procedure and what to expect to the child before administering.	Preparation by explanation encourages cooperation (specify action of drug).
Teach parents that daily bowel elimination is not necessary for a child and that straining is not always a symptom of constipation; that changes in bowel elimination pattern may be caused by illness.	Provides accurate information to replace beliefs or misinformation by expecting results that will frustrate child.
Discuss with parents that child may suppress defecation as a result of bad experiences during toilet training; if punished for accidental soiling of clothing; that an illness or discomfort when defecating may cause a child to suppress defecation.	Provides information about behavior common to toddlers and preschool age children and constipation is developed and perpetuated when bowel contents are retained.
Teach parents and child in dietary inclusion of high fiber foods including cereals, grains, fruit, and vegetables, or add fiber to foods for child.	Provides bulk to increase motility in child; fiber absorbs water to soften stool.
Instruct parents and child to avoid excessive milk products, rice, apples and apple juice, bananas, gelatin which are constipating foods.	Provides information about foods that prevent resolution of constipation.
Teach parents and child to increase fluids, age appropriate, and as child gets older and milk amount is reduced, replace with other fluids.	Provides adequate fluid intake to soften stool and maintain bowel elimination.
Teach parents and child to maintain activity and instruct child in abdominal and rectal exercises.	Promotes peristalsis and muscle strength involved in bowel elimination especially if child is ill and on bed rest or has poor anal sphincter control.

NIC: *Constipation Management*

Evaluation

(Date/time of evaluation of goal)

(Has goal been met? Not met? Partially met?)

(Describe pattern and consistency of bowel movements. Has constipation been relieved and the elimination pattern returned to prehospitalization or preoperative patterns? Describe.)

(Revisions to care plan? D/C care plan? Continue care plan?)

DEFICIENT FLUID VOLUME

Related to: (Specify: chemosensitive triggers medication, anesthesia, chemotherapy, toxins, increased ICP, inner ear disturbances, cerebral hypoxia, food intolerances, allergens, motion sickness.

Defining Characteristics: (Specify: nausea, vomiting, perspiration, weight loss or gain, pallor, dehydration, fluid and electrolyte imbalance, anxiety, hopelessness, loss of control, tachycardia, abdominal cramping, early morning vomiting (ICP and metabolic disease), fever and diarrhea (infection), decreased urine output, fatigue, hypotension, thirst.)

Related to: Emotional stimuli triggers (unpleasant sights, odors, fright, anorexia, eating disorders).

Defining Characteristics: (Specify: weight loss, change in level of consciousness or headache, malnutrition, weight gain [overeating], psychogenic vomiting [after meals], nausea, perspiration, pallor, dehydration, fluid and electrolyte imbalance, anxiety, tachycardia.

Related to: Visceral stimuli triggers (specify: irritation, inflammation, mechanical disturbance in GI tract or other related viscera, or GI pain).

Defining Characteristics: (Specify: chronic intermittent vomiting [malrotation], green bilious vomiting [bowel obstruction], curdled mucus or food, vomiting many hours after eating [poor gastric emptying or high intestinal obstruction], constipation [anatomic or functional obstruction], forceful vomiting [pyloric stenosis], localized abdominal pain, vomiting soon after meals [peptic ulcer disease], weight loss, nausea, perspiration, tachycardia, anxiety, pallor, dehydration, fluid and electrolyte imbalance, fatigue, decreased urinary output.)

Goal: Client will experience adequate fluid volume by (date/time to evaluate).

Outcome Criteria

✔ Denies nausea and vomiting.

✔ Intake increased to (specify).

✔ Elastic skin turgor and capillary refill <2 seconds.

NOC: *Fluid Balance*

INTERVENTIONS	RATIONALES
Assess food frequency and 24 hour recall, oral fluids, medications, food likes and dislikes, financial and cultural influences, food allergies, food preparation methods.	Provides information to evaluate nutritional status, patterns, habits, and environmental influences on diet.
Assess onset of nausea and vomiting, quality, quantity and presence of blood, bile, food, and odor.	Provides information about emesis and defining characteristics.
Assess relationship of nausea and vomiting to meals, time of day or activities, and associated triggers.	Provides information to identify factors related to time of fluid deficit.
Assess for presence of associated symptoms: diarrhea, fever, ear pain, UGI symptoms, vision changes, headache, seizures, high pitched cry, polydipsia, polyuria, polyphagia, anorexia, and so forth; record intake and output, including all body fluid losses, IVs and oral fluids (specify frequency).	Provides information to identify associated medical conditions; indicates fluid status; increased output and decreased intake indicate a fluid deficit and need for replacement.
Assess skin turgor, mucous membranes, weight, fontanelles of an infant, last void, and behavior changes.	Provides information about hydration status; including extracellular fluid losses, decreased activity levels, malaise, weight loss, poor skin turgor, concentrated urine.
Maintain NPO status, if prescribed (specify).	Provides rest for the gastrointestinal tract because of nausea and vomiting and associated medical conditions.
Initiate and monitor IV administration of nutrients as prescribed (specify).	Provides fluid and nutritional support to replace active fluid loss and prevention of fluid overload.
Assess vital signs, including apical pulse (specify when).	Provides monitoring of cardiovascular response to dehydration (weak, thready pulse, drop in blood pressure). Increased respiratory rate may contribute to fluid loss.

INTERVENTIONS	RATIONALES
Initiate small amounts of clear liquids, as tolerated when nausea and vomiting subside; offer oral hydration fluids; breast-fed babies need frequent short feedings at the breast: Infant: 70 to 100 ml/kg in 24 hours, toddler: 50 to 70 ml/kg in 24 hours, school-age: 20 to 50 ml/kg in 24 hours.	Provides fluids in minimal amounts until nausea and vomiting resolved.
Gradually reintroduce other fluids and regular diet.	Allows for the gradual return to the expected dietary intake.
Monitor urine specific gravity, color, and amount every voiding or as ordered.	Concentrated urine with an increased specific gravity indicates lack of fluids to dilute urine.
Monitor laboratory data results, as ordered (electrolytes, BUN, CBC, pH, etc.).	Allows identification of fluid losses and electrolyte imbalances.
Administer medications (specify drug, dose, route, and times) as ordered and evaluate effects/side effects.	Specify action.
Position child on side or sitting up when vomiting; keep suction available.	Avoids aspiration of emesis.
Provide comfort measures (e.g., cool cloth, clean linens, etc.).	Promotes comfort level and distraction.
Administer or assist with good oral hygiene (brushing teeth, mouthwash or oral swabs).	Provides moisture and comfort for drying oral mucosa.
Explain all interventions to child and parents and provide psychological support.	Provides comfort, information, relieves anxiety, and decreases feeling of powerlessness.
Assist child with activity and position changes.	Prevents injury and provides safety because of possible postural hypertension.
Instruct parents regarding causes of nausea and vomiting, signs of dehydration, and when to report them to the physician (specify).	Provides information for immediate treatment of excessive loss of fluids and electrolytes caused by nausea and vomiting.
Teach parents to position child safely during vomiting episodes and to provide oral hygiene.	Provides information to promote safety, oral hydration and hygiene.

NIC: *Fluid Management*

Evaluation

(Date/time of evaluation of goal)

(Has goal been met? Not met? Partially met?)

(Does client/parent deny nausea and vomiting? What is intake in time frame criteria? Is skin turgor elastic? What is capillary refill time?)

(Revisions to care plan? D/C care plan? Continue care plan?)

CHAPTER 4.1

APPENDICITIS

Appendicitis is the inflammation of the appendix, a blind sac connected to the end of the cecum. It is caused most commonly by a fecalith (hard feces) and may result in obstruction which leads to ischemia, necrosis, perforation, and peritonitis. Surgical removal of the appendix (appendectomy) is performed as treatment for this disorder, preferably before rupture for a positive outcome. Surgery after rupture requires external drainage and management to reduce the spread of peritonitis. The condition commonly occurs in children over 2 years of age.

MEDICAL CARE

Narcotic Analgesics: after diagnosis has been made and postoperatively.

Analgesics (non-narcotic analgesics): acetaminophen given postoperatively to control moderate pain.

Antibiotics: ampicillin or other anti-infectives to prevent or treat peritonitis.

Abdominal X-ray: reveals presence of fecalith or other material in the appendix.

Abdominal Ultrasound: reveals abscess location if present.

Complete Blood Count: reveals increased WBC of 15,000 to 20,000/cu mm and increased neutrophils.

COMMON NURSING DIAGNOSES

See RISK FOR DEFICIENT FLUID VOLUME

Related to: (Specify: excessive losses, NPO status postoperatively.)

Defining Characteristics: (Specify: vomiting, deviations affecting intake of fluids, elevated temperature, reduced urinary output, diaphoresis.)

See HYPERTHERMIA

Related to: Illness.

Defining Characteristics: (Specify: increase in body temperature above normal range, warm to touch, increased pulse and respiratory rate, flushing, abrupt rise in temperature with rupture of appendix.)

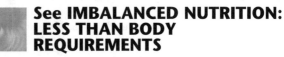 See IMBALANCED NUTRITION: LESS THAN BODY REQUIREMENTS

Related to: Inability to ingest food.

Defining Characteristics: (Specify: vomiting, anorexia, nausea, abdominal pain, presence of nasogastric function postoperative.)

See CONSTIPATION

Related to: Less than adequate physical activity.

Defining Characteristics: (Specify: bed rest following surgery, decreased or absent bowel sounds, frequency less than usual pattern, hard formed stool, abdominal pain.)

ADDITIONAL NURSING DIAGNOSES

PAIN

Related to: Biologic injuring agents, inflammation.

Defining Characteristics: (Specify: verbal descriptor of pain, guarding and protective behavior of painful area, irritability, refusal to move or change position, crying, muscular rigidity, clinging behavior, side-lying position with knees flexed.)

Goal: The client will experience less pain by (date/time to evaluate).

Outcome Criteria

✔ Client rates pain less than (specify using an appropriate rating scale for age and development).

NOC: *Pain Level*

INTERVENTIONS	RATIONALES
Assess severity of pain, generalized abdominal pain descending to lower right quadrant and localized at McBurney's point with rebound tenderness, reduced bowel sounds; behaviors indicating pain with psoas and/or obturator signs positive. Ask child to rate the pain using an appropriate scale for the child's age and development.	Provides information symptomatic of appendicitis with pain being the most common presenting complaint; behaviors manifested by pain vary with age with infant responding with crying, facial expression of pain and physical resistance; young children responding with crying loudly, clinging, irritability, uncooperation, rigid position, side-lying position with knees flexed up to abdomen, refusal to move.
Assess for severity of postoperative pain (specify when).	Provides information needed to administer most effective analgesic therapy.
Assess for acuteness of abdominal pain that progresses to abdominal rigidity, abdominal distention, tachycardia, shallow respirations, fever, pallor.	Indicates rupture of appendix and peritonitis.
Administer narcotic or non-narcotic analgesic preoperatively or postoperatively as ordered (specify drug, dose, route, and times).	Promotes relief of pain depending on severity, age and general condition (action of drug).
Avoid palpation of abdomen and unnecessary movements and care procedures of child.	Prevents increased pain and possible rupture of appendix.
Apply ice packs to abdomen.	Provides relief of pain.
Place in position of comfort; right side-lying or low to semi-Fowler's.	Promotes comfort to reduce pain; postoperatively will facilitate drainage if appendix has ruptured and prevent spread of infection.
Provide toys, games for quiet play.	Promotes diversionary activity to detract from pain.
Inform child that palpation will cause some pain and inform of any other procedures that cause pain.	Warns child of discomfort to expect and promotes trust of caretaker.

INTERVENTIONS	RATIONALES
Explain cause of pain to parents and child and measures that are taken to relieve pain.	Promotes understanding of condition and reasons for treatments and medication.
Inform parents of behavioral responses to pain that child is manifesting and that as pain subsides, child will return to usual behavior patterns.	Promotes understanding of behavior changes common to an age group in presence of pain.

NIC: *Pain Management*

Evaluation

(Date/time of evaluation of goal)

(Has goal been met? Not met? Partially met?)

(What is pain rating?)

(Revisions to care plan? D/C care plan? Continue care plan?)

RISK FOR INFECTION

Related to: Inadequate primary defenses (e.g., ruptured appendix), invasive procedure (surgery).

Defining Characteristics: (Specify: spread of infection in peritoneal cavity, absent bowel sounds, diffuse abdominal pain followed by an absence of pain, abdominal distention, vomiting, increased pulse and respirations, fever, redness, swelling, drainage at incision site whether closed by primary intension (appendectomy) or open and draining (ruptured appendix).

Goal: Client will not experience infection by (date and time to evaluate).

Outcome Criteria

✔ Incision will be clean and dry, without redness, edema, or odor.

NOC: *Risk Control*

INTERVENTIONS	RATIONALES
Assess closed incision site for redness, swelling pain, drainage, approximation of edges, healing (specify when).	Provides information indicating incision infection.

INTERVENTIONS	RATIONALES
(Assess open incision site for drainage and characteristics, drain placement and patency, need for dressing change, specify when.)	(Provides information about effectiveness of wound drainage to prevent abscess formation and spread of peritonitis.)
Administer antibiotic therapy IV as ordered (specify).	Destroys infectious agent with selection of medications based on culture and sensitivities of wound drainage.
Position in side-lying or semi-Fowler's.	Facilitates drainage through wound drain and prevents spread of infection upward in abdomen.
Redress incision wound using sterile technique as ordered.	Promotes cleanliness of wound and prevents introduction of pathogens.
(Change dressings on open wound or reinforce as needed, use Montgomery straps to hold dressings in place.)	(Maintains clean, dry dressings and allows for frequent changes without removing tape.)
(Apply warm, wet pack to open incision as ordered; specify.)	(Promotes circulation to the area and reduces inflammation.)
(Irrigate open wound with antibiotic solution as ordered; specify.)	(Cleanses wound and destroys pathogens.)
Initiate wound isolation precautions.	Prevents transmission of infectious agents to or from the child.
Inform parents and child of reason for infection and risk of spread of infection.	Promotes understanding and cooperation in treatments to prevent spread of existing infection or risk of infection of appendectomy incision.
Teach parents about incision care, dressing changes, removal of drainage, healing process.	Promotes understanding of wound healing and progression to infection resolution.
Teach parents and child that isolation is needed to prevent spread of infection and length of time isolation is carried out.	Promotes understanding of isolation techniques.

NIC: *Incision Site Care*

Evaluation

(Date/time of evaluation of goal)

(Has goal been met? Not met? Partially met?)

(Describe incision for: redness, edema, odor. Is incision clean and dry?)

(Revisions to care plan? D/C care plan? Continue care plan?)

ANXIETY

Related to: Change in health status of child, hospitalization of child, possible surgery of child (specify).

Defining Characteristics: (Specify: increased apprehension that condition might worsen and appendix rupture, expressed concern and worry about impending surgery, need for IV, NPO and NG tube and other treatments and procedures while hospitalized, lack of information about postoperative care.)

Goal: Clients will experience less anxiety by (date and time to evaluate).

Outcome Criteria

✔ Clients report decreased anxiety (specify, e.g., no anxiety or mild anxiety only).

NOC: *Anxiety Control*

INTERVENTIONS	RATIONALES
Assess source and level of anxiety and how anxiety is manifested; need for information that will relieve anxiety. Ask parents and child to rank their feelings of anxiety as none, mild, moderate, severe, or feelings of panic.	Provides information about anxiety level and need for interventions to relieve it; sources for the parents include fear and uncertainty about treatment and recovery, guilt for presence of illness; sources for child include separation from parents, procedures, fear of mutilation or death, unfamiliar environment; anxiety in the child may be manifested by crying, inability to play or sleep or eat, clinging aggression.
Encourage expression of concerns and questions about condition, procedures, recovery surgery by parents and child.	Provides opportunity to vent feelings and fears and secure information to reduce anxiety.
Communicate with parents and answer questions calmly and honestly; use pictures, drawings, and models for explanations to child (specify).	Promotes calm and supportive trusting environment (development level).

(continues)

(continued)

INTERVENTIONS	RATIONALES
Allow parents to stay with child and encourage to assist in care or open visitation.	Allows parents to care for and support child and continue parental role.
Give parents and child as much input in decisions about care and routines as possible.	Allows for more control over situation.
Teach parents and child about disease process, physical effects and symptoms of illness.	Provides information to relieve anxiety by knowledge of what to expect.
Explain reason for each pre and postoperative procedure or type of therapy, diagnostic tests, surgical procedure and rationales including IV, NG tube and dressings to parents and child as appropriate for age (specify).	Reduces fear which decreases anxiety.
Demonstrate and teach about wound care and dressing changes; allow for return demonstration; inform to protect dressing from diaper.	Ensures wound healing without complication of infection or recurrence of infection.

INTERVENTIONS	RATIONALES
Inform parents and child of activity restrictions and length of time before returning to school.	Ensures wound healing without complication of infection or recurrence of infection.
Teach to report changes in wound indicating infection (redness, swelling, pain, drainage).	Allows for immediate treatment in presence of infectious process.
Teach parents about dietary progression following removal of NG tube (specify).	Promotes return to nutritional baseline and bowel elimination.

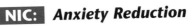 **NIC:** *Anxiety Reduction*

Evaluation

(Date/time of evaluation of goal)

(Has goal been met? Not met? Partially met?)

(How does client rank feelings of anxiety?)

(Revisions to care plan? D/C care plan? Continue care plan?)

APPENDICITIS

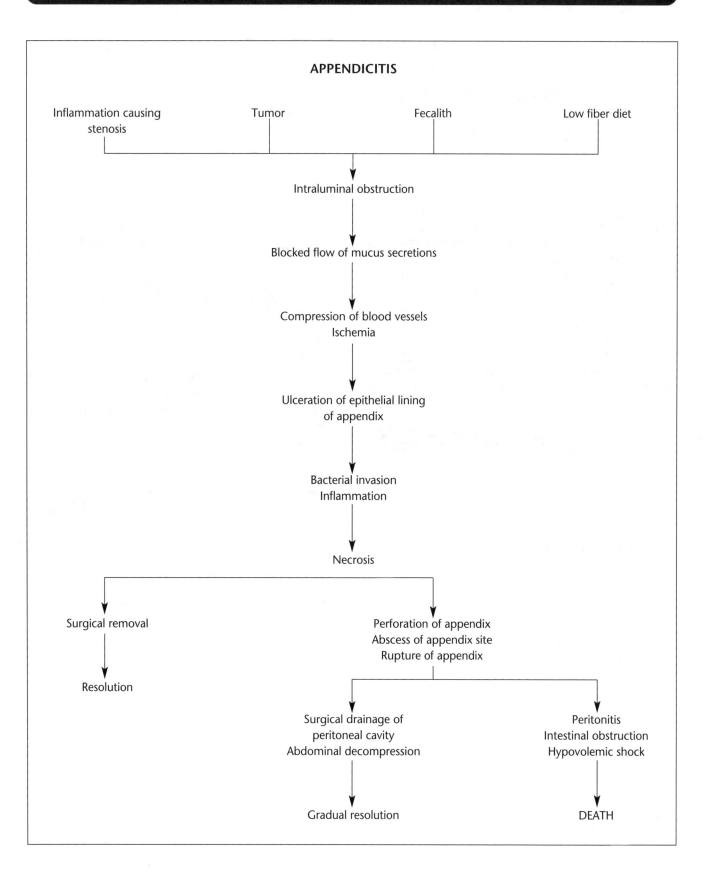

CHAPTER 4.2

CLEFT LIP/PALATE

Cleft lip and/or palate is a defect caused by failure of the soft and bony tissue to fuse in utero. They may occur singly or together and often occur with other congenital anomalies such as spina bifida, hydrocephalus, or cardiac defects. Treatment consists of surgical repair, usually of the lip first between 6 and 10 weeks of age, followed by the palate between 12 and 18 months of age. The surgical procedures are dependent on condition of the child and physician preference. Management involves a multidisciplinary approach that includes the surgeon, pediatrician, nurse, orthodontist, propthodontist, otolaryingologist, and speech therapist.

MEDICAL CARE

Surgical Repair: Cleft lip: Z-plasty between 6 to 10 weeks with Logan bow taped to cheeks to protect incision. Cleft palate: repair between 12 to 18 months of age.

Analgesics (narcotic analgesics): codeine or morphine sulfate postoperatively to control pain.

Analgesics (non-narcotic analgesics): acetaminophen given postoperatively to control moderate pain.

Complete Blood Count (CBC): done as a routine preoperative examination.

Urinalysis: done as a routine preoperative examination.

Follow-up: speech therapy, orthodontia, prosthodontia.

COMMON NURSING DIAGNOSES

See IMBALANCED NUTRITION: LESS THAN BODY REQUIREMENTS

Related to: Inability to ingest food.

Defining Characteristics: (Specify: presence of cleft lip/palate, sore, inflamed buccal cavity, inability to suck, weakness of sucking and swallowing muscles.)

See INEFFECTIVE AIRWAY CLEARANCE

Related to: Tracheobronchial aspiration of feedings, trauma of surgery.

Defining Characteristics: (Specify, e.g., abnormal breath sounds, dyspnea, tachypnea, cyanosis, changes in rate or depth of respirations, cough with or without sputum, postoperative edema.)

ADDITIONAL NURSING DIAGNOSES

ANXIETY

Related to: Situational crisis of congenital defect of infant.

Defining Characteristics: (Specify: severe reaction to appearance of infant with a facial defect, responses to imperfect infant [shock, denial and grief], expression of guilt, blame and helplessness, feelings of inadequacy and uncertainty, worried and anxious about impending surgery.)

Goal: Clients will experience decreased anxiety by (date and time to evaluate).

Outcome Criteria

✔ Clients report decreased anxiety (specify, e.g., no anxiety or mild anxiety only).

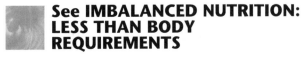 **NOC:** *Anxiety Control*

INTERVENTIONS	RATIONALES
Assess level of anxiety and need for information that will relieve anxiety. Ask parents to rank their feelings of anxiety as none, mild, moderate, severe, or feelings of panic.	Provides information to allay anxiety manifested by the infant's appearance at birth with level increased with the location and extent of the defect (lip and/or palate defect).
Encourage expression of concerns and questions about condition, to discuss feelings about appearance of infant.	Provides an environment conducive to venting of feelings to facilitate adjustment to the infant's defect.
Provide an accepting environment and attitude and handle the infant in a gentle, caring way.	Promotes trust and conveys to parents that infant is a valuable human baby deserving of love and caring.
Communicate with parents in a calm, honest, way, discuss the surgical procedures for correction of the defects using pictures and models, and allow to view pictures of children with successful defect repair.	Promotes a calm and supportive environment to reduce anxiety and instill hope.
Allow parents to stay with infant and encourage to assist in care as appropriate.	Reduces anxiety and promotes bonding that may be blocked by infant's appearance.
Emphasize the infant's positive features when providing information.	Promotes positive feelings for infant.
Suggest visits with parents who have a child with a similar defect.	Provides support and information to reduce anxiety.
Inform parents of usual ages for cleft lip repair and/or cleft palate, stages of surgery and type of procedure performed.	Provides information to reduce fear and anxiety and to know what to expect.

NIC: *Anxiety Reduction*

Evaluation

(Date/time of evaluation of goal)

(Has goal been met? Not met? Partially met?)

(How do parents rank feelings of anxiety?)

(Revisions to care plan? D/C care plan? Continue care plan?)

DEFICIENT KNOWLEDGE

Related to: Lack of information about preoperative care.

Defining Characteristics: (Specify: request for information about cause of defects, feeding techniques, prevention of complications caused by defects preoperatively.)

Goal: Clients will obtain knowledge about preoperative care by (date and time to evaluate).

Outcome Criteria

✔ Clients verbalize understanding of preoperative care and demonstrate proper feeding techniques for their infant (specify).

NOC: *Knowledge: Infant Care*

INTERVENTIONS	RATIONALES
Assess parents' ability to feed infant with a defect and acceptance of methods used, knowledge, cause and type of defects, preoperative needs and care, ability of infant to swallow (specify).	Provides information about defect that may be inherited or congenital, partial or complete, unilateral or bilateral cleft of lip and/or palate; adequate nutritional status and freedom from infection before surgery done.
Teach and observe parents to hold infant while feeding with the head in an upright position, use a nipple or feeding device, allow feeder to control the flow or the infant to express the formula, apply gentle, steady pressure on the bottom of the bottle and avoid removing the nipple frequently; instruct in feeding method that will be used postoperatively (specify).	Holding head upright reduces possibility of aspiration, pressure at the base of the bottle prevents choking or coughing, special nipples or devices are used because the cleft interferes with the ability to suck and liquid often flows into the nose when taken into the mouth, use of a nipple encourages development of sucking muscles.
Teach and observe to feed slowly and in small amounts, burping frequently (tends to swallow air), and extend nipple or feeding device well back into the mouth.	Prevents choking, abdominal distention, possible flow of liquid into nose or aspirated into lungs causing pneumonia or otitis media or upper respiratory infections.
Inform parents that feeding should not last any longer than 20 to 30 minutes.	Prolonged feedings may deplete an infant's energy and cause fatigue.
(Instruct in use and care of preoperative orthodontic device [plastic palate mold] for infant with cleft palate including removing and cleaning daily, replacing, preventing infant from removing palate.)	Promotes the alignment of maxilla and more normal speech sounds and prevents food from entering nasal cavity.

(continues)

(continued)

INTERVENTIONS	RATIONALES
Instruct parents to cleanse lip, oral cavity and nose with water before and after feeding.	Prevents infection or skin breakdown with cleft lip or palate.
Teach parents to avoid prone position and place child on back or side (use arm restraints, use cup for feeding if palate repair to be done, feed upright if lip repair is to be done for the period preoperatively).	Prepares the child to treatments that will be done postoperatively.
Inform parents of procedure for correction of defect(s), medications and procedures done to prepare infant for surgery, what to expect postoperatively.	Prepares parents for surgical correction of defect(s) and what to expect during convalescence.

NIC: *Teaching: Infant Care*

Evaluation

(Date/time of evaluation of goal)

(Has goal been met? Not met? Partially met?)

(Did clients verbalize understanding of preoperative care? Use quotes. Describe how parents feed their infant.)

(Revisions to care plan? D/C care plan? Continue care plan?)

RISK FOR INJURY

Related to: Surgery (broken skin).

Defining Characteristics: (Specify: trauma to suture line, use of protective device, formula or drainage at suture site, improper mouth care and teeth brushing, hands or other objects in mouth, redness, swelling and drainage from incision site, crying caused by pain of incision, improper feeding method.)

Goal: Infant will not experience injury to incision by (date and time to evaluate).

Outcome Criteria

✔ Suture line free of trauma, accumulation of substances, infection.

✔ Sutures intact and healing with protective device in place.

NOC: *Risk Control*

INTERVENTIONS	RATIONALES
Assess suture line for cleanliness, redness, swelling or drainage (frequency).	Provides information indicating possible infection and need for cleansing away formula or drainage.
Assess for respiratory distress following palate surgery (specify frequency).	Monitors breathing through a smaller airway caused by edema and breathing through nose.
Cleanse suture site of lip repair with gauze or cotton tipped applicator with saline, apply ointment after cleansing as prescribed (specify); rinse mouth with water before and after each feeding.	Removes material to prevent inflammation or sloughing and final cosmetic result expected.
Provide air humidification or place in mist tent for a short time following surgery, as ordered.	Decreases dry mouth and nose mucous membranes.
Monitor lip protective device taped on operative site.	Relaxes the site and prevents tension on sutures caused by facial movement or crying.
Provide ordered analgesics (specify) for pain, hold, cuddle or rock child, anticipate needs to prevent crying.	Promotes comfort and prevents crying caused by pain which creates tension on suture line.
Apply soft elbow restraints and remove periodically to perform ROM on arms and allow for some movement and holding; a child may need a jacket restraint to prevent rolling over.	Prevents child from touching or injuring operative site.
Remove sharp objects or toys, avoid use of forks, straws or other pointed objects.	Prevents trauma to mouth and suture line.
Feed with a cup or spoon if palate repair done; avoid placing spoon in mouth.	Prevents damage to suture line.
Accompany child when playing or ambulating.	Prevents trauma caused by accidental falls.
Teach parents about cleansing suture site and to apply antibiotic ointment.	Prevents infection and enhances comfort and healing.
Teach parents in feeding method of infant and allow to practice appropriate technique using a syringe soft tube in mouth away from any suture line or using a cup for older child (specify).	Promotes nutrition following surgery without sucking on a nipple.

INTERVENTIONS	RATIONALES
Instruct parents in soft diet inclusions and avoidance of toast, hard cookies or foods, as ordered.	Provides nutritional needs until incision heals completely.
Explain to parents and child to keep hands and objects away from mouth or to maintain use of restraints with removal until incision is healed.	Prevents trauma to suture line.
Advise parents not to allow child to play with small toys or those that are sharp or require sucking or blowing; suggest soft, stuffed toys for infant.	Removes possibility of placing toy in mouth or damage incision.
Explain to parents that usual feeding patterns may be resumed in 2 weeks for lip repair or in 4 to 6 weeks for palate repair.	Provides estimated times based on suture removal and healing to resume regular bottle feeding or return to baseline dietary status.

NIC: *Wound Care*

Evaluation

(Date/time of evaluation of goal)

(Has goal been met? Not met? Partially met?)

(Describe suture line)

(Revisions to care plan? D/C care plan? Continue care plan?)

COMPROMISED FAMILY COPING

Related to: Inadequate information and temporary family disorganization caused by defect(s) and future correction.

Defining Characteristics: (Specify: expression of concern about defect(s), long-term care required for successful outcome, confirmation of worry about normal growth and development, limited family support and assistance.)

Goal: Family will increase coping ability by (date and time to evaluate).

Outcome Criteria

✔ Family will identify short term and long-term goals (specify number).

✔ Family members will work together to identify 3 coping mechanisms.

NOC: *Family Coping*

INTERVENTIONS	RATIONALES
Assess family coping methods used and their effectiveness; family ability to cope with child that needs long-term care and guidance; stress on family relationships; developmental level of family; perception of crisis situation by family, response of siblings.	Provides information identifying coping methods that work and need to develop new coping skills, family attitudes directly affect child's feeling of self-worth, child with special needs may strengthen or strain family relationships.
Encourage family members to express problem areas and explore solutions together.	Reduces anxiety and enhances understanding; provides opportunity to identify problems and problem solving strategies.
Assist family members to identify 3 healthy coping mechanisms they can use.	Empowers the family to find solutions appropriate for them.
Assist family to establish short- and long-term goals for child and importance of integrating child into family activities.	Promotes involvement and control over situations and maintains parental role.
Encourage to follow home routines and meet child's needs with participation of family members.	Increases child's sense of security and sense of belonging.
Give positive feedback to family and praise family efforts in development of coping and problem solving techniques in caring for child.	Encourages family to continue involvement in long-term care.
Teach family that overprotective behavior may hinder growth and development and to treat the child as normally as it is possible.	Enhances family understanding of importance of making child one of the family and adverse effects of overprotection of child.
Discuss the long-term treatment of speech therapy, hearing impairment preventions, dental corrections for crossbite or malocclusion or other therapies.	Promotes a positive outcome when family collaborates with the health team.
Inform parents to observe for hearing deficits and to schedule hearing tests as prescribed.	Provides preventive therapy for permanent changes in ear caused by frequent otitis media.
Teach parents to stimulate speech after sutures removed by playing games, encourage use of words beginning with F, P, S, T, and encourage chewing and swallowing of foods.	Promotes speech development.

(continues)

(continued)

INTERVENTIONS	RATIONALES
Refer family to community agencies, March of Dimes, American Cleft Palate Association (specify).	Provides information and support services for families of children with cleft defect.

NIC: *Coping Enhancement*

Evaluation

(Date/time of evaluation of goal)

(Has goal been met? Not met? Partially met?)

(What goals did family identify? What coping mechanisms?)

(Revisions to care plan? D/C care plan? Continue care plan?)

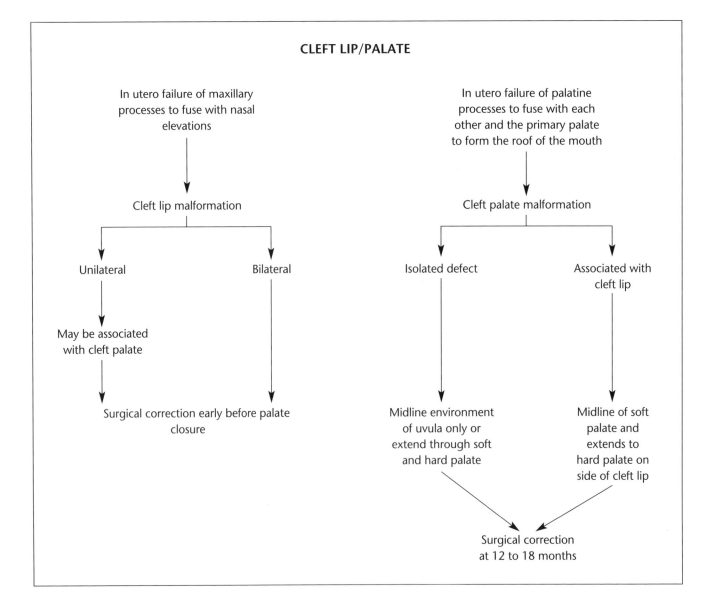

CLEFT LIP/PALATE

In utero failure of maxillary processes to fuse with nasal elevations

↓

Cleft lip malformation

Unilateral   Bilateral

Unilateral → May be associated with cleft palate → Surgical correction early before palate closure

Bilateral → Surgical correction early before palate closure

In utero failure of palatine processes to fuse with each other and the primary palate to form the roof of the mouth

↓

Cleft palate malformation

Isolated defect   Associated with cleft lip

Isolated defect → Midline environment of uvula only or extend through soft and hard palate

Associated with cleft lip → Midline of soft palate and extends to hard palate on side of cleft lip

→ Surgical correction at 12 to 18 months

CHAPTER 4.3

GASTROENTERITIS

Gastroenteritis is an acute infectious process affecting the gastrointestinal tract caused by bacteria or viruses. Younger children are most commonly affected with specific organisms found in different age groups. At highest risk are those in daycare centers and schools, and those with immune system abnormalities. The disease is transmitted by ingestion of contaminated food, water, or by contaminated hands, linens, equipment, and supplies. Its most serious complication is dehydration and electrolyte losses which may lead to metabolic acidosis and death.

MEDICAL CARE

Antibiotics: selection depends on identification and sensitivity to organism revealed by culture, whether therapy is prophylactic and term of treatment with use of doxycycline (Vibramycin) in children over 8 years of age.

Stool Examination: reveals toxins, culture reveals ova and parasites, specific pathogen for treatment mode.

Electrolyte Panel: reveals decreases in electrolyte levels (K) in persistent diarrhea.

Complete Blood Count: reveals decreased RBC, Act, Hgb with blood loss in persistent diarrhea, and inflammation of bowel mucosa; increased WBC in severe infectious process of tract.

COMMON NURSING DIAGNOSES

 ### See RISK FOR DEFICIENT FLUID VOLUME

Related to: Excessive losses through normal routes, NPO status.

Defining Characteristics: (Specify: vomiting, diarrhea, decreased skin turgor, dry skin and mucous membranes, weakness, fever, decreased urinary output, decreased pulse volume, increased pulse rate.)

 ### See RISK FOR IMPAIRED SKIN INTEGRITY

Related to: External factor of excretions and secretions.

Defining Characteristics: (Specify: redness, excoriation at anal site and perineum, presence of persistent diarrhea.)

 ### See IMBALANCED NUTRITION: LESS THAN BODY REQUIREMENTS

Related to: Inability to ingest and digest foods.

Defining Characteristics: (Specify: NPO status, nausea, vomiting, diarrhea, weight loss, anorexia, abdominal cramps.)

See HYPERTHERMIA

Related to: Illness (infectious process).

Defining Characteristics: (Specify: increase in body temperature above normal range, warm to touch, increased pulse and respirations.)

See DIARRHEA

Related to: (Specify: dietary intake, contaminants, toxins, inflammation and irritation of bowel.)

Defining Characteristics: (Specify: abdominal pain, cramping, increased frequency of bowel sounds, increased frequency, loose, liquid stools, changes in color, urgency.)

ADDITIONAL NURSING DIAGNOSES

DEFICIENT KNOWLEDGE

Related to: Lack of information about disease and treatment.

Defining Characteristics: (Specify: request for information about effect and treatment of the disease and preventions of transmission of disease.)

Goal: Clients will obtain information about gastroenteritis by (date and time to evaluate).

Outcome Criteria

✔ Parents verbalize understanding of the cause and treatment (specify).

✔ Clients demonstrate proper handwashing techniques.

NOC: *Knowledge: Treatment Regimen*

INTERVENTIONS	RATIONALES
Assess knowledge of causes of types of enteritis, methods to treat and control disease.	Promotes effective plan of instruction that is realistic, prevents repetition of information.
Provide parents and child with information and clear explanations in understandable language, include teaching aids and encourage questions.	Ensures understanding based on interest and need to know to promote compliance.
Instruct to offer rehydration fluids (Pedialyte) and avoid those fluids high in Na$^+$ (milk, broth). Encourage to reintroduce normal diet of easily-digested foods as child tolerates.	Provides and replaces fluids and electrolytes lost in frequent diarrheal stools, Na$^+$ increases removal of fluid from cells by osmosis.
Instruct in collection of stool specimens for culture: collect stool specimens from other family members and inform to take to laboratory for examination (specify).	Reveals identification of specific organism responsible for enteritis as a basis for treatment; reveals occult blood in stool in severe inflammation of bowel.

INTERVENTIONS	RATIONALES
Teach about enteric precautions and effective handwashing.	Prevents transmission of organisms.
Inform to take temperature by axillary method.	Prevents additional irritation to rectum.
Instruct to avoid over-the-counter drugs to treat diarrhea or vomiting.	Prevents use of medications that may exacerbate condition.
Demonstrate and instruct to insert antiemetic or sedative suppository (specify).	Treats vomiting and additional fluid loss and promotes rest.
Instruct to measure I&O and determine imbalance to report (specify).	Prevents possible fluid imbalance complication which leads to dehydration.
Instruct in antibiotic or other medication administration (specify).	(Action of drug.)

NIC: *Teaching: Disease Process*

Evaluation

(Date/time of evaluation of goal)

(Has goal been met? Not met? Partially met?)

(What did parents verbalize about the cause and treatment of the illness? Did clients demonstrate proper handwashing techniques?)

(Revisions to care plan? D/C care plan? Continue care plan?)

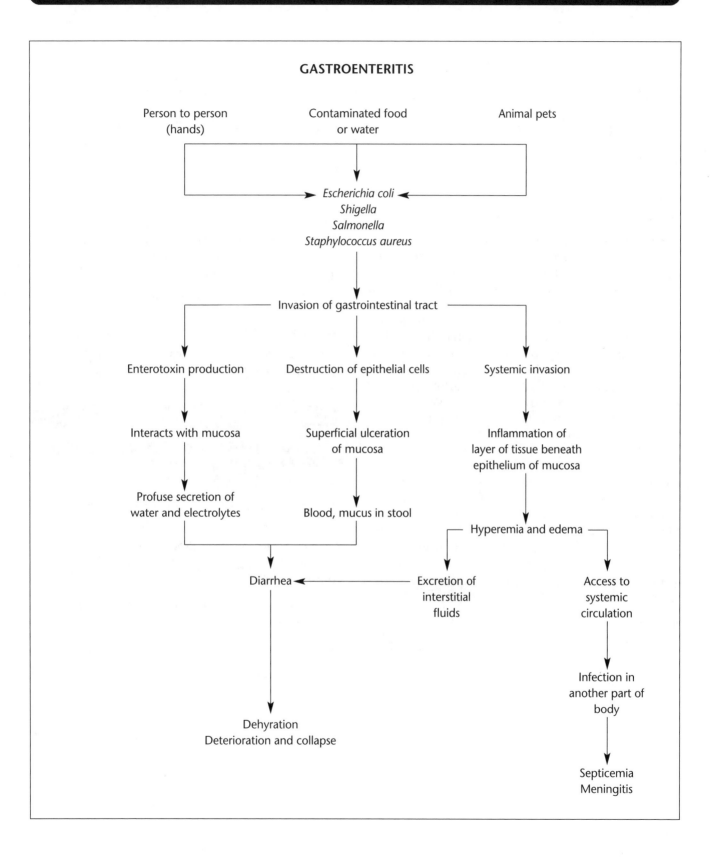

GASTROENTERITIS

Person to person
(hands)

Contaminated food
or water

Animal pets

Escherichia coli
Shigella
Salmonella
Staphylococcus aureus

Invasion of gastrointestinal tract

Enterotoxin production

Destruction of epithelial cells

Systemic invasion

Interacts with mucosa

Superficial ulceration
of mucosa

Inflammation of
layer of tissue beneath
epithelium of mucosa

Profuse secretion of
water and electrolytes

Blood, mucus in stool

Hyperemia and edema

Diarrhea

Excretion of
interstitial
fluids

Access to
systemic
circulation

Dehyration
Deterioration and collapse

Infection in
another part of
body

Septicemia
Meningitis

CHAPTER 4.4

GASTROESOPHAGEAL REFLUX DISEASE (GERD)

Gastroesophageal reflux (chalasia, cardiochalasia) is the return of gastric contents into the esophagus and possibly the pharynx. It is caused by dysfunction of the cardiac sphincter at the esophagus-stomach juncture. Reasons for this incompetence include an increase of pressure on the lower esophageal sphincter; following esophageal surgery; or immature lower esophageal neuromuscular function. The result of the persistent reflux is inflammation, esophagitis, and bleeding causing possible anemia and damage to the structure of the esophagus as scarring occurs. It also may predispose to aspiration of stomach contents causing aspiration pneumonia and chronic pulmonary conditions. Most commonly affected are infants and young children. As the condition becomes more severe or does not respond to medical treatment and the child experiences failure to thrive, surgical fundoplication to create a valve mechanism or other procedures may be done to correct the condition.

MEDICAL CARE

Proton Pump Inhibitors: lansoprazole (Previcid) or omeprazole (Prilosec) to suppress gastric acid secretion.

H₂ Receptor Antagonists: cimetidine (Tagamet), or ranitidine (Zantac) to reduce gastric acidity and pepsin secretion.

Barium Esophagram: reveals reflux of barium into the esophagus under fluoroscopy if done at time reflux occurs.

Manometry: reveals esophageal sphincter pressure of less than 6 mm Hg.

Intraesophageal pH Monitoring: reveals pH measurements of the distal esophagus reflux contents.

Gastroesophageal Scintigraphy: reveals reflux or aspiration following ingestion of a radioactive compound and scanning the esophagus.

Gastroscopy: endoscopic examination that reveals view of esophagus to note esophagitis or to remove tissue for biopsy.

Complete Blood Count: reveals decreased RBC, Hgb, Hct in persistent blood loss.

COMMON NURSING DIAGNOSES

See IMBALANCED NUTRITION: LESS THAN BODY REQUIREMENTS

Related to: Inability to ingest or digest food because of biologic factors.

Defining Characteristics: (Specify: weight loss, vomiting, increased appetite, heartburn (older child), failure to thrive, gastric bloating.)

See RISK FOR DEFICIENT FLUID VOLUME

Related to: Excessive losses through normal route.

Defining Characteristics: (Specify: vomiting, diarrhea (postoperatively), decreased urine output, dehydration.)

See INEFFECTIVE AIRWAY CLEARANCE

Related to: Tracheobronchial aspiration and infection.

Defining Characteristics: (Specify: abnormal breath sounds, dyspnea, changes in rate or depth of respirations, fever, cough that is effective or ineffective and with or without sputum.)

ADDITIONAL NURSING DIAGNOSES

RISK FOR ASPIRATION

Related to: Increased intragastric pressure with an incompetent cardiac sphincter.

Defining Characteristics: (Specify: laryngospasm, choking, coughing, apnea, cyanosis, wheezing, pneumonitis.)

Goal: Client will not aspirate by (date and time to evaluate).

Outcome Criteria

✔ Absence of aspiration with breathing pattern maintained at baseline parameters (specify).

✔ Absence of recurrent pulmonary infection.

NOC: *Risk Control*

INTERVENTIONS	RATIONALES
Assess respiratory status for rate, depth and ease, breath sounds before and after feedings.	Provides information about respiratory pattern changes caused by aspiration.
Assess vomiting, activity, and position before and after feeding.	Predisposes to aspiration of contents of reflux which is precipitated by factors associated with feeding.
Place in prone position (flat prone or with head elevated 30 degrees) or in an infant seat.	Maintains prone position to prevent reflux and risk of reflux.
Offer frequent, small feedings (of thickened formula, if ordered).	Prevents reflux and minimizes symptoms.
Administer medications ordered (specify).	(Action of drug.)
Maintain suction and O$_2$ equipment at hand.	Removes aspirate and promotes airway patency and tissue oxygenation.
Inform parents of risk for aspiration and consequences of recurring aspiration associated with the condition.	Provides information about potential for complications.
Instruct parents in feeding modifications, positions before and after feedings. Reassure parents that it is best for their child to sleep prone, not on the back like others.	Minimizes risk for reflux and aspiration.
Reassure parents that most children outgrow GERD. Praise parents' efforts to prevent complications.	Reassurance and praise provide positive reinforcement to parents.

NIC: *Airway Management*

Evaluation

(Date/time of evaluation of goal)

(Has goal been met? Not met? Partially met?)

(Describe breathing pattern. Has child experienced any respiratory infection?)

(Revisions to care plan? D/C care plan? Continue care plan?)

RISK FOR INJURY

Related to: (Specify: malnutrition, abnormal blood profile.)

Defining Characteristics: (Specify: decreased Hgb with esophageal bleeding leading to anemia, severe reflux disorder leading to failure to thrive.)

Goal: Client will not experience injury by (date and time to evaluate).

Outcome Criteria

✔ No esophageal bleeding (negative Guaiac tests) is found.

✔ Child exhibits appropriate growth (specify).

NOC: *Risk Detection*

INTERVENTIONS	RATIONALES
Assess for severity of reflux, weight loss or gain, failure to thrive, stool and vomit for occult blood (specify when).	Provides information about complication of esophagitis or esophageal structure, anemia or failure to thrive.
Prepare parents and infant for diagnostic procedures and possible surgical procedure (specify).	Reveals severity of reflux and need for surgical interventions.
Inform parents that infant usually outgrows the disorder and achieves normal function by 6 weeks of age and those with a continuing problem of reflux usually improve by 6 months of age.	Provides reassurance to parents that medical regimen may be successful and complication may not occur.
Teach to perform Guaiac test on stool and vomitus and allow to return demonstration.	Reveals presence of occult blood in esophagitis.

(continues)

(continued)

INTERVENTIONS	RATIONALES
Inform that severe reflux may require NPO status and naso-gastric tube insertion with suction.	Prevents distention and continuing reflux activity of stomach contents.

NIC: *Bleeding Precautions*

Evaluation

(Date/time of evaluation of goal)

(Has goal been met? Not met? Partially met?)

(What are results of Guaiac testing? What is child's weight gain? Is that appropriate for age?)

(Revisions to care plan? D/C care plan? Continue care plan?)

ANXIETY

Related to: Change in health status of infant, possible surgery of infant.

Defining Characteristics: (Specify: increased apprehension that condition might worsen and that surgery be required, expressed concern and worry about impending surgery, pre and postoperative care, gastrostomy and treatments while hospitalized and complications following surgery.)

Goal: Clients will experience less anxiety by (date and time to evaluate).

Outcome Criteria

✔ Clients report a decrease in their anxiety level to none or mild.

NOC: *Anxiety Control*

INTERVENTIONS	RATIONALES
Assess source of level of anxiety and how anxiety is manifested: need for information that will relieve anxiety. Ask clients to rate anxiety from none, to mild, moderate, severe, or panic level.	Provides information about anxiety level and need for interventions to relieve it; sources for the parents include fear and uncertainty about treatment and recovery, guilt for presence of illness.
Encourage expression of concerns and to ask questions about condition, procedures, recovery surgery by parents.	Provides opportunity to vent feelings and fears and secure information to reduce anxiety.

INTERVENTIONS	RATIONALES
Communicate frequently with parents and answer questions calmly and honestly; use pictures, drawings, and models for explanations.	Promotes calm and supportive trusting environment.
Encourage parents to stay with child and to assist in care.	Allows parents to care for and support child and continue parental role.
Give parents as much input in decisions about care and routines as possible.	Allows for more control over situation.
Provide consistent care of infant with familiar staff assigned for care.	Promotes trust and reduces anxiety.
Inform parents of disease process, physical effects, and symptoms of illness.	Provides information to relieve anxiety by knowledge of what to expect.
Explain reason for each pre and postoperative procedure or type of therapy, diagnostic test, surgical procedure and rationales including IV, NG tube, dressings and gastrostomy tube (specify).	Reduces fear which decreases anxiety.
(Inform parents that NG tube is removed when postoperative ileus is resolved and gastrostomy tube is removed 2 or more weeks after surgery.)	Reduces anxiety that the tube placements and care evokes.
(Instruct in care of and feeding via gastrostomy tube and inform of complications of choking, delayed gastric emptying, inability to vomit, gas bloating that may occur following surgery; specify.)	Information of what to expect will reduce anxiety.
(Demonstrate and instruct in wound care and dressing changes; allow for return demonstration, inform to protect dressing from diaper.)	Ensures wound healing without complication of infection or recurrence of infection.
Instruct parents in feeding techniques, allowing infant to take a long time to feed and to report any feeding problems.	Familiarizes parents with changes in feeding patterns to prevent complications of choking, aspiration.
Instruct to report changes in wound indicating infection (redness, swelling, pain, drainage).	Allows for immediate treatment in presence of infectious procedure.

NIC: *Anxiety Reduction*
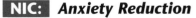

Evaluation

(Date/time of evaluation of goal)

(Has goal been met? Not met? Partially met?)

(How do parents rate their anxiety?)

(Revisions to care plan? D/C care plan? Continue care plan?)

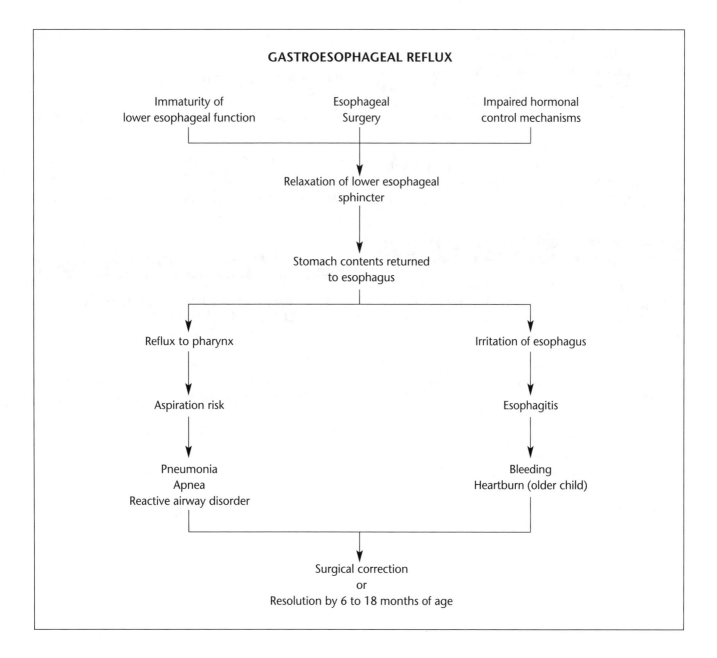

GASTROESOPHAGEAL REFLUX

Immaturity of lower esophageal function   Esophageal Surgery   Impaired hormonal control mechanisms

Relaxation of lower esophageal sphincter

Stomach contents returned to esophagus

Reflux to pharynx   Irritation of esophagus

Aspiration risk   Esophagitis

Pneumonia
Apnea
Reactive airway disorder   Bleeding
Heartburn (older child)

Surgical correction
or
Resolution by 6 to 18 months of age

CHAPTER 4.5

HEPATITIS

Hepatitis is the inflammation of the liver usually caused by a virus. Four viruses that may cause it are: hepatitis A (HAV), hepatitis B (HBV), hepatitis D (HDV) and hepatitis non-A, non-B (NANB). Most common of the types found in children is hepatitis A which is transmitted by the fecal-oral route. The incidence in children is increased in those living in crowded housing. The disorder is usually self-limiting with resolution within 2 to 3 months or may develop into chronic hepatitis. Symptomology varies with severity of the disease.

MEDICAL CARE

Immunizing Agents: immune globulin (Gamma globulin) given IM as prophylaxis to provide passive immunity or modify severity of hepatitis A; hepatitis B immune globulin (H-BIG) given IM as prophylaxis after exposure to hepatitis B or to provide passive immunity if exposed to contaminated materials (blood serum); hepatitis B vaccine given to newborns IM to immunize against hepatitis B.

Metabolic Enzymes: alanine aminotransferase (ALT), aspartate aminotransferase (AST), lactic dehydrogenase (LDH) reveal increases as liver damage occurs and cells release enzymes; alkaline phosphatase reveals increase in liver disease.

Immunoglobulins: reveal IgM antibodies indicating hepatitis A virus antibodies for diagnosis of hepatitis A, IgG indicates susceptibility or past exposure to hepatitis A. Hepatitis B surface antigen (HBsAg); titer that reveals antibodies or antigens that are produced in response to hepatitis B and indicates chronic hepatitis B if present longer than 6 months or improvement as the antigen is decreased or disappears.

Bilirubin: reveals increases in indirect bilirubin if liver damaged.

Ammonia: reveals increases in poorly functioning liver.

Protein: reveals increased globulins and decreased albunin.

Prothrombin Time: reveals increases in severe liver disease.

Urine Urobilinogen: reveals increases in liver disease whether the serum bilirubin level changes or not.

Stool: reveals changes in color if bile is not produced as a result of liver disease.

COMMON NURSING DIAGNOSES

See IMBALANCED NUTRITION: LESS THAN BODY REQUIREMENTS

Related to: Inability to ingest, digest food.

Defining Characteristics: (Specify: anorexia, nausea, vomiting, weight loss, fatigue, abdominal discomfort.)

See RISK FOR DEFICIENT FLUID VOLUME

Related to: Excessive losses through normal routes.

Defining Characteristics: (Specify: vomiting, diarrhea, reduced intake of fluids, reduced urinary output, signs and symptoms of dehydration, gastrointestinal bleeding.)

See RISK FOR IMPAIRED SKIN INTEGRITY

Related to: External factors of excretions and secretions, internal factor of altered pigmentation.

Defining Characteristics: (Specify: redness, irritation of perianal area with diarrhea, jaundice with pruritis.)

ADDITIONAL NURSING DIAGNOSES

RISK FOR ACTIVITY INTOLERANCE

Related to: Generalized weakness, bed rest.

Defining Characteristics: Easy fatigue, malaise, preference for inactivity, deconditioning with bed rest.

Goal: Client will tolerate appropriate levels of activity by (date and time to evaluate).

Outcome Criteria

✔ (Specify level of activity for client, e.g., quiet play in bed.)

NOC: *Energy Conservation*

INTERVENTIONS	RATIONALES
Assess intolerance to activity and manifestations.	Provides information about extent of fatigue.
Maintain bed rest while illness is in acute stage but allow for quiet play and progress as condition allows.	Allows for time for liver to heal and prevents any further damage.
Provide access to needed articles within reach, aids to assist in performing ADL.	Preserves energy which improves endurance.
Provide increasing activity participation as tolerated on a daily basis (specify).	Promotes recovery without compromising energy or causing fatigue.
Help parents devise a rest and activity schedule which can be adjusted to child's tolerance and allow child to regular activity at own pace (specify).	Provides information to improve activity tolerance without causing fatigue or remission or disease.
Inform parents and child of level of activity necessary to return to school.	Permits return to normal activity when possible.

NIC: *Activity Therapy*

Evaluation

(Date/time of evaluation of goal)
(Has goal been met? Not met? Partially met?)
(Describe client's activity)

(Revisions to care plan? D/C care plan? Continue care plan?)

DEFICIENT KNOWLEDGE

Related to: Lack of information about transmission of disease.

Defining Characteristics: (Specify: request for information about spread of disease, measures to take to prevent spread of disease and possible relapse of condition.)

Goal: Parents will obtain information about hepatitis by (date and time to evaluate).

Outcome Criteria

✔ Parents verbalize understanding of the cause and treatment of hepatitis.

NOC: *Knowledge: Disease Process*

INTERVENTIONS	RATIONALES
Assess knowledge of disease and isolation precautions to take to prevent transmission.	Promotes knowledge and understanding of disease.
Instruct parents and child in proper handwashing and teach to perform before meals, after using bathroom.	Prevents transmission of microorganisms for type A which is carried via the oral-fecal route.
Teach parents and child that toys may become contaminated and that they should not be shared.	Prevents transmission to others via handling of toys.
Instruct to use disposable gloves when handling blood, excrete any other body fluids.	Prevents transmission of microorganisms.
Instruct parents to use disposable dishes, wash linens in hot soapy water and rinse well and dry, separate child's personal hygiene articles from other members of household.	Prevents transmission of microorganisms to others.
Teach parents and child of signs and symptoms of disease, how disease is transmitted, dietary inclusions of protein and carbohydrate, activity program and signs, symptoms of disease recurrence (pain, anorexic fever, nausea and vomiting, jaundice) to report.	Provides information about disease and treatments to prevent transmission or relapse.

(continues)

(continued)

INTERVENTIONS	RATIONALES
Inform parents of immune globulins available (for hepatitis A if given before exposure or after exposure if during early incubation period, or hyper-immune gamma globulin for hepatitis B if given after exposure but reserved for those at risk).	Provides information about prophylactic measures available.
Teach parents and child to avoid over-the-counter drugs without physician advice to prevent toxicity if liver is unable to detoxify drugs.	Provides information.

NIC: *Teaching: Disease Process*

Evaluation

(Date/time of evaluation of goal)

(Has goal been met? Not met? Partially met?)

(What do parents verbalize about hepatitis?)

(Revisions to care plan? D/C care plan? Continue care plan?)

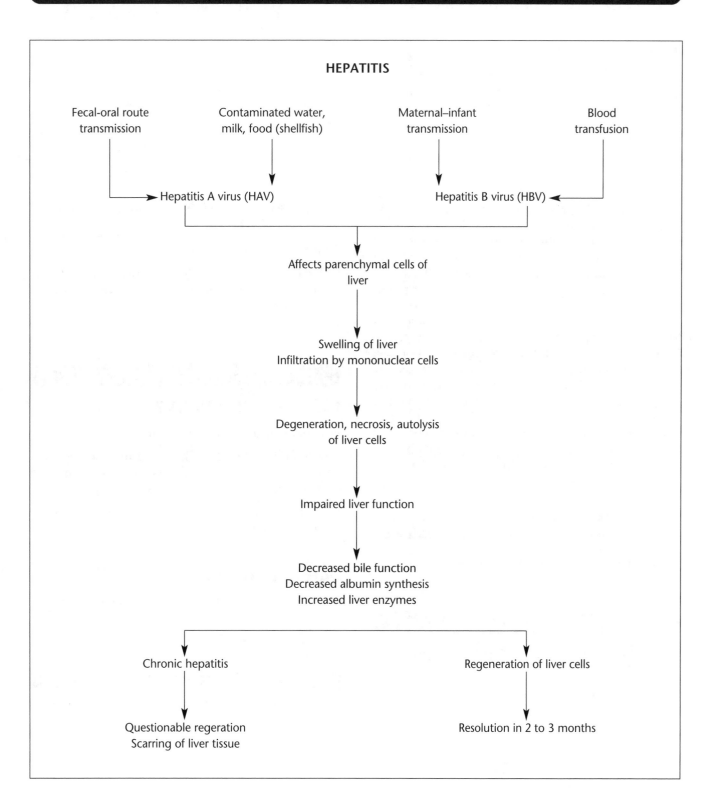

HEPATITIS

Fecal-oral route transmission

Contaminated water, milk, food (shellfish)

Maternal–infant transmission

Blood transfusion

Hepatitis A virus (HAV)

Hepatitis B virus (HBV)

Affects parenchymal cells of liver

Swelling of liver
Infiltration by mononuclear cells

Degeneration, necrosis, autolysis of liver cells

Impaired liver function

Decreased bile function
Decreased albumin synthesis
Increased liver enzymes

Chronic hepatitis

Regeneration of liver cells

Questionable regeration
Scarring of liver tissue

Resolution in 2 to 3 months

CHAPTER 4.6

HERNIA

A hernia results from a protrusion of abdominal contents through an opening in a weakened musculature. An umbilical hernia is the protrusion of intestine and omentum through the umbilical ring caused by a failure of complete closure after birth. Inguinal hernia is the protrusion of intestine through the inguinal ring caused by a failure of the processus vaginalis to atrophy to close before birth allowing for a hernial sac to form along the inguinal canal. Umbilical hernia usually resolves by 4 years of age; those that do not by school age are corrected by surgery. Inguinal hernia becomes apparent in the infant by 2 to 3 months of age when intra-abdominal pressure increases enough to open the sac. It is usually associated with a hydrocele. Both are corrected by surgical repair (herniorrhaphy) to prevent obstruction and eventual incarceration of a loop of bowel.

MEDICAL CARE

Surgical reduction and repair of defect.

COMMON NURSING DIAGNOSES

See INEFFECTIVE BREATHING PATTERN

Related to: Pain, decreased lung expansion.

Defining Characteristics: (Specify: dyspnea, tachypnea, respiratory depth changes, altered chest excursion.)

See RISK FOR DEFICIENT FLUID VOLUME

Related to: Postoperative status.

Defining Characteristics: (Specify: NPO status, altered intake, signs and symptoms of dehydration, I&O imbalance.)

See RISK FOR IMPAIRED SKIN INTEGRITY

Related to: Surgical incision.

Defining Characteristics: (Specify: disruption of skin surface, invasion of body structures, excreta in diaper contaminating the incision area.)

ADDITIONAL NURSING DIAGNOSES

RISK FOR INJURY

Related to: Intestinal obstruction.

Defining Characteristics: (Specify: irreducible loop of bowel, incarceration of the bowel with complete obstruction.)

Goal: Client will not experience injury by (date and time to evaluate).

Outcome Criteria

✔ Child appears comfortable, denies pain (specify).

NOC: *Risk Detection*

INTERVENTIONS	RATIONALES
Assess by palpation for umbilical or inguinal swelling that appears when infant cries or when child strains or coughs, and ability to reduce swelling with gentle compression if bowel forced into sac.	Reveals hernia that is reducible.
Assess tenderness at hernia site with abdominal distention, anorexia, irritability and defecation changes.	Indicates partial or complete obstruction caused by incarceration and strangulation.

INTERVENTIONS	RATIONALES
Instruct parents to report signs and symptoms to physician; inform of reason for disorder and what signs are expected and those that indicate obstruction.	Prevents more severe complication of eventual gangrene of bowel.
Teach parents of surgical procedure to repair hernia and possible hydrocele and course of progress to expect.	Corrects and repairs hernia and hydrocele if present before complication arises.
Encourage parents to prevent infant from crying as much as possible; hold and feed when hungry as preventive measures.	Prevents bowel from being forced into sac.
Teach about dietary inclusions and restrictions to prevent straining (specify).	Modification of diet to prevent constipation, decreased straining and increased intra-abdominal pressure that forces bowel into sac.
Reassure parents that hernia usually resolves itself and if not, surgery may be required to repair.	Provides information regarding prognosis of disorder.

NIC: *Teaching: Prescribed Activity*

Evaluation

(Date/time of evaluation of goal)

(Has goal been met? Not met? Partially met?)

(What did parents verbalize about caring for their child?)

(Revisions to care plan? D/C care plan? Continue care plan?)

PAIN

Related to: Surgical repair.

Defining Characteristics: (Specify: irritability in infant, crying, moaning, guarding behavior, verbal descriptor of pain, refusal to move, change in facial expression in child.)

Goal: Client will experience less pain by (date and time to evaluate).

Outcome Criteria

✔ Client rates pain less than (specify) on the (specify scale used for developmental level).

NOC: *Pain Level*

INTERVENTIONS	RATIONALES
Assess incision pain and associated symptoms.	Provides information about need for analgesic therapy.
Administer analgesic appropriate for severity of pain and age as ordered (specify drug, route, dose, and time).	Relieves pain and discomfort caused by incision. (Specify action of drug.)
Maintain position of comfort.	Promotes comfort and reduces pain caused by strain on incision.
Support buttocks when lifting or changing position.	Prevents strain and pull on incision site.
Apply ice bag to scrotal area if hydrocele corrected and apply scrotal support if applicable (specify).	Promotes comfort by decreasing edema.
Provide toys, games for quiet play (specify).	Promotes diversionary activity to detract from pain.
Teach parents to hold infant when feeding or when irritable, burp frequently to remove swallowed air.	Reduces strain on incision and promotes comfort.
Encourage parents to change diapers frequently.	Prevents irritation and pain at incision area caused by damp diapers.
Explain cause of pain to parents and child and measures taken to relieve it.	Promotes understanding of treatments for pain postoperatively.

NIC: *Pain Reduction*

Evaluation

(Date/time of evaluation of goal)

(Has goal been met? Not met? Partially met?)

(How does child rate pain (or use infant scale and report findings)?)

(Revisions to care plan? D/C care plan? Continue care plan?)

DEFICIENT KNOWLEDGE

Related to: Lack of knowledge about postoperative care.

Defining Characteristics: (Specify: request for information about activity allowed, wound care, diet, bathing and comfort measures.)

Goal: Parents will obtain knowledge about postoperative care by (date and time to evaluate).

Outcome Criteria

✔ Parents verbalize understanding of postoperative care for their child.

NOC: *Knowledge: Treatment Procedure*

INTERVENTIONS	RATIONALES
Assess knowledge of causes of hernia, surgical procedure performed, willingness and interest to implement treatment regimen.	Promotes effective plan of instruction to ensure compliance.
Provide parents and child as appropriate with information and clear explanations in understandable language, include teaching aids and encourage questions.	Ensures understanding based on learning ability and age.
Inform to maintain incision dressing until it peels off and to apply diaper so that it does not cover incision.	Maintains dry and clean incision site.
Teach to give sponge baths until incision heals.	Maintains incision integrity.
Encourage to hold infant when crying and to feed; activity is not usually restricted; advise child to refrain from lifting, pushing, or engaging in strenuous play or gym classes at school.	Reduces strain on incision and possible recurrence of hernia.

INTERVENTIONS	RATIONALES
Advise parents to increase diet and fluids as ordered (specify).	Promotes return to nutritional status without causing gastrointestinal strain on incision.
Reassure parents that infant usually tolerates surgery well and progresses to wellness without incident and that this condition is one of the most common surgeries in infancy.	Provides assurance and comfort to parents in giving care.

NIC: *Teaching*

Evaluation

(Date/time of evaluation of goal)

(Has goal been met? Not met? Partially met?)

(Does child appear comfortable? Does child deny abdominal discomfort?)

(Revisions to care plan? D/C care plan? Continue care plan?)

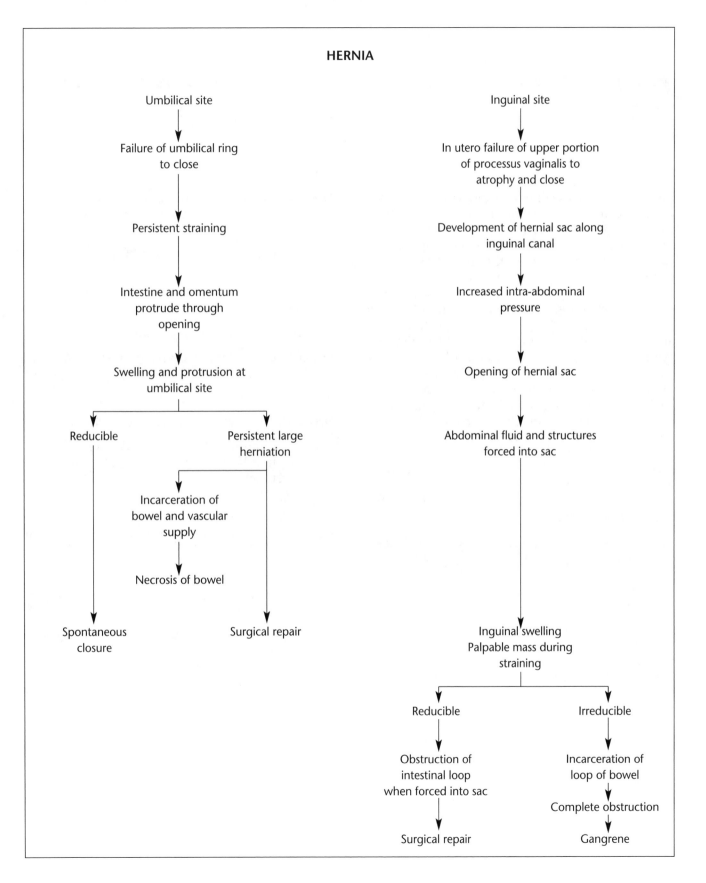

HERNIA

Umbilical site

Failure of umbilical ring
to close

Persistent straining

Intestine and omentum
protrude through
opening

Swelling and protrusion at
umbilical site

Reducible

Persistent large
herniation

Incarceration of
bowel and vascular
supply

Necrosis of bowel

Spontaneous
closure

Surgical repair

Inguinal site

In utero failure of upper portion
of processus vaginalis to
atrophy and close

Development of hernial sac along
inguinal canal

Increased intra-abdominal
pressure

Opening of hernial sac

Abdominal fluid and structures
forced into sac

Inguinal swelling
Palpable mass during
straining

Reducible

Irreducible

Obstruction of
intestinal loop
when forced into sac

Incarceration of
loop of bowel

Complete obstruction

Surgical repair

Gangrene

CHAPTER 4.7

INFLAMMATORY BOWEL DISEASE

Inflammatory bowel disease includes Crohn's disease and ulcerative colitis with similar signs and symptoms but with different intestinal pathology. Actual cause of either disease is unknown but they are associated with immunologic, nutritional, and infectious disturbances with psychogenic factors responsible for severity and exacerbation of the disease. Crohn's disease affects the small and/or large intestine with the terminal ileus the most common site. It involves all layers of the bowel and results in a thickening and eventual obstruction. Lesions from this disease are patchy with areas of normal tissue while lesions from ulcerative colitis are continuous in the affected bowel. Ulcerative colitis also affects the mucosa and submucosa of the large intestine and rectum in a hyperemia and edema of which effects absorption of nutrients and eventually a narrowed, inflexible, scarred bowel. Both diseases are characterized by remissions and exacerbations and occur in children of school age but are most commonly found in the adolescent age group.

MEDICAL CARE

Anti-inflammatories: corticosteroids, azathioprine, mercaptopurine.

Anti-infectives: sulfasalazine (Azulfidine) to prevent recurrences administered with folic acid supplement as it interferes with utilization of this substance; metronidazole (Flagyl) given to treat perianal condition, intestinal amebiasis.

Analgesics: codeine given to control pain.

Gastrointestinal X-ray (Barium enema): reveals colon abnormalities.

Gastrointestinal X-ray (Barium swallow): reveals small intestine abnormalities.

Colonoscopy: reveals view of colon abnormalities such as intermittent mucosa involvement, mucosal erosion, cobblestoning, granularity.

Bowel biopsy: taken during colonoscopy or sigmoidoscopy at different sites reveals bowel pathology especially in Crohn's.

Sigmoidoscopy: reveals abnormalities in rectum, sigmoid colon.

Erythrocyte sedimentation rate (ESR): reveals increases in Crohn's disease.

Protein: reveals decreases in albumin.

Immunoglobulins: reveal decreases in IgG, IgA.

C-Reactive protein (CRP): reveals increases in presence of inflammatory disorder, especially Crohn's disease.

Electrolyte Panel: reveals decreased K^+ with diarrhea.

Complete Blood Count (CBC): reveals increased with inflammation WBC, decreased RBC, Hct with blood loss and anemia.

Stool: fecal culture reveals presence of pathologic organisms that may cause diarrhea; fecal analysis for fat content reveals absorption defect; fecal occult blood reveals bleeding from intestinal tract.

COMMON NURSING DIAGNOSES

 See IMBALANCED NUTRITION: LESS THAN BODY REQUIREMENTS

Related to: Inability to ingest and digest food, absorb nutrients.

Defining Characteristics: (Specify: anorexia, diarrhea, abdominal cramping, weight loss, growth retardation, abdominal distention, possible vomiting.

See RISK FOR DEFICIENT FLUID VOLUME

Related to: Excessive losses through normal routes.

Defining Characteristics: (Specify: diarrhea, output greater than intake, signs and symptoms of dehydration, electrolyte imbalance (K⁺).

 ### See DIARRHEA

Related to: Irritation, or malabsorption of bowel, dietary intake.

Defining Characteristics: (Specify: abdominal pain, cramping, increased frequency, increased frequency of bowel sounds, loose, liquid, watery stools, urgency, changes in color and constituents (blood, mucus), ingestion of high fiber foods.)

See RISK FOR IMPAIRED SKIN INTEGRITY

Related to: External factor of secretions and excretions, internal factor of extra-intestinal skin lesions.

Defining Characteristics: (Specify: irritation, redness, pain at perianal area, disruption of skin surfaces, chronic and excessive diarrhea.)

See DELAYED GROWTH AND DEVELOPMENT

Related to: Effects of physical disability.

Defining Characteristics: (Specify: altered physical growth, delay in sexual maturation, delay in bone age, weight loss, school absences during exacerbations.)

ADDITIONAL NURSING DIAGNOSES

 ### PAIN

Related to: Biologic injuring agents, inflammation and irritation of the bowel.

Defining Characteristics: (Specify: abdominal cramping, abdominal distention, intermittent pain aggravated by eating or pain that is constant and aching, verbalization of other pain descriptors, guarding and protective behavior towards abdomen.)

Goal: Child will experience less pain by (date and time to evaluate).

Outcome Criteria

✔ Child rates pain less than (specify) on a scale of (specify).

NOC: *Pain Level*

INTERVENTIONS	RATIONALES
Assess severity of pain, onset and precipitating factors, location, duration, remissions and exacerbations (specify when).	Provides information symptomatic of inflammatory bowel disease with pain common in Crohn's disease and less frequent in ulcerative colitis; pain is associated with dietary intake in both diseases.
Administer medications as ordered (specify drug, dose, route, and times); assess effect of medications in relieving discomfort.	(Action of drug)
Assist to assume position of comfort.	Promotes comfort to reduce pain.
Provide toys, TV, book, games for quiet play during painful episodes (specify).	Promotes diversionary activity to detract from pain.
Teach child relaxation exercises and guided imagery, use of music for relaxation.	Provides child with methods to control discomfort by diversion.
Explain cause of pain to child and measures taken to relieve pain.	Provides information for understanding of condition and reasons for treatments and medication.
Teach child about factors that exacerbate pain episodes and to express presence of pain at onset.	Promotes opportunity to avoid those foods or stressful situations that contribute to pain and provides for immediate relief.

NIC: *Pain Reduction*

Evaluation

(Date/time of evaluation of goal)

(Has goal been met? Not met? Partially met?)

(How does child rate pain?)

(Revisions to care plan? D/C care plan? Continue care plan?)

ANXIETY

Related to: Threat to self-concept (body image), change in health status.

Defining Characteristics: (Specify: expressed fear and uncertainty, feelings of inadequacy among peer group, feeling of helplessness about consequences, delayed growth and sexual maturation, feeling of being different or frequency of being ill, school absences, ongoing dietary restrictions, presence of a colostomy if colectomy performed.)

Goal: Child will experience decreased anxiety by (date and time to evaluate).

Outcome Criteria

✔ Verbalized reduction in anxiety.

✔ Child verbalizes reduction of anxiety to (specify level, e.g., none, mild, moderate, severe, or panic level).

NOC: *Anxiety Control*

INTERVENTIONS	RATIONALES
Assess level of anxiety of child and how it is manifested; the need for information that will relieve anxiety (specify when).	Provides information about source and level of anxiety and need for interventions to relieve it; sources for the child may be procedures, fear of mutilation or death, unfamiliar environment of hospital and may be manifested by restlessness, inability to play or sleep or eat, clinging, aggression, withdrawal.
Assess possible need for special counseling services for child.	Reduces anxiety and supports child dealing with a long-term illness and promotes adjustment to lifestyle changes.
Encourage expression of concerns about illness and procedures and treatments.	Provides opportunity to vent feelings and fears to reduce anxiety.
Communicate with child at appropriate age level and answer questions calmly and honestly; use pictures, models and drawings for explanations.	Promotes understanding and trust.
Encourage child's input in decisions about care and routines as possible.	Allows for more control and independence in situations.
Teach child disease process, physical effects, signs and symptoms of disease.	Provides information to promote understanding and relieve anxiety.
Explain reason for each procedure or type of therapy, diagnostic tests and what to expect.	Reduces fear of unknown which evokes anxiety.

NIC: *Anxiety Reduction*

Evaluation

(Date/time of evaluation of goal)

(Has goal been met? Not met? Partially met?)

(How does child rank anxiety?)

(Revisions to care plan? D/C care plan? Continue care plan?)

IMPAIRED ADJUSTMENT

Related to: Disability requiring change in lifestyle, inadequate support systems.

Defining Characteristics: (Specify: verbalization of nonacceptance of health status change, unsuccessful in ability to be involved in problem solving, lack of movement towards independence.)

Goal: Child will adapt to lifestyle changes by (date and time to evaluate).

Outcome Criteria

✔ Child and family verbalize strengths.

✔ Child and family identify 3 ways to cope with illness.

NOC: *Acceptance: Health Status*

INTERVENTIONS	RATIONALES
Assess for ability of child and family to adapt, willingness of family and child to support medical regimen and need to change lifestyle, ability to problem solve and utilize coping mechanisms.	Provides information about ability of family and child to modify lifestyle, make plans for a constructive lifestyle within limits imposed by change in health status.
Encourage to identify strengths and roles of family and child, coping mechanisms that have been successful in the past, resources and support groups available.	Allows for support needed to manage long-term illness of child.
Assist child and family to develop a health care regimen by making decisions regarding care, sharing goals and progress, accepting accountability for specific aspects of care.	Promotes independence and control over care and situations.
Assist child and family to deal with denial behavior and to differentiate between denial of	Permits realistic lifestyle changes that are congruent with health status changes.

INTERVENTIONS	RATIONALES
change in health status and denial of limits imposed by change in health status.	
Maintain a positive, hopeful attitude about lifestyle changes accomplished to promote health.	Promotes maximal use of personal resources and acceptance of support systems.
Provide information about disease process, treatment, potential disability, prognosis.	Promotes understanding of disease and effect on lifestyle.
Prepare child and family for colostomy or ileostomy surgery if indicated and emphasize the positive aspects of such a surgery and possibility of fairly normal life regardless of bowel diversion (permanent recovery, normal growth and sexual development).	Provides information that may begin to lead to acceptance of change in bowel elimination.
Refer to resources such as insurance assistance (government and private, support groups, social services, colitis and Ileitis Foundation, United Ostomy Association).	Assists family and child to seek out support and information over long period of time for current treatment development and research and economic and psychological assistance.

NIC: *Self-Awareness Enhancement*

Evaluation

(Date/time of evaluation of goal)

(Has goal been met? Not met? Partially met?)

(What strengths did child and family identify? How do child and family plan to cope with illness?)

(Revisions to care plan? D/C care plan? Continue care plan?)

DEFICIENT KNOWLEDGE

Related to: Lack of information about long-term medical regimen.

Defining Characteristics: (Specify: request for information about medication, dietary regimen, care of colostomy or ileostomy.)

Goal: Clients will obtain knowledge about care by (date and time to evaluate).

Outcome Criteria

✔ Clients verbalize plan of care for child.

NOC: *Knowledge: Treatment Regimen*

INTERVENTIONS	RATIONALES
Assess parents and child for knowledge of prescribed medical regimen and postoperative care if applicable.	Provides information of learning needs of parents and/or child.
Instruct in special nutritional needs including diet that is high in protein and calories and low in fat and fiber.	Provides replacement of nutritional losses caused by the disease and to promote metabolic function and energy levels.
Inform that mouth care before meals and bland foods should be encouraged if mouth pain is present.	Promotes comfort if stomatitis present.
Teach about long-term administration of medications, folic acid supplement including actions, dosages during acute and chronic stages, frequency, times, side effects, (specify) effect of discontinuing a steroid without tapering, signs and symptoms to report.	Provides information.
(Teach, demonstrate, and allow for return demonstration for ostomy care including, application and removal of appliance peristomal skin care, emptying and cleansing of ostomy bag, odor control; continent ileostomy care and catheterization of the pouch.)	Promotes independence in ostomy care with as normal a return to activities as possible; procedure done if child does not respond to medical treatment.
(Inform of nasogastric tube feedings or total parenteral nutrition if required.)	Provides information about alternate methods of nutritional support during acute state of disease.
Provide praise and encouragement to child and family as they learn new skills.	Positive reinforcement enhances understanding and skill.

NIC: *Teaching: Disease Process*

Evaluation

(Date/time of evaluation of goal)

(Has goal been met? Not met? Partially met?)

(What did clients verbalize about child's plan of care?)

(Revisions to care plan? D/C care plan? Continue care plan?)

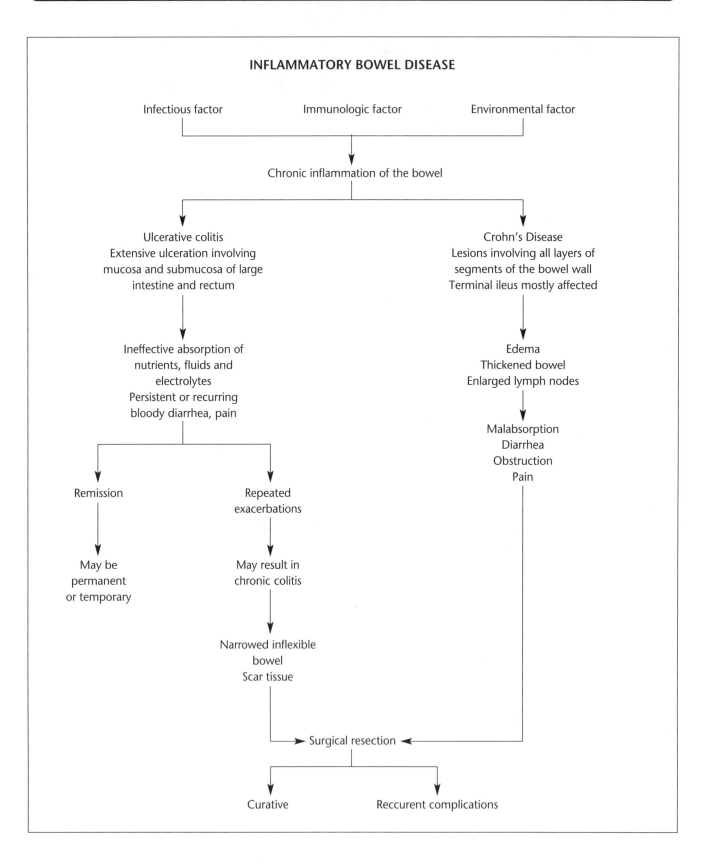

CHAPTER 4.8

INTUSSUSCEPTION

Intussusception is a telescoping of one section of the bowel into another section which results in obstruction to passage of the intestinal contents and inflammation and decreased blood flow to the parts of the intestinal walls that are pressing against one another. If left untreated, eventual necrosis, perforation, and peritonitis occurs. It occurs in infants most commonly between 3 to 12 months of age or in children 12 to 24 months of age. The actual cause is unknown but risk for the condition increased in children with Meckel's diverticulum, celiac disease, cystic fibrosis, diarrhea, or constipation. Surgical correction is indicated if the obstruction of the involved segment cannot be reduced manually or by hydrostatic pressure or if bowel becomes necrotic.

MEDICAL CARE

Analgesics (narcotic analgesics): codeine, morphine sulfate preoperatively before diagnostic test or postoperatively for pain.

Analgesics (non-narcotic analgesics): acetaminophen given for pain postoperatively.

Antibiotics: given to prevent or treat peritonitis.

Lower Gastrointestinal X-ray, Ultrasound: barium enema reveals an obstruction which prevents the flow of barium into the colon.

Reduction of the Intussusception: usually occurs as a result of the pressure of the barium enema, or may be accomplished by other methods of hydrostatic or air pressure reduction.

Surgical Reduction of the Intussusception: with possible resection for necrotic bowel.

COMMON NURSING DIAGNOSES

See IMBALANCED NUTRITION: LESS THAN BODY REQUIREMENTS

Related to: Inability to ingest and digest foods.

Defining Characteristics: (Specify: vomiting, abdominal pain, NPO status, NG tube pre and postoperatively.)

See RISK FOR DEFICIENT FLUID VOLUME

Related to: Excessive losses through normal routes.

Defining Characteristics: (Specify: vomiting, decreased urine output, altered intake with NPO status, signs and symptoms of dehydration or electrolyte imbalance.)

See CONSTIPATION

Related to: Specify: medications, diagnostic procedure using barium enema.

Defining Characteristics: (Specify: hard formed, barium colored stools, decreased bowel sounds, less frequent passage of stools and flatus, abdominal discomfort.)

ADDITIONAL NURSING DIAGNOSES

RISK FOR INJURY

Related to: Bowel dysfunction.

Defining Characteristics: (Specify: severe abdominal pain, bowel obstruction.)

Goal: Client will not experience injury by (date and time to evaluate).

Outcome Criteria

✔ Intussusception is reduced by hydrostatic pressure.

✔ Client passes normal brown stool.

 NOC: *Symptom Control*

INTERVENTIONS	RATIONALES
Assess presence of acute abdominal pain with loud crying and drawing knees up to chest which may be episodic, vomiting, passage of a brown stool followed by red, currant jelly-like stool, pallor, irritability.	Provides information that indicates that intussusception is present which may lead to obstruction and signs of peritonitis if not treated.
Assess presence of diarrhea, constipation, episodes of vomiting and colic in older child.	Indicates presence of intussusception and need for further evaluation.
Provide NG tube attached to suction, IV fluids to decompress bowel and maintain hydration status and maintain patency of therapy as ordered (specify).	Prevents vomiting and dehydration and prepares child for barium enema procedure to diagnose and reduce the invagination.
Note bowel elimination and stool characteristics and ability to eliminate barium following the procedure.	Indicates success of the procedure in reducing the affected bowel as the condition may recur within 36 hours.
Provide reassurance to parents and allow to accompany child during procedure.	Promotes trust and reduces anxiety.
Provide information about all care given and allow for opportunity to ask questions about procedures.	Reduces anxiety.
Teach parents about reasons for IV and NG tube, NPO status (specify).	Provides information about treatments for understanding and reduction of anxiety.
Inform parents that surgical reduction may be necessary if barium enema does not reduce the invagination.	Prepares parents for possibility of surgical correction.
Reinforce information given by physician.	Provides information about surgery intervention if barium enema reduction not successful or if bowel obstruction and gangrene is present.

NIC: *Surveillance*

Evaluation

(Date/time of evaluation of goal)

(Has goal been met? Not met? Partially met?)

(Was intussusception reduced by hydrostatic pressure? Did client pass a normal brown stool?)

(Revisions to care plan? D/C care plan? Continue care plan?)

DEFICIENT KNOWLEDGE

Related to: Lack of information about condition.

Defining Characteristics: (Specify: request for information about causes of condition, postoperative or post-procedural care.)

Goal: Parents will obtain information about intussusception by (date and time to evaluate).

Outcome Criteria

✔ Parents verbalize understanding of intussusception, the need for a barium enema, and possibility of surgical intervention.

NOC: *Knowledge: Disease Process*

INTERVENTIONS	RATIONALES
Assess knowledge of condition, causes, treatment regimen following procedure(s).	Promotes development of effective plan of instruction.
Provide parents with information and clear explanation in understandable language, include aids in teaching and encourage questions (specify).	Ensures understanding of care needs based on ability to learn.
(Inform parents of signs and symptoms of incision infection and demonstrate and allow for return demonstration of dressing change.)	Promotes awareness of signs and symptoms to report to treat complication of wound infection.
Teach to report any blood in stool, change in stool characteristics or diarrhea or constipation or absence of stools.	Indicates gastrointestinal bleeding and possible recurrence or chronicity of condition.
Teach parents about preparation procedures for reduction by barium enema or surgery and antibiotic and postoperative care given to child.	Provides information regarding care to expect during hospitalization.
Teach parents that child will be NPO and when advisable, will be offered clear fluids and slowly progress to usual diet.	Prevents vomiting or abdominal distention until condition resolved.
Inform parents of activity restrictions (specify).	Allows condition and/or wound to heal and resolve itself without complications.

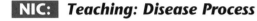

INTERVENTIONS	RATIONALES
Inform parents that bowel elimination of brown stools indicate that condition has been corrected.	Provides parents with baseline expected with successful resolution of problem.

NIC: *Teaching: Disease Process*

Evaluation

(Date/time of evaluation of goal)

(Has goal been met? Not met? Partially met?)

(What did parents verbalize about intussusception, barium enema, and possibility of surgery? Use quotes.)

(Revisions to care plan? D/C care plan? Continue care plan?)

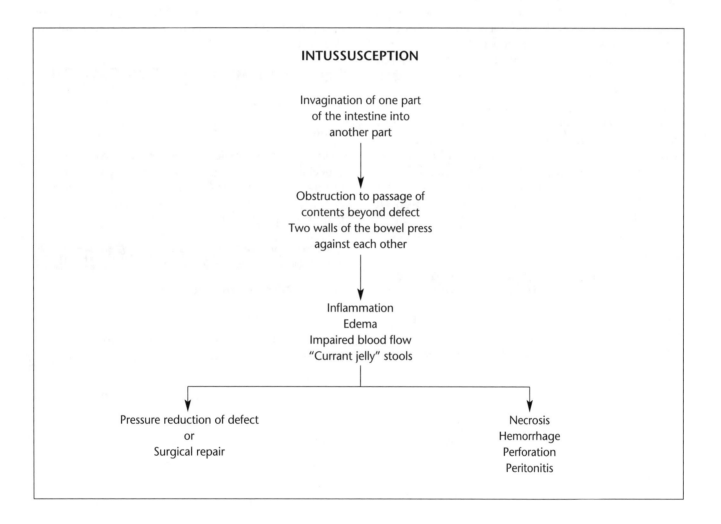

INTUSSUSCEPTION

Invagination of one part of the intestine into another part

↓

Obstruction to passage of contents beyond defect
Two walls of the bowel press against each other

↓

Inflammation
Edema
Impaired blood flow
"Currant jelly" stools

Pressure reduction of defect
or
Surgical repair

Necrosis
Hemorrhage
Perforation
Peritonitis

CHAPTER 4.9

PYLORIC STENOSIS

Pyloric stenosis is a hypertrophic disorder of the circular muscle of the pylorus in which the pylorus is greatly enlarged and hyperplasic and causes progressive narrowing of the canal between the stomach and duodenum. As the canal becomes obstructed over time, associated inflammation and edema result in complete obstruction. The enlarged pylorus muscle may be felt as an "olive-like" mass in the upper abdomen. The infant appears very hungry but exhibits projectile vomiting soon after eating and fails to gain appropriate weight. Metabolic alkalosis is a possibility from loss of hydrochloric acid.

The exact cause is unknown although heredity is suspected. The abnormality is most common in young children between 1 to 6 months of age. Pyloric obstruction is treated successfully with surgical correction.

MEDICAL CARE

Pyloromyotomy: surgical enlargement of the pyloric lumen.

Analgesics (narcotic analgesics): postoperatively for pain control.

Analgesics (non-narcotic analgesics): acetaminophen postoperatively for moderate pain.

Upper Gastrointestinal X-ray: reveals delayed gastric emptying with an elongated canal between stomach and duodenum.

Ultrasound: reveals narrowed canal between stomach and duodenum without the use of barium swallow.

Electrolyte Panel: reveals increased Hgb, Hct as hemoconcentration occurs with fluid depletion.

COMMON NURSING DIAGNOSES

See RISK FOR DEFICIENT FLUID VOLUME

Related to: (Specify: excessive losses through normal routes, NPO status pre and postoperatively.

Defining Characteristics: (Specify: vomiting with an eventual projectile character, electrolyte losses, signs and symptoms of dehydration, hemoconcentration, decreased urine output.)

See IMBALANCED NUTRITION: LESS THAN BODY REQUIREMENTS

Related to: Inability to ingest, digest food.

Defining Characteristics: (Specify: excessive vomiting especially after eating, chronic hunger, weight loss, failure to gain weight, diminished stools, abdominal distention, NG tube pre and postoperatively for stomach decompression.)

ADDITIONAL NURSING DIAGNOSES

RISK FOR INJURY

Related to: GI obstruction.

Defining Characteristics: (Specify: vomiting that increases in severity leading to dehydration, hunger, and weight loss.)

Goal: Infant will not experience injury by (date and time to evaluate).

Outcome Criteria

✔ Absence of vomiting, weight gain (specify for infant) per week.

✔ Skin turgor elastic, mucous membranes moist, intake equals output.

NOC: *Risk Control*

INTERVENTIONS	RATIONALES
Assess pattern of vomiting, development of projectile vomiting, vomiting that occurs	Provides information about presence of hypertrophic pyloric stenosis causing obstruction as

INTERVENTIONS	RATIONALES
after feeding or hours after feeding, weight loss, diminished stools, palpable mass in the epigastrium to the right of the umbilicus, presence of visible gastric peristaltic waves across the epigastrium.	the canal to the duodenum narrows.
Maintain NPO status and NG tube connected to suction, position with head slightly elevated.	Decompresses stomach for 24 to 36 hours in preparation for surgery.
Assess skin for decreased turgor, elasticity, loss of subcutaneous tissue, sunken eyeballs, urinary output (specify frequency).	Provides information about the presence of dehydration caused by excessive vomiting.
Maintain IV fluids and electrolytes (Na$^+$, K$^+$, CA$^-$, Cl$^-$), glucose for nutritional support (specify fluid and rate).	Provides hydration and replaces lost glycogen stores and electrolytes for 24 to 36 hours in preparation for surgery or when needed.
Weigh daily at same time on same scale.	Reveals losses or gains related to fluid and nutritional.
Teach parents about diagnostic tests and procedures done and reason for them.	Provides information needed to reduce anxiety.

NIC: *Surveillance*

Evaluation

(Date/time of evaluation of goal)

(Has goal been met? Not met? Partially met?)

(Has infant vomited? What is weight gain per week? What is intake and output? Describe skin turgor and mucous membranes.)

(Revisions to care plan? D/C care plan? Continue care plan?)

ANXIETY

Related to: Change in health status of infant, surgical correction of condition.

Defining Characteristics: (Specify: increased apprehension and expressed concern and worry about impending surgery, pre and postoperative care, treatments while hospitalized and complications following surgery.)

Goal: Clients will experience decreased anxiety by (date and time to evaluate).

Outcome Criteria

✔ Parents verbalize decreased anxiety (use a scale; specify).

NOC: *Anxiety Control*

INTERVENTIONS	RATIONALES
Assess source and level of anxiety and how anxiety is manifested; need for information that will relieve anxiety (use a scale).	Provides information about anxiety level and need for interventions to relieve it; sources for the parent(s) include fear and uncertainty about treatment and recovery, guilt for presence of illness.
Encourage expression of concerns and questions about condition, procedures, and surgery.	Provides opportunity to vent feelings and fears and secure information to reduce anxiety.
Communicate with parents and answer questions calmly and honestly; use pictures, drawings, and models for explanations.	Promotes calm and supportive trusting environment.
Encourage parents to stay with child and assist in care and feeding.	Allows parents to care for and support child and continue parental role.
Give parents as much input in decisions about care and routines as possible.	Allows for more control over situation.
Provide consistent care of infant with familiar staff assigned for care.	Promotes trust and reduces anxiety.
Inform parents of disease process, physical effects and symptoms of illness.	Provides information to relieve anxiety by knowledge of what to expect.
Explain reason for each pre and postoperative procedure or type of therapy, diagnostic tests, surgical procedure and rationales including IV, NG tube, dressings that will be in place.	Reduces fear which decreases anxiety.
Teach parents about surgical procedure (pyloromyotomy).	Reduces anxiety and concern about surgery and outcome.
Demonstrate and teach parents about wound care and dressing changes and allow for return demonstration; apply and pin diaper low or use a urine collecting system to maintain dry dressing and wound.	Ensures wound healing without complication of infection.

(continues)

(continued)

INTERVENTIONS	RATIONALES
Teach parents to report redness, swelling, or drainage at wound site.	Indication that infectious process is present.
Teach parents about feeding after NG tube removed and allow to feed clear liquids slowly and frequently and progress to formula or breast milk expressed by mother or to limit nursing to 5 minutes and gradually increase until previous pattern established, as ordered.	Promotes comfort and bonding with infant with continuation of parenting role until feeding pattern returns; prevents overdistention of stomach and vomiting.
Instruct parents to hold infant upright and use nipple that does not flow too rapidly, burp frequently, and place on right side or abdomen after feeding.	Facilitates feeding postoperatively and prevents vomiting and possible aspiration.

INTERVENTIONS	RATIONALES
Inform parents to sponge bathe infant until incision heals.	Promotes comfort and cleanliness of infant.
Reassure parents and offer praise for their care of infant.	Positive reinforcement reduces anxiety associated with learning new skills.

NIC: *Anxiety Reduction*

Evaluation

(Date/time of evaluation of goal)

(Has goal been met? Not met? Partially met?)

(What do parents verbalize about their feelings of anxiety?)

(Revisions to care plan? D/C care plan? Continue care plan?)

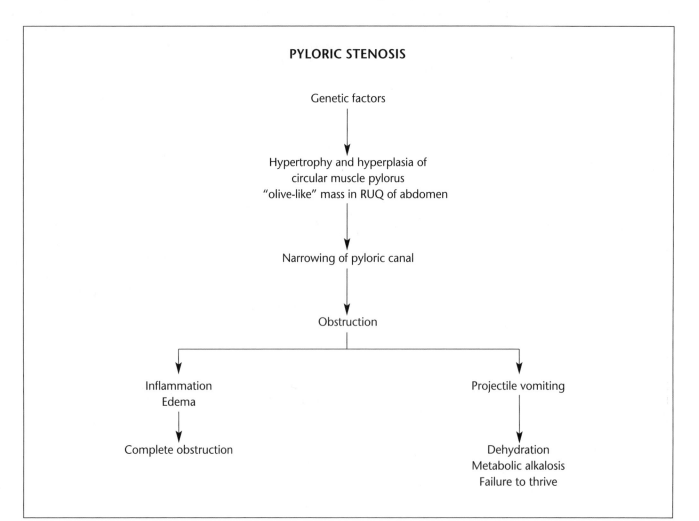

PYLORIC STENOSIS

Genetic factors

↓

Hypertrophy and hyperplasia of circular muscle pylorus "olive-like" mass in RUQ of abdomen

↓

Narrowing of pyloric canal

↓

Obstruction

Inflammation Edema

↓

Complete obstruction

Projectile vomiting

↓

Dehydration
Metabolic alkalosis
Failure to thrive

UNIT 5

GENITOURINARY SYSTEM

CHAPTER 5.0

GENITOURINARY SYSTEM: BASIC CARE PLAN

The genitourinary system is made up of the reproductive organs, the kidneys, ureters, urethra, and bladder. The kidneys regulate fluid and electrolyte balance, maintain the pH of the body, and provide for the excretion of the end product of protein metabolism in the form of urea. Fluid and electrolyte balance is controlled by filtration, reabsorption, and secretion of these substances during urine formation in the glomeruli and renal tubules. The kidneys produce erythropoietin-stimulating factor in response to lowered oxygen levels, which increases red blood cell production in the bone marrow. They also release renin in response to hypotension, which initiates the renin-angiotensin pathway to increase blood pressure.

Urine descends through the ureters to the bladder, where it is stored until it is excreted via the urethra. Disease processes may cause inflammation, tissue damage, and scarring with resultant dysfunction of the organs or structures of the genitourinary system. Structural defects may be either congenital or acquired and can obstruct urine flow causing renal damage and possibly lead to kidney failure. The kidneys of infants and children are immature in regard to fluid and electrolyte balance because of their limited ability to concentrate urine. This creates increased risk for fluid and electrolyte fluctuations and the possibility of dehydration during illness. Renal function matures as the child grows.

GENITOURINARY GROWTH AND DEVELOPMENT

ORGAN STRUCTURE

- Infant kidney size is, proportionately, three times larger than adult size
- The number of nephrons increase until 1 year of age with continued maturation of the nephrons throughout development of the young child.

- Tubules and glomeruli continue to form and enlarge after birth; tubular length is highly variable but glomeruli size is less variable; tubular length increases until 3 months of age.
- The loop of Henle is short in the infant which affects ability to reabsorb water and sodium causing urine to be dilute.
- The length of the urethra in children is proportionately shorter according to their growth and age.
- The urinary bladder increases in size with growth and development and is considered an abdominal organ in infancy; it becomes a pelvic organ with growth.
- Urinary output and bladder capacity increase with growth:

  Infant: 350 to 550 ml/24 hr
  Child: 500 to 1000 ml/24 hr
  Adolescent: 700 to 1400 ml/24 hr

GROWTH AND DEVELOPMENTAL CHANGES

- Glomerular filtration and absorption values are reached between 1 to 2 years of age.
- The kidneys' ability to concentrate urine increases at 3 months of age with urea synthesis and excretion reaching adult levels by this time; by age 2, urine is concentrated at the adult level.
- Excretion of water and hydrogen ion is reduced during infancy and excretion of sodium is also reduced during the first month of life with an inefficient reabsorption of sodium.
- The volume of urinary output varies with age:

  Infant: 5 to 10 ml/hr
  10 yr old: 10 to 25 ml/hr

- The number of voidings/day vary but decrease with age as urine becomes more concentrated.

- Voluntary control of the urethral sphincter is achieved between 18 to 24 months of age with night control of bladder usually achieved by 3 years of age; by 4 years of age, bladder capacity reaches 250 ml which allows the child to remain dry at night.

- The amount of total body water varies with age, growth, and sex and decreases as the child grows and develops

  Birth: 75 to 80% of weight
  3 yr old: 63% of weight
  12 yr old: 58% of weight

- Extracellular fluid levels decrease within the first year. Intracellular fluid volume increases with the growth of muscles and organs.

- The infant and young child have greater intake and output relative to size than older children, and water loss or decreased intake are more likely to cause dehydration as this age group is more vulnerable to fluid and electrolyte alterations.

- The increased amount of extracellular fluid results in a high water turnover (50% of the extracellular fluid is exchanged daily) and higher tendency to develop dehydration.

- Water loss through respirations, increased metabolism is greater in children; the greater surface area increases water loss through the skin.

- Acid–base balance is maintained by a buffer system that is less mature in children.

- The newborn is at risk of developing severe metabolic acidosis because hydrogen ion excretion is reduced, immature kidneys cannot conserve water efficiently, high metabolic levels produce increased acid, and plasma bicarbonate levels are low.

- Sodium excretion is reduced in the immediate newborn period, and the kidneys are less able to adapt to deficiencies and excesses of sodium.

- Infants have a diminished capacity to reabsorb glucose and, during the first few days of life, to produce ammonium ions.

NURSING DIAGNOSES

 ### RISK FOR DEFICIENT FLUID VOLUME

Related to: Excessive losses.

Defining Characteristics: (Specify: vomiting, diarrhea, excessive renal excretion, dry skin and mucous membranes, weight loss, decreased urinary output, altered intake, sunken fontanels in infant, decrease of tears and saliva, sunken soft eyeballs, nasogastric suction, fistula.)

Related to: Factors influencing fluid needs.

Defining Characteristics: (Specify: hypermetabolic states, temperature elevation [diaphoresis], increased insensible loss [respirations, perspirations], failure to absorb or reabsorb water, excessive renal excretion, extremes of age, water output exceeds intake.)

Related to: Medications.

Defining Characteristics: (Specify: use of diuretics, administration of IV fluids containing NaCl.)

Goal: Client will maintain fluid balance by (date and time to evaluate).

Outcome Criteria

✔ Intake equals output.

✔ Mucous membranes are moist, elastic skin turgor (specify for infant: fontanels flat).

NOC: *Fluid Balance*

INTERVENTIONS	RATIONALES
Assess fluid losses, sources, amounts, and effects; urinary output (should be 1–2 ml/kg/hr; weigh diapers for infant and calculate as 1 ml/gm); vomiting (include spitting up); diarrhea (include watery or bloody); stoma drainage (liquid); nasogastric aspirate (suctioning); insensible losses (respirations, diaphoresis from body temperature or ambient temperature); wound damage hemorrhage (fluid volume reduced); injury (burns).	Provides information about body fluid losses and depletion which can lead to serious consequences in the infant/child; include output analysis when comparing to intake; causes include failure to absorb or reabsorb water, reduced intake or NPO status, excessive renal excretion, inappropriate ADH secretion, increased temperature or respirations, over-use of diuretic therapy, improper fluid replacement.
Assess intake and accurately compare to losses (q 2–8h) for I&O determination and balance; oral intake (liquids, fluid content of foods/formula, foods that become liquid at body temperature, fluids given with medications); parenteral (IV, IM, TPN); enteral (NG, gastrostomy tube feedings).	Provides strict I&O to determine positive or negative balance and potential for fluid deficit/ dehydration; mild dehydration: less than 50 ml/kg fluid loss; moderate dehydration: 50 to 90 ml/kg; severe dehydration: about 100 ml/kg.

(continues)

(continued)

INTERVENTIONS	RATIONALES
Assess infant's weight (undressed without diaper) on the same scale.	Determines losses related to fluid deficit and potential for dehydration; mild dehydration: loss of 5% in infant, 3% in older child; moderate: loss of 10% in infant, 6% in older child; severe: loss of 15% in infant, 9% in older child.
Assess for presence of dehydration (q 2–8h) including decreased urinary output, poor skin turgor, dry skin and mucous membranes, gray or mottled color to skin, reduced or absent tears and saliva, sunken, soft eyeballs (sunken fontanels in infants), increased sp. gr. and serum osmolality, blood urea nitrogen (BUN), creatinine, hemoglobin, creatinine hematocrit, thirst in the older child, vital signs changes (tachycardia, lowered blood pressure, postural changes in blood pressure).	Reveals signs and symptoms of dehydration and hydration status; dehydration occurs when output exceeds intake and is classified as isotonic dehydration (water and electrolyte deficits equal); hypertonic dehydration (water loss is greater than sodium loss); hypotonic dehydration (sodium loss is greater than water loss).
Assess (and teach parents) for presence of electrolyte depletion (specify).	Reveals signs and symptoms of electrolyte imbalance which are related to specific diseases; provides information regarding fluid/electrolyte imbalances, kidney function and risk for acidosis or alkalosis.
Potassium (K^+): muscle weakness and cramping, irritability, fatigue, hypotension, arrhythmias.	K^+: excessive urinary output, diuretic therapy, vomiting, diarrhea, NG aspirate (functions in neural transmission in smooth, skeletal and cardiac muscle).
Sodium (Na^+): nausea, abdominal cramps, weakness, dizziness, apathy.	Na^+: excessive water loss via any route, fever, diaphoresis, vomiting, diarrhea, NG aspirate, fistula or wounds (functions to control movement of fluid between fluid compartments).
Calcium (Ca^{++}): tingling of fingertips, toes, hypotension, muscle irritability, tetany.	Ca^{++}: renal insufficiency, loss through gastrointestinal route, inadequate Ca^{++} intake or vitamin D deficiency (functions to prevent metabolic acidosis).
Assess urinalysis, electrolyte panel, serum and urine osmolality, blood urea nitrogen, creatinine, arterial blood gases, as indicated.	Provides information regarding fluid/electrolyte imbalances, kidney function and risk for acidosis or alkalosis.

INTERVENTIONS	RATIONALES
Encourage increased oral fluid intake in proportion to losses; provide a varied selection of beverages (specify); if the fluid volume deficit is caused by diarrhea, allow child to request oral fluid preferences or provide ORT solutions; start with rapid replacement for 4 to 6 hours and continue over 24 hours for maintenance therapy as tolerated: Infant: 150 ml/kg/day Toddler: 120 ml/kg/day Preschool: 100 ml/kg/day School-age: 75 ml/kg/day	Provides replacement of lost fluids if able to retain PO; child requires 750 to 2000 ml/day fluids depending on age and weight and calculation of losses; fluids with a high carbonation content, usually have a low electrolyte content; the caffeine in caffeinated soft drinks acts as a mild diuretic and may lead to increased loss of water and sodium; chicken or beef broth contains excessive sodium and inadequate carbohydrates.
Provide oral rehydration therapy (i.e., Pedialyte, Rehydralyte, Infalyte) for infant.	Promotes fluid and electrolyte replacement and prevents risk of dehydration and electrolyte deficits.
Prepare child and initiate IV fluid therapy with (specify: solution rate and amount).	Provides immediate replacement and ongoing prevention of losses for those who are unable to ingest fluids PO.
Teach parents (and child) about need for IV fluids, how the pump works, what alarms mean. Reassure the child that the IV is not a punishment.	Teaching helps parents and child cope with IV therapy.
Use infusion pump or volume control chamber for IV with a pediatric infusion set with long tubing and restrain body parts as needed.	Provides regulated and accurate fluid rate and volume with a microdrip IV infusion set (60 gtt/ml); long tubing allows for movement in bed, and proper restraining and monitoring provides safe IV administration.
Monitor IV hourly for amount, site infiltration, tube patency or displacement; change fluid bag and tubing (q 24h), use a transparent occlusive dressing over IV site.	Ensures safe fluid administration; allows for ROM of restrained parts, prevents complication of IV therapy.
Provide non-nutritive sucking for infant, hold and cuddle child, mouth care (spray water into mouth) for oral dryness.	Provides support and comfort to infant/child.
During IV therapy, note presence of headache, cramps, vomiting, crackles, muscle twitching, lethargy, decreased urine output.	Indicates overhydration.

INTERVENTIONS	RATIONALES
Discontinue IV when fluids are tolerated orally; begin with small amounts of clear fluids, gradually increase in amounts and frequency as tolerated to regular diet; baby food for infants.	Resumes oral fluid intake when condition improves; oral intake may be resumed as soon as 5 to 50 hours after surgery.
Employ play at developmental level including games, use of straws, small cup (medicine or animal image cup, specify).	Promotes oral intake of fluids when child is ill and doesn't fulfill fluid goals.
Place water and cup in room and allow to take frequent sips; praise child for drinking fluids.	Promotes adequate intake of fluids and promotes independence.
Allow child to participate in the fluid selection and scheduling, to record intake using symbols or checks with colors.	Promotes independence and control over the situations and enhances compliance.
Teach parents and child the amount of fluid needed by the infant/child daily and therapeutic need based on disorder or illness.	Provides information about fluid needs as a basic need and increase of fluid need as treatment for deficit.

INTERVENTIONS	RATIONALES
Teach to measure I&O and allow for return demonstration by calculating and measuring for 24 hours.	Permits accurate monitoring of I&O to determine risk for dehydration.
Suggest referral to a nutritionist for administration of electrolyte formula, dilution of fluids, caloric and sodium content of commercial fluids.	Provides information and instruction and support to parents for safe fluid administration PO.

NIC: *Fluid and Electrolyte Management*

Evaluation

(Date/time of evaluation of goal)

(Has goal been met? Not met? Partially met?)

(What has been intake [specify time]? What has the output been [time]? Describe moisture of mucous membranes and skin turgor. Describe infant's fontanels.)

(Revisions to care plan? D/C care plan? Continue care plan?)

CHAPTER 5.1

CHRONIC RENAL FAILURE

Chronic renal failure (CRF) is the progressive deterioration of kidney function that reaches 50% or more loss or a creatinine level of less than 2 mg/dl. Causes include congenital kidney and urinary tract abnormalities in children less than 5 years of age, and glomerular and hereditary kidney disorders in children 5 to 15 years of age. The disease involves all body systems as abnormalities include water, Na^+, Ca^{++} losses, K^+, HPO^{2-}_4, Mg^{++} increases, and reduced Hgb and Hct that result in metabolic acidosis, anemia, growth retardation, hypertension, and bone demineralization. Eventually, if untreated, uremic syndrome develops as the kidneys are not able to maintain fluid and electrolyte balance. End stage renal disease (ESRD) is defined as loss of kidney function at 90% or greater. ESRD is the term applied when the kidneys are no longer able to clear wastes from the body. Eventually the disease terminates in death unless kidney transplantation or dialysis is performed.

MEDICAL CARE

Electrolyte Panel: at diagnosis lab results will reveal decreased Ca^{++}, Cl^-, CO_2, and *increased* K^+, HPO^{2-}_4, Na^+, and hydrogen ions. With diuretic therapy and increased K^+ intake, lab results may display decreased K^+ and Na^+.

Diuretics: furosemide, or hydrochlorothiazide to promote excretion of water and electrolytes to reduce edema associated with renal failure.

Antihypertensives: for severe hypertension.

Alkalizing Agents: metabolic acidosis is treated with oral alkalizing agents, such as sodium bicarbonate or a combination of sodium and potassium citrate (Bicitra).

Antibiotics: specific to identified microorganisms and sensitivity to specific antimicrobials to prevent or treat infection with dosage adjusted to renal function to prevent toxicity.

Vitamins/Minerals: water-soluble vitamins may be prescribed (B, C, folic acid, niacin) and vitamin D is prescribed. Folic acid (and sometimes ferrous sulfate) is prescribed to enhance iron absorption.

Renal Scan/Renal Ultrasound: may reveal renal abnormality.

Calcium Carbonate Preparations: used as phosphate binders, also act as a calcium supplement and as an alkalizing agent.

Aluminum Hydroxide Gels: are effective phosphorus binders. Only used for severe or unresponsive hyperphosphatemia due to risk of aluminum toxicity.

Epogen: recombinant human erythropoietin (rHuEPO) is prescribed to treat anemia.

Growth Hormone: recombinant human growth hormone is used to treat growth retardation secondary to CRF and following renal transplant.

Blood Urea Nitrogen (BUN): reveals increases as renal failure progresses and protein catabolism increases.

Serum Creatinine: reveals increases as renal failure progresses and glomerular filtration rate is reduced.

Electrolyte Panel: reveals decreased Na^+, Ca^{++}, Cl^- and increased K^+, CO_2.

Complete Blood Count: reveals decreased RBC, Hct, Hgb, WBC, reticulocyte count.

Prothrombin Time (PT): Activated Partial Thromboplastin Time (APPT): reveals prolonged time as erythropoietin production is reduced.

COMMON NURSING DIAGNOSES

See EXCESS FLUID VOLUME

Related to: Compromised regulatory mechanism.

Defining Characteristics: (Specify: edema, water and Na retention, weight gain, clothes begin to feel tight, decreased urine output, facial puffiness, altered electrolyte, shortness of breath, crackles, hypertension, vascular congestion.)

See IMBALANCED NUTRITION: LESS THAN BODY REQUIREMENTS

Related to: Loss of appetite.

Defining Characteristics: (Specify: anorexia, nausea, fatigue, weight loss, limited K^+, HPO^{2-}_4 and protein food intake, poor absorption of Ca^{++}, iron by intestines, growth retardation; may observe weight gain [caused by fluid retention and oliguria] or weight loss (caused by anorexia and electrolyte disturbances].)

See HYPERTHERMIA

Related to: Renal failure.

Defining Characteristics: (Specify: frequent infections, increase in body temperature malaise.)

See RISK FOR IMPAIRED SKIN INTEGRITY

Related to: Chronic renal failure.

Defining Characteristics: (Specify: dryness, pruritis, uremic frost, sallow color, disruption of skin surfaces from scratching secondary skin breakdown [caused by edema].)

See DELAYED GROWTH AND DEVELOPMENT

Related to: (Specify: loss of appetite, depletion of body protein, decreased erythropoietin production, and related metabolic disturbances.)

Defining Characteristics: (Specify: altered physical growth, delay in sexual maturation, frequent absences from school and disruptions in socialization, inability to participate in activities, frequent hospitalizations.)

ADDITIONAL NURSING DIAGNOSES

ACTIVITY INTOLERANCE

Related to: Weakness.

Defining Characteristics: (Specify: complaints of fatigue on exertion, preference for quiet play, lack of energy.)

Goal: Child will progress to increased tolerance for activity by (date and time to evaluate).

Outcome Criteria

✔ (Specify an activity level appropriate for child; e.g., child will go to playroom for 15 minutes each afternoon.)

NOC: *Activity Tolerance*

INTERVENTIONS	RATIONALES
Assess degree of weakness, fatigue, ability to participate in activities (active and passive).	Provides information about effect of activities on fatigue and energy reserves.
Schedule care and provide rest periods following an activity; encourage child to set own limits in amount of exertion tolerated.	Promotes independence and control of situations as the presence of a chronic disease may encourage independence.
Provide for quiet play, reading, TV, games during times of fatigue.	Provides diversion, stimulation and requires minimal energy expenditure.
Explain to child reason for restrictions; explain when to stop activity and rest to child.	Promotes understanding of the need to conserve energy and rest.
Teach parents and child that full participation in activities is important and should be encouraged for as long as possible (within capabilities and disease restriction).	Promotes an active and normal life for the child with a chronic illness.

NIC: *Activity Therapy*

Evaluation

(Date/time of evaluation of goal)

(Has goal been met? Not met? Partially met?)

(What has been child's activity level? How does it compare with the outcome criteria?)

(Revisions to care plan? D/C care plan? Continue care plan?)

RISK FOR INFECTION

Related to: (Specify: pulmonary edema, metabolic acidosis, uremia, loss of appetite.)

Defining Characteristics: (Specify: changes in respiratory pattern, productive cough with yellow or other abnormal color, adventitious sounds, elevated temperature, cloudy, foul smelling urine, dysuria, urgency, frequency.)

Goal: Child will not experience infection by (date and time to evaluate).

Outcome Criteria

✔ Temperature remains <99° F, WBC count < (specify for age), urine and/or blood cultures negative.

NOC: *Risk Control*

INTERVENTIONS	RATIONALES
Assess lab results for infection (elevated WBC and positive blood cultures).	To prevent and treat infection.
Assess temperature, respiratory and urinary system changes as disease progresses (specify frequency).	Provides information about presence of infection caused by progressive chronic disease and its deteriorating effect on all systems.
Administer antibiotic therapy as ordered (specify drug, dose, route, and times).	Prevents or treats infection (action of drug).
Perform handwashing, medical or surgical asepsis during procedures or care as appropriate. Instruct child and parents in handwashing technique, proper disposal of tissues and used articles.	Prevents transmission of pathogens to child.
Secure urine or sputum cultures for analysis.	Identifies presence and type of microorganism responsible for infection and specific sensitivities to antibiotic therapy.
Teach parents and child to decrease growth of microorganisms by bathing daily, wiping from front to back after toileting, and wearing loose cotton underwear.	Information empowers parents and child to help prevent infection.
Teach child to avoid contact with persons with upper respiratory infections.	Prevents transmission of infectious agents that may lead to pneumonia.

NIC: *Infection Control*

Evaluation

(Date/time of evaluation of goal)

(Has goal been met? Not met? Partially met?)

(What is child's temperature and WBC count? What are results of any urine/blood cultures?)

(Revisions to care plan? D/C care plan? Continue care plan?)

DISTURBED BODY IMAGE

Related to: Biophysical and psychosocial factors.

Defining Characteristics: (Specify: verbal and nonverbal responses to change in body appearance, disruptions in school attendance and participation in school activities and socialization, negative feelings about body, multiple stressors and change in daily living, severe growth retardation [in height and weight]; dry skin, facial puffiness.)

Goal: Child will experience improved body image by (date and time to evaluate).

Outcome Criteria

✔ Verbalization of positive feelings about self.

NOC: *Self-Esteem*

INTERVENTIONS	RATIONALES
Assess child for feelings about abilities, chronic illness, difficulty in school and social situations, short stature, inability to keep up with peers.	Provides information about status of self-concept and special needs.
Encourage expression of feelings and concerns and support communication with parents, teachers, and peers.	Provides opportunity to vent feelings and reduce negative feelings about change in appearance.
Stress positive activities and accomplishments, avoid negative comments.	Enhances sense of positive body image, confidence, self-esteem.
Teach parents to maintain support for child.	Encourages acceptance of the child with special needs (dialysis, dietary requirements, urinary device, medications).
Encourage parents to be flexible in care of child and to integrate care and routines into family routines.	Promotes well-being of child and sense of belonging.
Teach child and parents about food selections which can be tolerated when eating out with friends.	Promotes social interactions with peers within limitations imposed by disease.

NIC: *Self-Esteem Enhancement*

Evaluation

(Date/time of evaluation of goal)

(Has goal been met? Not met? Partially met?)

(What did child verbalize about self?)

(Revisions to care plan? D/C care plan? Continue care plan?)

ANTICIPATORY GRIEVING

Related to: (Specify: perceived potential loss of child by parents; perceived potential loss of physiopsychosocial well-being by child.

Defining Characteristics: (Specify: expression of distress of potential loss, inevitable kidney failure, kidney dialysis, premature death of child.)

Goal: Parents and child will begin to work through the grief process by (date and time to evaluate).

Outcome Criteria

✔ Parents will verbalize stages of grief.

✔ Parents and child will identify 3 positive coping methods.

NOC: *Family Coping*

INTERVENTIONS	RATIONALES
Assess stage of grief process, problems encountered, feelings regarding long-term illness and potential loss of child.	Provides information about stage of grieving as time to work through the process varies with individuals; the longer the illness, the better able the parents and family will be able to move towards acceptance.
Provide emotional and spiritual comfort in an accepting environment and avoid conversations that will cause guilt or anger.	Provides for emotional needs of parents and assists them to cope with ill child without adding stressors that are difficult to resolve.
Allow for parental and child responses and expression of feelings.	Allows for reactions necessary to work through grieving.
Assist to identify and use effective coping mechanisms and to understand situations over which they have no control.	Promotes use of coping mechanisms over long period of time of illness; chronic disease causes physical and emotional stress on family members which may be positive or negative.

INTERVENTIONS	RATIONALES
Refer to social worker and/or counseling as appropriate (specify).	Offers information and support to parents and family in need of psychologic, economic assistance.
Teach parents of stages of grieving and behaviors that are common in resolving grief.	Promotes understanding of feelings and behaviors that are manifested by grief.
Assist parents and child to develop coping skills, problem solving skills and approaches that may be used.	Promotes coping ability over prolonged period of illness and assists in resolution of family stress.
Refer to clergy, local support groups for kidney diseases, National Kidney Foundation (specify).	Provides support and assistance in adapting and accepting chronic illness and services and information for care.

NIC: *Grief-Work Facilitation*

Evaluation

(Date/time of evaluation of goal)

(Has goal been met? Not met? Partially met?)

(What did parents say about the stages of grief? What 3 coping mechanisms were identified? Use quotes.)

(Revisions to care plan? D/C care plan? Continue care plan?)

RISK FOR INJURY

Related to: Renal failure.

Defining Characteristics: (Specify: complications of impaired renal function, hypertension, anemia, metabolic acidosis, osteodystrophy, neurologic manifestations, uremic syndrome if disorder untreated.)

Goal: Child will not experience injury by (date and time to evaluate).

Outcome Criteria

✔ BP remains (specify range for child).

✔ Hgb and Hct remain > (specify lower limit).

✔ Child denies bone pain or sensory loss.

NOC: *Risk Control*

INTERVENTIONS	RATIONALES
Assess blood pressure for alterations; administer antihypertensives ordered (specify).	Provides data regarding hypertension evident in advanced renal disease (action of drug).
Assess I&O, electrolyte panel, and creatinine; administer diuretics as ordered (specify).	Provides indication of renal function affecting output with water and electrolyte retention as disease progresses and nephrons are destroyed (action of drug).
Assess RBC, Hct, Hgb and administer iron and transfusion of packed red blood cells, as ordered (specify).	Provides indication of anemia caused by the reduced production of erythropoietin by the failing kidneys and inadequate intake of iron in a restricted diet.
Assess bone pain and deformities affecting ambulation and activities; administer supplemental vitamin D, calcium and alkalizing agents, as ordered.	Provides indication of osteodystrophy caused by a calcium phosphorus imbalance resulting in bone demineralization and growth retardation; kidney disease results in the inability to synthesize vitamin D needed to absorb Ca^{++}; acidosis causes dissolution of alkaline salts of bone, phosphate is increased, and calcium decreased as glomerular filtration is reduced.
Assess presence of acidosis by pH, bicarbonate losses and administer alkalizing agents (specify).	Provides indication of impending metabolic acidosis caused by the inability of the failing kidneys to excrete metabolic acids that are byproducts of metabolism; the hydrogen ion is retained and bicarbonate is lost as the tubules are unable to reabsorb it.
Assess for sensory loss, confusion and changes in consciousness.	Reveals possible changes in neurologic status as kidney function deteriorates and uremic syndrome appears.

INTERVENTIONS	RATIONALES
Teach parents medication administration including actions, dosage, frequency, side effects to report.	Ensures compliance of correct medication administration; long-term of many medications are given for disease to prevent complications and uremic syndrome.
Instruct parents and child in dietary regimen, to restrict Na^+, K^+, HOP^{2-}_4 and include Ca^{++}, iron in diet, to restrict protein and water intake if appropriate and amounts allowed; offer lists of foods and sample menus for planning (specify).	Promotes compliance with dietary inclusions or restrictions depending on degree of renal failure.
Teach parents and child of dialysis procedure and frequency if appropriate; include biologic, psychological and social effects.	Provides information if renal dialysis is needed; usually based on creatinine level which indicated the ability of the kidneys to excrete waste materials and the degree of renal failure.

NIC: *Surveillance*

Evaluation

(Date/time of evaluation of goal)

(Has goal been met? Not met? Partially met?)

(What is BP? Hgb and Hct? What does child say about bone pain? Give examples of sensory ability.)

(Revisions to care plan? D/C care plan? Continue care plan?)

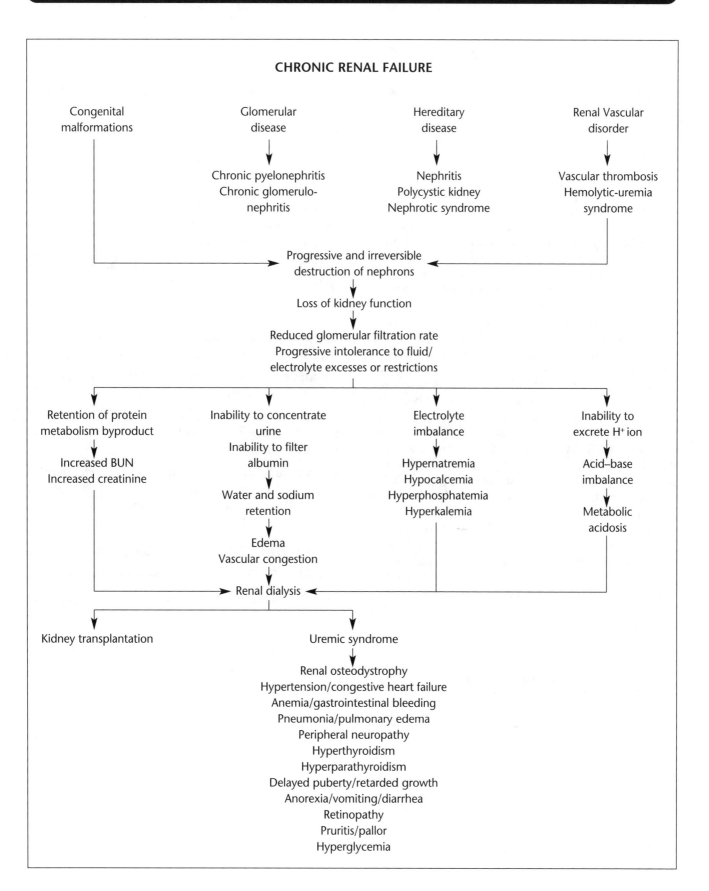

CHAPTER 5.2

GLOMERULONEPHRITIS

Acute glomerulonephritis (AGN) is an alteration in renal function caused by glomerular injury, which is displayed by the classic symptoms of gross hematuria, mild proteinuria, edema (usually periorbital), hypertension, and oliguria. AGN is also classified as either: a primary disease, associated with group A, beta-hemolytic streptococcal infection; or a secondary disease, associated with various systemic diseases (i.e., systemic lupus erythema, sickle cell disease, Henoch's chorea purpura). The most common type of AGN is the primary disease, described as an immune-complex disease (or an antigen-antibody complex formed during the streptococcal infection which becomes entrapped in the glomerular membrane, causing inflammation 8 to 14 days after the onset of this infection). AGN is primarily observed in the early school-age child, with a peak age of onset of 6 to 7 years. The onset of the classic symptoms of AGN is usually abrupt, self-limiting (unpredictable), and prolonged hematuria and proteinuria may occur. AGN results in decreased glomerular filtration rate causing retention of water and sodium (edema); expanded plasma and interstitial fluid volumes that lead to circulatory congestion and edema (hypervolemia); hypertension (cause is unexplained; plasma renin activity is low during the acute phase, hypervolemia is suspected to be the cause).

MEDICAL CARE

DIAGNOSTIC EVALUATION

Urinalysis: reveals gross hematuria, and some proteinuria, increased specific gravity. Microscopic examination of the urine sediment will reveal: red blood cells, leukocytes, epithelial cells, granular and red blood cast cells. Bacteria not present, urine cultures negative.

Creatinine Clearance: reveals increase in AGN. Determines presence of severe renal impairment.

Blood Urea Nitrogen (BUN): determines presence of renal disease, dehydration, hemorrhage, high protein intake, corticosteroids therapy.

Electrolyte Panel: will reveal normal electrolytes (sodium, potassium, and chloride ions) and carbon dioxide levels (unless the AGN has progressed to renal failure).

Complete Blood Count: reveals decreased RBC, Hct, Hgb and increased WBC.

Throat Culture: positive cultures of the pharynx (occur in only a few cases).

Antistreptolysin O (ASO): an ASO titer of 250 Todd units or higher is diagnostic for AGN, as is a rising titer in 2 samples taken a week apart.

Erythrocyte Sedimentation Rate (ESR), C-Reactive Protein (CRP), and Serum Mucoprotein Test: are all elevated during the early stages of AGN and then gradually return to normal as healing occurs.

MEDICAL MANAGEMENT

Diuretics: to treat edema and fluid overload.

Antihypertensives: with diuretics to decrease blood pressure.

Hyperkalemia Treatment: if hyperkalemia is present, administration of calcium, glucose and insulin, or a sodium polystyrene sulfonate (Kayexalate) enema may be required.

COMMON NURSING DIAGNOSES

See EXCESS FLUID VOLUME

Related to: Compromised regulatory mechanism.

Defining Characteristics: (Specify: dependent edema, periorbital edema, pleural effusion, puffiness in the face, moderate blood pressure increases, intake greater than output, weight gain, azotemia, crackles and pleural effusion (occasionally is seen if pulmonary congestion occurs), decreased Hgb and Hct, altered electrolytes, decreased urinary output.)

See IMBALANCED NUTRITION: LESS THAN BODY REQUIREMENTS

Related to: Loss of appetite.

Defining Characteristics: (Specify: anorexia fatigue, nausea, vomiting, malaise, no added-salt diet, lethargy, abdominal discomfort.)

See INEFFECTIVE TISSUE PERFUSION: CEREBRAL

Related to: (Specify: hypervolemia, hypertensive encephalopathy, cerebral ischemia.)

Defining Characteristics: (Specify: early signs of hypertensive encephalopathy: headache, dizziness, abdominal discomfort, and vomiting; if hypertensive encephalopathy worsens: transient loss of vision and/or hemiparesis, disorientation, generalized convulsions (tonic/clonic type), coma.)

See RISK FOR IMPAIRED SKIN INTEGRITY

Related to: Edema, altered circulation.

Defining Characteristics: (Specify: bed rest, impaired tissue perfusion, pressure on skin and bony prominences, pink or redness of skin, disruption of skin from IV infusions.)

ADDITIONAL NURSING DIAGNOSES

ACTIVITY INTOLERANCE

Related to: Generalized weakness, bed rest.

Defining Characteristics: (Specify: expressed weakness and fatigue, anemia, lethargy.)

Goal: Child will progress to increased tolerance for activity by (date and time to evaluate).

Outcome Criteria

✔ (Specify an activity level appropriate for child; e.g., child will play with a puzzle.)

NOC: *Activity Tolerance*

INTERVENTIONS	RATIONALES
Assess weakness, fatigue, ability to move about in bed and participate in play activities.	Provides information about energy reserves during the acute phase of the disease and acceptance of bed rest status.
Schedule care and provide rest periods following any activity in a quiet environment.	Provides adequate rest and reduces stimuli and fatigue.
Maintain bed rest during the acute stage, disturb only when necessary.	Conserves energy and decreases production of waste materials which increases work of the kidneys.
Provide for quiet play, reading, TV, games as symptoms subside.	Provides diversion, stimulation and requires minimal energy expenditures.
Explain reason for activity restriction to parents and child.	Promotes understanding of the need to conserve energy and rest to promote recovery.
Inform parents and child to rest following ambulation or any activity.	Prevents fatigue and conserves energy during recovery.
Instruct parents and child to rest when feeling tired.	Prevents fatigue and promotes recovery.

NIC: *Activity Therapy*

Evaluation

(Date/time of evaluation of goal)

(Has goal been met? Not met? Partially met?)

(What has been child's activity level? How does it compare with the outcome criteria?)

(Revisions to care plan? D/C care plan? Continue care plan?)

RISK FOR INFECTION

Related to: Chronic disease.

Defining Characteristics: (Specify: persistent streptococcal infections.)

Goal: Child will not experience infection by (date and time to evaluate).

Outcome Criteria

✔ Child denies sore throat.

✔ Throat cultures are negative.

NOC: *Risk Detection*

INTERVENTIONS	RATIONALES
Assess temperature, chills, sore throat, cough (presence or recurrence).	Indicates persistence of streptococcal infection.
Obtain throat culture for analysis and sensitivities.	Identifies streptococcal microorganism and sensitivity to specific antibiotic therapy.
Administer antibiotic therapy to child and to family members if ordered (specify).	Destroys microbial agents by preventing cell wall synthesis and prevents transmission to family members.
Instruct parents about antibiotic therapy and to administer full course of medication.	Promotes parental understanding and prevents development of super-infection.
Provide for disposal of used tissues and articles properly.	Prevents transmission of microorganisms to others or reinfection.
Instruct child and family to wash hands after sneezing/coughing and to dispose of used tissues.	Prevents spread of disease.
Instruct parents to avoid exposure of child to others with upper respiratory infection.	Prevents respiratory infections in the susceptible child.
Inform parents to report fever, cough, sore throat.	Indicates infection and provides for early intervention.

NIC: *Infection Control*

Evaluation

(Date/time of evaluation of goal)

(Has goal been met? Not met? Partially met?)

(Does child deny sore throat? What are results of throat cultures?)

(Revisions to care plan? D/C care plan? Continue care plan?)

RISK FOR INJURY

Related to: Impaired renal function.

Defining Characteristics: (Specify: complications of impaired renal function, hypertension, cardiac failure, renal failure; risk of complications (i.e., encephalopathy, congestive heart failure, acute renal failure).)

Goal: Child will not experience injury by (date and time to evaluate).

Outcome Criteria

✔ BP remains (specify range for child).

✔ Child denies headache, appears calm.

NOC: *Risk Detection*

INTERVENTIONS	RATIONALES
Assess BP, pulse, respirations q 4h (monitor BP q 1h if diastolic is more than 90, pulse and respirations q 1h if tachycardia, tachypnea or dyspnea present).	Provides information about complication of hypertension which may lead to encephalopathy, pulse and respirations that change with heart failure and pulmonary edema.
Assess changes in I&O, extent of edema, decreased urinary output, headache, pallor, electrolyte balance.	Indicates signs and symptoms of possible renal failure.
Administer antihypertensives, diuretic therapy, cardiac glycoside (specify) and monitor for expected results (specify).	Provides therapy for complications if a more severe renal impairment is present (action of drugs).
Limit fluids as ordered; allow intake of the amount lost via urine and insensible losses (specify).	Prevents further fluid retention and edema in the presence of renal damage.
Limit foods high in Na$^+$, K$^+$ and protein during the acute phase of AGN; encourage a diet with the increased carbohydrates and fats (only during acute phase of AGN), as ordered.	Provides nutrition during the acute period with limitation of K$^+$ during oliguria, Na$^+$ with presence of edema, protein limitation if oliguria is prolonged.
Note behavior changes including lethargy, irritability, restlessness associated with hypertension and administer anticonvulsives if ordered (specify).	Indicates need for safety precautions associated with seizure activity as a result of cerebral changes.
Teach parents about potential for complications and signs and symptoms to report (increased weight, blood in urine with decreased amount of output, complaints of headache and anorexia).	Provides for early intervention to prevent severe renal impairment.

INTERVENTIONS	RATIONALES
Teach about dietary inclusions and restrictions; offer a list of foods to include and avoid that comply with Na+, K+, protein allowances.	Provides nutrition while disease is being resolved.
Encourage to allow activity/rest periods as energy and fatigue requires; progressively increase as condition warrants.	Prevents fatigue and conserves energy during acute stage and convalescence.
Reinforce to parents the need for follow-up care and supervision.	Ensures ongoing monitoring of child for chronic renal disease or persistent streptococcal infection.

NIC: *Surveillance*

Evaluation

(Date/time of evaluation of goal)

(Has goal been met? Not met? Partially met?)

(What is child's BP? Describe child's behavior. Does child deny headache?)

(Revisions to care plan? D/C care plan? Continue care plan?)

GLOMERULONEPHRITIS

Post-streptococcal infection
(group A, beta-hemolytic)
↓
Release of material from the organism into the
circulation (antigen)
↓
Formation of antibody
↓
Immune-complex reaction in the
glomerular capillary
↓
Inflammatory response
↓
Proliferation of endothelial cells lining
glomerulus and cells between endothelium and
epithelium of capillary membrane
↓
Swelling of capillary membrane and infiltration
with leukocytes
Increased permeability of base membrane
↓
Occlusion of the capillaries of glomeruli
Vasospasm of afferent arterioles
↓
Decreased glomerular filtration rate
↓
Decreased ability to form filtrate from
glomeruli plasma flow
↓
Retention of water and sodium
Reduced circulatory volume (hypovolemia)
Circulatory congestion
↓
Edema (peripheral and periorbital)
Hypertension
Decreased urinary output (hematuria, proteinuria)
Urine dark in color
Anorexia
Irritability lethargy
↓
Acute glomerulonephritis

CHAPTER 5.3

HYPOSPADIAS/EPISPADIAS

Hypospadias and epispadias are congenital defects of the penis that result in incomplete development of the anterior urethra. The congenital defect results in an abnormal urethral opening at any place along the shaft of the penis and may even open onto the scrotum or perineum. The incidence of this defect in the United States is approximately 3.2 in 1,000 live male births or about 1 in every 300 male children. The etiology of this defect is unknown but is associated with a higher familial tendency and by race/ethnic background (more common in whites, Italians, and Jews). Chordee, an abnormal curvature of the penis, is frequently associated with hypospadias. Other associated anomalies/diseases include: undescended testes (9%–32%); inguinal hernia (9%–17%); and Wilms' tumor.

The goal of treatment of this defect is to reconstruct a straight penis with a meatus close to the normal anatomic location. Repair is being performed at progressively younger ages to avoid emotional distress in the young child. Currently, the recommended age for repair is between 3 and 12 months (for hypospadias/epispadias or urethroplasty); and during the first year (for chordee repair or orthoplasty). Three objectives of surgical correction of this defect are: to ensure the child's ability to void in the standing position with a straight stream (will minimize child and parent anxiety); to improve the child's physical appearance and ensure a positive body image; and to preserve sexual function.

MEDICAL CARE

Analgesics: postoperatively to control pain.

Antibiotics: to prevent infection or treat infection postoperatively.

Complete Blood Count: reveals increased WBC if infection present.

Chromosome Analysis: testosterone level reveals male hormone if ambiguous genitalia is present.

COMMON NURSING DIAGNOSES

See RISK FOR IMPAIRED SKIN INTEGRITY

Related to: Surgical incision.

Defining Characteristics: (Specify: disruption of skin surface, surgical correction of defect, catheter site irritation, poor wound healing or wound infection, edema within the urethra.)

See RISK FOR DEFICIENT FLUID VOLUME

Related to: (Specify.)

Defining Characteristics: (Specify: NPO preoperatively, temperature elevation with infection, decreased urinary output, inadequate fluid replacement postoperatively, risk of intraoperative hemorrhage and postoperative bleeding.)

See HYPERTHERMIA

Related to: Presence of postoperative wound infection or UTI (specify).

Defining Characteristics: (Specify: increase in body temperature above normal range, warm to touch, increased pulse and respiratory rate, evidence of infection at surgical site, evidence of lower urinary tract infection.)

ADDITIONAL NURSING DIAGNOSES

ANXIETY

Related to: (Specify: threat to self-concept, change in health status, change in environment [hospitalization].)

Defining Characteristics: (Specify: expressed apprehension and concern about correction of defect by surgery and the imperfect appearance of the penis following surgery, preoperative and postoperative care.)

Goal: Parents will experience less anxiety by (date and time to evaluate).

Outcome Criteria

✔ Parents state they feel less anxious.

NOC: *Coping*

INTERVENTIONS	RATIONALES
Assess source and level of anxiety and need for information that will relieve anxiety.	Provides information about anxiety level and need to relieve it; concerns include the type of procedure and appearance of penis after surgery; whether the penis will be sexually adequate; possibility that correction may need to be done in stages if child is old enough; fear of castration and change in body image.
Encourage expression of concerns and time for parents (and child) to ask questions about condition, procedures, recovery.	Provides opportunity to vent feelings and fears and secure environment.
Answer questions calmly and honestly; use pictures, drawings, and models for information.	Promotes trust and a calm, supportive environment.
Encourage parents to stay with child during hospitalizations and to assist in care.	Allows parents to care for and support child and continue parental role.
Ask for parents' input into decisions about care and usual routines.	Allows for control over situations and maintains familiar routines for care.
Inform parents of cause of defect, and extent of defect to be corrected, whether a mild defect or severe defect, that correction is best done between 3 to 9 months, placement of meatus on penis, and possible number of procedures necessary to correct defect (specify).	Provides information that will enhance understanding of the defect to relieve anxiety.
Teach parents of reason for surgery (urethroplasty), type of procedure, appearance of penis following surgery and cosmetic results to expect; inform older	Provides rationale for surgery which includes voiding in a standing position with ability to direct stream, improve appearance of penis and preserve

INTERVENTIONS	RATIONALES
child that penis will not be cut off and that procedure is not a form of punishment.	self-image, and to develop a sexually adequate penis.
Teach parents about postoperative care (indwelling meatal or suprapubic catheter or stents will be in place; restraints may be in place; medications will be administered to control pain and promote sedation; specify).	Provides information about postoperative care and what to expect following surgery.
Teach parents relaxation techniques.	Reduces anxiety and promotes ability to provide calm and supportive care.
Reassure parents and child (if appropriate) that defect or surgery will not affect sexual activity or orientation and will not affect reproductive ability.	Relieves anxiety produced by fear caused by misinformation.

NIC: *Anxiety Reduction*

Evaluation

(Date/time of evaluation of goal)

(Has goal been met? Not met? Partially met?)

(How do parents evaluate their anxiety now?)

(Revisions to care plan? D/C care plan? Continue care plan?)

PAIN

Related to: Surgery.

Defining Characteristics: (Specify: communication of pain descriptors, crying, irritability, restlessness, withdrawal, increased P, increased R, increased BP.)

Goal: Infant will experience decreased pain by (date and time to evaluate).

Outcome Criteria

✔ Infant will score less than (specify pain scale to be used and expected score after interventions).

NOC: *Comfort Level*

INTERVENTIONS	RATIONALES
Assess verbal and nonverbal behavior; type, location and severity of pain depending on child's age. (Specify pain scale to be used.)	Provides information about pain as basis for analgesic therapy.
Administer analgesic and sedative, as ordered (specify).	Reduces pain and promotes rest which reduces stimuli and pain (action).
Place in position of comfort; position catheter to avoid tension and kinking.	Promotes comfort and prevents pain from pulling on or manipulating catheter.
Apply ice pack if ordered.	Reduces edema and pain.
Inform parents that medications will prevent pain and restlessness and allow for healing.	Provides information about need for pain medications for child's comfort.

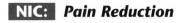 **Pain Reduction**

Evaluation

(Date/time of evaluation of goal)

(Has goal been met? Not met? Partially met?)

(What is score on pain scale now?)

(Revisions to care plan? D/C care plan? Continue care plan?)

▓▓▓ RISK FOR INFECTION

Related to: (Specify: inadequate primary defenses [surgical incision]; invasive procedure [catheter].)

Defining Characteristics: (Specify: redness, swelling, drainage at incision site; cloudy, foul-smelling urine, elevated temperature, positive urine or wound culture.)

Goal: Infant will not become infected by (date and time to evaluate).

Outcome Criteria

✔ Wound is clean and intact without redness, edema, odor or drainage.

✔ Urine culture negative.

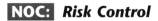 **Risk Control**

INTERVENTIONS	RATIONALES
Assess wound for redness, swelling, drainage on dressing, healing (specify when).	Provides information indicating presence of infection or poor healing.
Assess catheter insertion site for redness, irritation, swelling; assess urine collected in drainage system for cloudiness, foul odor, sediment (specify frequency).	Indicates infectious process at catheter site or in urinary bladder.
Collect urine specimen for culture and sensitivities (as ordered).	Provides information about specific organism and sensitivity to antibiotic.
Administer anti-infective if culture results are 100,000 ml/mm or more as ordered (specify).	Treats specific organism causing urinary infection or prevents infection when catheter is in place.
Use sterile technique when changing dressings or giving catheter care or emptying drainage bag.	Prevents contamination by introducing organisms into sterile wound or cavity.
Encourage to increase fluid intake according to age needs (specify).	Promotes dilution of urine to prevent urinary infection and after catheter removed will encourage voiding.
Maintain catheter and collection bag below level of bladder and a closed drainage system free of kinks in the tubing (if a drainage device is used) then maintain catheter and collection bag—marked in red.	Provides information that will enhance understanding of the defect to relieve anxiety.
Immobilize arms and legs with restraints, remove periodically; use a bed cradle following surgery.	Prevents accidental removal or disturbance of catheter or contamination of wound if surgical correction done for a more severe defect.
Avoid change of dressing, reinforce as needed, and secure catheter to penis with dressing and tape, and to leg or abdomen with tape.	Promotes comfort and prevents infection and catheter displacement.
Note urinary output of at least 1 ml/kg/hr and report if less.	Indicates that catheter obstruction may be present with urinary retention which leads to infection.
Demonstrate to parents catheter care, irrigation, emptying of drainage bag or use of diaper for urine drainage, how to tape catheter and bag to leg; allow for return demonstration.	Provides information and skill in caring and maintaining patency for catheter as child may be discharged with a catheter or stent in place.

(continues)

(continued)

INTERVENTIONS	RATIONALES
Teach parents to avoid allowing child to straddle toys, play in a sandbox, swim, or engage in rough activities until advised by physician.	Prevents trauma to or dislodging of catheter or infection.
Teach parents to sponge bathe the child and use loose fitting clothing, avoiding contact of feces with wound, and instruct in cleansing after each bowel elimination.	Promotes cleanliness and comfort without constriction.
Teach parents in signs and symptoms of infection to report.	Provides information about need for reporting to allow for early treatment.

NIC: *Infection Control*

Evaluation

(Date/time of evaluation of goal)

(Has goal been met? Not met? Partially met?)

(Describe wound. What are results of urine culture?)

(Revisions to care plan? D/C care plan? Continue care plan?)

 ## IMPAIRED URINARY ELIMINATION

Related to: (Specify: mechanical trauma [urethroplasty].)

Defining Characteristics: (Specify: dysuria, frequency, urgency, retention, bladder spasms, inadequate output, edema of the urethra.)

Goal: Client will experience improved urinary elimination by (date and time to evaluate).

Outcome Criteria

✔ Client voids through new or corrected urinary meatus after catheter is removed.

✔ Unable to palpate bladder after voiding.

NOC: *Urinary Elimination*

INTERVENTIONS	RATIONALES
Assess I&O ratio, voiding stream, color and amount of urine on first voiding and each subsequent voiding.	Provides information about voiding pattern after clamping or removal of catheter.
Assess for pain, abdominal distention, inability to void for 8 hours after catheter.	Indicates urinary dysfunction and possible obstruction or continuing edema of meatus.
Support child after catheter is removed and provide privacy for voiding.	Prevents embarrassment which is common in an older child.
Encourage increased fluid intake after catheter removed, offer preferred liquids q 1h.	Promotes micturition.
Instruct parents to notify physician if urinary pattern changes or if child is unable to void.	Allows for early intervention to prevent complications.

NIC: *Urinary Elimination Management*

Evaluation

(Date/time of evaluation of goal)

(Has goal been met? Not met? Partially met?)

(Describe client's ability to void through new or corrected meatus. Is bladder palpable above symphysis after voiding?)

(Revisions to care plan? D/C care plan? Continue care plan?)

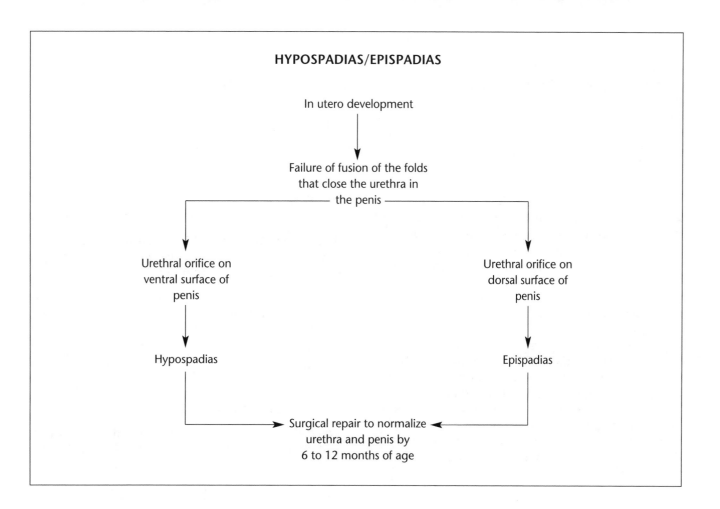

CHAPTER 5.4

NEPHROTIC SYNDROME

Nephrotic syndrome is an alteration of renal function caused by increased glomerular basement membrane permeability to plasma protein (albumin). Alterations to the glomerulus result in classic symptoms of gross proteinuria, hypoalbuminemia, generalized edema (anasarca), oliguria, and hyperlipidemia. Nephrotic syndrome is classified either by etiology or the histologic changes in the glomerulus. Nephrotic syndrome is also classified into 3 types: primary minimal change nephrotic syndrome (MCNS), secondary nephrotic syndrome, and congenital nephrotic syndrome. The most common type of nephrotic syndrome is MCNS (idiopathic type) and it accounts for 80% of cases of nephrotic syndrome. MCNS can occur at any age but usually the age of onset is during the preschool years. MCNS is also seen more in male children than in female children. Secondary nephrotic syndrome is frequently associated with secondary renal involvement from systemic diseases. Congenital nephrotic syndrome (CNS) is caused by a rare autosomal recessive gene which is localized on the long arm of chromosome 19. Currently, CNS has a better prognosis because of early treatment of protein deficiency, nutritional support, continuous cycling peritoneal dialysis (CCPD), and renal transplantation. The prognosis for MCNS is usually good, but relapses are common, and most children respond to treatment.

MEDICAL CARE

Diagnostic Evaluation: Evaluation is based on the history and the presence of classic clinical manifestations of MCNS.

Urinalysis: reveals great increases of protein (proteinuria) of 3+ to 4+ or 300 to 1000 mg/dl; increased sp. gr.; hyaline-casts and few RBC.

Renal Biopsy: provides information regarding the glomerulus status, type of nephrotic syndrome, expected response to steroids and prognosis.

Creatinine Clearance: reveals increase in MCNS. It will determine presence of severe renal impairment.

Blood Urea Nitrogen (BUN): determines presence of renal disease, dehydration, hemorrhage, high protein intake, corticosteroids therapy.

Serum Protein: reveals decreases in total proteins (albumin and globulin) with electrophoresis revealing a great decrease in albumin.

Serum Lipids: reveals increases with a great increase in cholesterol to 450 to 1500 mg/dl.

Electrolyte Panel: reveals decreased Na$^+$ and Ca^{++} and K$^+$ at normal level.

Complete Blood Count: reveals normal Hct and Hgb and increased platelet count of 500,000 to 1,000,000 cu/mm resulting from hemoconcentration.

MEDICAL MANAGEMENT

Corticosteroid Therapy: continues until the urine is free from protein and remains normal for 10 days to 2 weeks. A positive response to therapy usually occurs in 1 to 3 weeks.

Plasma Expanders: human albumin for severe edema to increase plasma protein level and promote diuresis.

Diuretics: typically not used; used for edema which interferes with respirations or results in secondary skin breakdown.

Diet: salt is restricted by a no-added salt diet and a diet generous in protein. A high-protein diet is a contraindication with the presence of azotemia and renal failure.

COMMON NURSING DIAGNOSES

See EXCESS FLUID VOLUME

Related to: Compromised regulatory mechanism.

Defining Characteristics: (Specify: edema [pitting], periorbital and facial puffiness in morning and dependent in the evening, abdominal ascites, scrotal or labial edema, edema of mucous membranes of intestines, anasarca, slow weight gain, decreased urine output, altered electrolytes, sp. gr., BP, R.)

See IMBALANCED NUTRITION: LESS THAN BODY REQUIREMENTS

Related to: (Specify: inability to ingest and digest foods and absorb nutrients.)

Defining Characteristics: (Specify: anorexia, edema of intestinal tract affecting absorption, weight loss, loss of protein [negative nitrogen balance], rejection of low salt diet.)

See RISK FOR IMPAIRED SKIN INTEGRITY

Related to: Edema.

Defining Characteristics: (Specify: disruption of skin surface, waxy pallor, stretched and shiny appearance, muscle wasting, decreased tissue perfusion, pressure on edematous area, irritation of anal area with diarrhea.)

See DIARRHEA

Related to: Inflammation, edema, malabsorption.

Defining Characteristics: (Specify: increased frequency, loose, liquid stools, abdominal discomfort.)

See RISK FOR DEFICIENT FLUID VOLUME

Related to: (Specify: medications, intravascular fluid loss.)

Defining Characteristics: (Specify: diuretic therapy, increased fluid output, urinary frequency, rapid weight loss, hypotension, hypovolemia, protein and fluid loss, edema.)

ADDITIONAL NURSING DIAGNOSES

FATIGUE

Related to: Discomfort.

Defining Characteristics: (Specify: extreme edema, lethargy, easily fatigued with any activity.)

Goal: Child will conserve energy by (date and time to evaluate).

Outcome Criteria

✔ Child alternates activity with rest periods (specify).

NOC: *Energy Conservation*

INTERVENTIONS	RATIONALES
Assess degree of weakness, fatigue, extent of edema and difficult movement or activity in bed.	Provides information about fatigue and tendency of lying in prone position and not moving or changing position.
Maintain bed rest during most acute stage.	Prevents energy expenditure when edema is severe.
Provide selected play activities as tolerated and adjust schedule to allow for rest periods and after activity.	Provides stimulation and activity within endurance level as edema is relieved.
Plan activities with discretion and observe for behavior changes after activity.	Prevents fatigue while improving endurance; inactivity and steroid therapy and disease result in mood swings and irritability in the child.
Allow for quiet play followed by unrestricted activity and encourage child to set own limits when feasible.	Promotes independence and control of situations.
Inform child to rest when feeling tired.	Reduces fatigue and conserves energy.
Inform parents and child that full participation in activities will be allowed as the disease is resolved.	Promotes return to active life for child.

NIC: *Energy Management*

Evaluation

(Date/time of evaluation of goal)

(Has goal been met? Not met? Partially met?)

(Describe child's activity and rest pattern.)

(Revisions to care plan? D/C care plan? Continue care plan?)

RISK FOR INFECTION

Related to: Inadequate secondary defenses.

Defining Characteristics: (Specify: fluid overload, edema, elevated temperature, immunosuppression, suppressed inflammatory response, leukopenia.)

Goal: Child will not become infected by (date and time to evaluate).

Outcome Criteria

✔ Temperature remains <99° F.
✔ Breath sounds clear bilaterally.
✔ Urine is clear without foul odor.

NOC: *Risk Detection*

INTERVENTIONS	RATIONALES
Assess temperature elevation, respiratory changes (dyspnea, productive cough with yellow sputum), urinary changes (cloudy, foul-smelling urine), skin changes (redness, swelling, pain in an area) (specify when).	Indicates presence of infectious process resulting from steroid and immunosuppressant therapy given to enhance body defenses and reduce relapse rate.
Provide private room or share room with children who are free from infections.	Protects child from pathogen transmission.
Maintain and teach medical aseptic techniques and handwashing when giving care.	Promotes measures to prevent infection.
Maintain warmth for child, regulate room environmental temperature and humidity.	Prevents chilling and predisposition to upper respiratory infection.
Administer antibiotic therapy if ordered (specify).	Prevents or treats infection based on culture and sensitivities (action of drug).
Instruct parents and child to avoid exposure to those with infections.	Provides understanding of susceptibility to infections.
Instruct parents to report any sign or symptom of infection to physician immediately.	Allows for immediate medical intervention to prevent relapse.

NIC: *Infection Control*

Evaluation

(Date/time of evaluation of goal)
(Has goal been met? Not met? Partially met?)

(What is temperature? Describe breath sounds and urine)
(Revisions to care plan? D/C care plan? Continue care plan?)

DEFICIENT KNOWLEDGE

Related to: Lack of exposure to information about disease.

Defining Characteristics: (Specify: expressed need for information about disease, medication administration, follow-up care and procedures, anxiety associated with relapse of disease.)

Goal: Parents will obtain information about child's illness by (date and time to evaluate).

Outcome Criteria

✔ Parents verbalize understanding of cause and treatment for illness.

NOC: *Knowledge: Disease Process*

INTERVENTIONS	RATIONALES
Assess knowledge of disease, signs and symptoms of relapse, dietary and activity aspects of care, medication administration and side effects, monitoring urine and VS.	Provides information about teaching needs for follow-up care.
Assess level of anxiety and need for support in care of ill child and possible relapse.	Anxiety will interfere with learning process.
Teach parents and child about the cause of the child's illness and treatment to expect. Encourage questions and allow time for discussion.	Teaching provides needed information about the disease and treatment.
Teach about medication administration including side effects of steroids and immunosuppressives; that these are reversible when discontinued and must be discontinued gradually.	Promotes compliance of accurate medication administration and what can be expected from drug therapy.
Inform parents that immunizations may be postponed.	Provides safety measure to prevent complications in a child that is immunosuppressive.

INTERVENTIONS	RATIONALES
Teach parents and child of potential for relapse to avoid infection.	Prevents risk of infection that may precipitate a relapse.
Demonstrate and allow for parents to return demonstrate urine testing by dipstick for albumin, monitor for edema, taking daily weights and BP, and to report changes of increased weight or presence of albumin in urine to physician immediately.	Allows for monitoring of possible relapse of disease.
Offer praise and encouragement to parents and child as they learn skills.	Positive reinforcement enhances desire to learn new skills.
Reinforce physician instructions about Na$^+$ restriction, activity progression and pacing.	Promotes return to usual patterns of living.
Provide information about disease, its causes, need for frequent hospitalizations if disease becomes prolonged or is a relapsing type with remissions and exacerbations.	Promotes understanding of disease process and importance of compliance with therapy to prevent exacerbation.

NIC: *Teaching: Disease Process*

Evaluation

(Date/time of evaluation of goal)

(Has goal been met? Not met? Partially met?)

(What did parents verbalize about the cause and treatment of the child's illness? Use quotes.)

(Revisions to care plan? D/C care plan? Continue care plan?)

NEPHROTIC SYNDROME (NEPHROSIS)

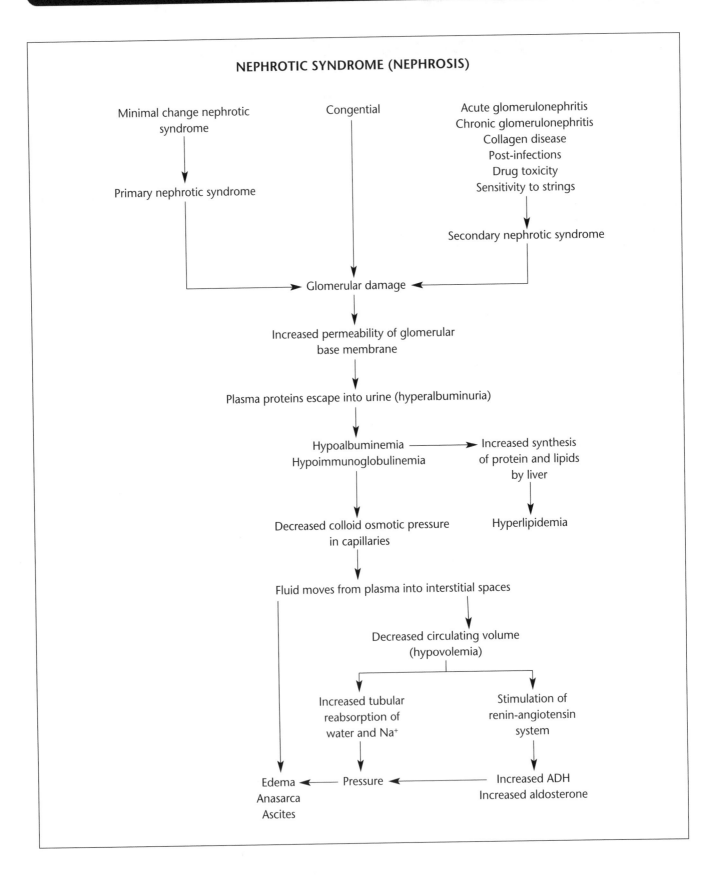

CHAPTER 5.5

SEXUALLY TRANSMITTED DISEASES

Sexually transmitted diseases (STD) are a diverse group of viral, bacterial, protozoal, and ectoparasitic infections that have a common route of transmission through sexual intercourse. Infectious organisms associated with STDs include: *Chlamydia trachomatis*; *Neisseria gonorrhoeae*; bacterial vaginosis, vulvovaginal candidiasis, trichomoniasis; syphilis; herpes simplex; papillomavirus (genital warts); genital herpes and HIV. Infection by each of the above organisms has its own pattern of clinical patterns; medications/treatments; prognosis; transmission dynamics/host response to infection; and patterns of sexual contact.

STDs are identified as one of the major causes of morbidity during adolescence.

MEDICAL CARE

DIAGNOSTIC EVALUATION

Diagnosis is completed by identification of the organism from direct smear or culture techniques.

Venereal Disease Research Laboratory (VDRL): reveals presence of *Treponema pallidum* (syphilis) by antibody tests (FTA-ABS and TPI).

Cultures: Urethral and/or cervical smears for microorganism identification in gonorrhea, Chlamydia, urethritis; lesion smear to detect herpes, syphilis.

MEDICAL MANAGEMENT

Antibiotics: specific for the infectious organism.

Anti-viral Medications: to decrease severity and possible prevent recurrent outbreaks.

COMMON NURSING DIAGNOSES

See RISK FOR IMPAIRED SKIN INTEGRITY

Related to: External factor of excretions and secretions, internal factor of infectious agent invasion.

Defining Characteristics: Disruption of skin surface, invasion of body structures, pus from urethra or cervix, vesicles on genitalia, buttocks, thighs, penile or vaginal discharge, chancre lesion on penis or female genitalia, skin rash, popupapules on skin, blisters and ulcerations on genitalia, itching and burning of lesions or sores, conjunctivitis, pharyngitis, dermatitis.

See HYPERTHERMIA

Related to: Pelvic inflammatory disease.

Defining Characteristics: (Specify: increase in body temperature above normal range, warm to touch, increased pulse and respiratory rate, evidence of infectious process.)

ADDITIONAL NURSING DIAGNOSES

DEFICIENT KNOWLEDGE

Related to: Lack of information about disease.

Defining Characteristics: (Specify: expressed need for information about treatment and prevention of recurrence of sexually transmitted disease.)

Goal: Child will obtain information about sexually transmitted diseases and how to prevent them by (date and time to evaluate).

Outcome Criteria

✔ Client verbalizes understanding of mode of transmission for STDs and identifies 2 ways to avoid becoming infected.

NOC: *Knowledge: Disease Process*

INTERVENTIONS	RATIONALES
Assess knowledge of signs and symptoms of specific diseases, risk factors in acquiring or transmitting disease, and potential complications.	Provides information about the disease causes, treatment and preventive measures.

(continues)

(continued)

INTERVENTIONS	RATIONALES
Teach about type of culture and blood testing done for diagnosis of disease.	Provides information about need to identify specific organisms by culture of discharge from lesions, urethra, vagina, and cervix.
Teach to report pain, tingling, burning, dysuria, frequency, purulent discharge or leukorrhea, itching of genitalia.	Indicates active disease caused by lesion, inflammation.
Teach about treatment: antibiotics, analgesics, topical agents as ordered (specify); emphasize need to take full course of ordered antibiotic and follow-up exam for syphilis, gonorrhea, pelvic inflammation, chlamydial infection; (application of topical chemical agent and removing the drug by washing off in 4–6 hours to remove warts); (topical application of topical antiviral to treat herpes) (specify).	Provides treatment of choice for specific disease and instructions for administration (action of drug).
Inform that disease is contracted and transmitted by sexual contact and to avoid sexual contact with an infected partner and during active phase of the disease; instruct to use male or female condom protection if sexually active.	Prevents spread of the disease to others and recurrence in the infected person.
Instruct in handwashing technique to be used following toileting and to avoid touching face with hands.	Prevents transmission of infectious agents to genitalia or other body parts.
Explain consequences of disease if left untreated or follow-up evaluation avoided.	Prevents progression or complications of the disease; may lead to infertility or second stage syphilis.
Reassure that information will be kept confidential according to state laws.	Promotes environment conducive to instruction and that is nonjudgmental and accepting.

INTERVENTIONS	RATIONALES
Teach about causes of flare-ups of herpes and to avoid changes in environment extremes, tight clothing, colds, exposure to sun.	Prevents recurrence of herpes lesions that commonly occur with illnesses, trauma, or changes that may lower resistance.
Encourage to report the disease and inform contacts.	Promotes control of disease by tracing and treating contacts as well as the infected person.
Teach about the recommended use of spermicide-coated latex condoms.	Usage helps prevent transmission of infections (action of spermicide).
Reinforce that the best form of prevention is avoiding exposure (by sexual activity).	This information may decrease incidence and reoccurrence of STDs in the adolescent.
Provide education to the adolescent that STDs are not contracted from toilet seats, drinking glasses or bath towels; also, that hormonal contraceptive methods do not provide protection against STDs.	Adolescents are often uninformed or lack accurate information regarding how STDs are contracted.

NIC: *Teaching: Disease Process*

Evaluation

(Date/time of evaluation of goal)

(Has goal been met? Not met? Partially met?)

(What did client say about the mode of transmission of STDs? What 2 methods to prevent STDs did the client identify?)

(Revisions to care plan? D/C care plan? Continue care plan?)

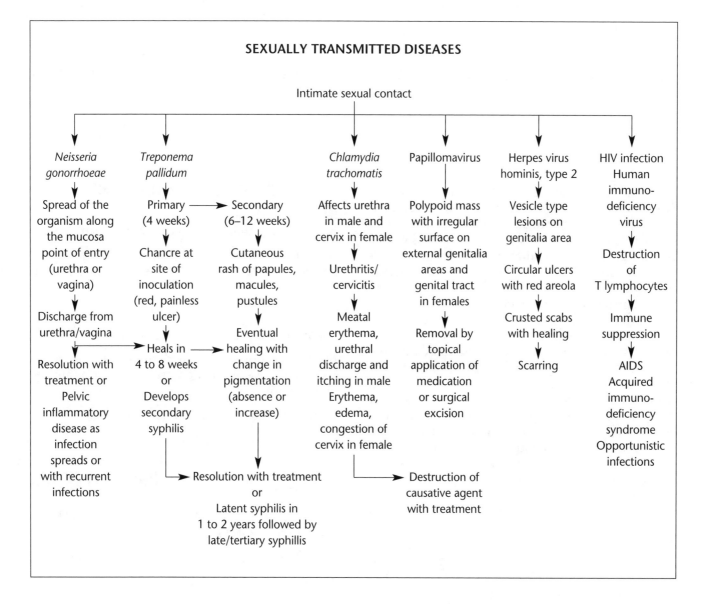

SEXUALLY TRANSMITTED DISEASES

Intimate sexual contact

| *Neisseria gonorrhoeae* | *Treponema pallidum* | *Chlamydia trachomatis* | Papillomavirus | Herpes virus hominis, type 2 | HIV infection Human immuno-deficiency virus |

Neisseria gonorrhoeae

Spread of the organism along the mucosa point of entry (urethra or vagina)

Discharge from urethra/vagina

Resolution with treatment or Pelvic inflammatory disease as infection spreads or with recurrent infections

Treponema pallidum

Primary (4 weeks) → Secondary (6–12 weeks)

Chancre at site of inoculation (red, painless ulcer)

Cutaneous rash of papules, macules, pustules

Heals in 4 to 8 weeks or Develops secondary syphilis

Eventual healing with change in pigmentation (absence or increase)

Resolution with treatment or Latent syphilis in 1 to 2 years followed by late/tertiary syphillis

Chlamydia trachomatis

Affects urethra in male and cervix in female

Urethritis/ cervicitis

Meatal erythema, urethral discharge and itching in male Erythema, edema, congestion of cervix in female

Destruction of causative agent with treatment

Papillomavirus

Polypoid mass with irregular surface on external genitalia areas and genital tract in females

Removal by topical application of medication or surgical excision

Herpes virus hominis, type 2

Vesicle type lesions on genitalia area

Circular ulcers with red areola

Crusted scabs with healing

Scarring

HIV infection Human immuno-deficiency virus

Destruction of T lymphocytes

Immune suppression

AIDS Acquired immuno-deficiency syndrome Opportunistic infections

CHAPTER 5.6

CRYPTORCHIDISM

Undescended testes (cryptorchidism) is a condition present at birth in which one or both testes fail to descend through the inguinal canal into the scrotal sac. The testes usually descend spontaneously by 1 year of age. If not, a child may receive human chorionic gonadotropin therapy or surgery (orchiopexy) performed between 1 to 2 years of age. Surgery prevents damage to the testes that may be affected by exposure to a higher temperature in the abdomen. Repair at a younger age also prevents the adverse effect on body image and embarrassment caused by the difference in the appearance of the empty smaller scrotal sac. Undescended testes that are associated with the presence of an inguinal hernia are repaired at the time of herniorrhaphy. Failure of the testes to descend can occur at any point along the normal path of descent into the scrotum. Symptoms of undescended testes rarely cause discomfort. The entire scrotum, or one side, will appear smaller than normal and may appear incompletely developed. Congenital inguinal hernias are frequently present with this defect.

MEDICAL CARE

DIAGNOSTIC EVALUATION

Retractile Testes: testes can be manually pushed back down (or milked) into the scrotum. True undescended testes cannot be manually pushed back down into the scrotum.

Cremasteric Reflex: (after 6 months of age and peaks by 4 to 5 years of age). Procedure: drawing up of the scrotum and testicle when the skin over the front and inside thigh is stimulated; will result in spontaneous retraction of testes back into the pelvic cavity.

Diagnostic Tests, may include: testicular ultrasonography, computed tomography, and laparoscopy. All can be performed to confirm undescended testes prior to surgical intervention and to rule out masses, tumors, or cysts.

MEDICAL MANAGEMENT

By 1 year of age, the undescended testes will spontaneously descend into the scrotum in 75% of cases.

Surgical Intervention (Orchiopexy): recommended for undescended testes repair before the child's second birthday.

Analgesics: postoperatively to control pain.

Antibiotics: to prevent infection at operative site.

Hormones: chorionic gonadotropin to enhance testicular descent in the absence of an anatomic impediment.

Complete Blood Count: reveals increased WBC if infection present.

COMMON NURSING DIAGNOSES

See RISK FOR IMPAIRED SKIN INTEGRITY

Related to: External factor of surgical incision.

Defining Characteristics: (Specify: disruption of skin surface, surgical invasion.)

ADDITIONAL NURSING DIAGNOSES

ANXIETY

Related to: (Specify: threat to self-concept, change in health status of child, hospitalization and surgery of child.)

Defining Characteristics: (Specify: increased apprehension and expressed concern about future infertility and effect on body image, presence of empty scrotum and smaller size, expressed concern about impending surgery or need for future surgery and procedure performed to correct abnormality.)

Goal: Client will experience decreased anxiety by (date and time to evaluate).

Outcome Criteria

✔ Parents verbalize decreased anxiety about child's undescended testes.

NOC: *Anxiety Control*

INTERVENTIONS	RATIONALES
Assess source and level of anxiety and how it is manifested; need for information that will relieve anxiety.	Provides information about anxiety level and need for interventions to relieve it; source for the parents include fear and uncertainty about treatment and recovery; source for child include embarrassment by different shape and size of scrotum after school age.
Allow expression of concerns and opportunity to ask questions about diagnosis, procedures, effect of abnormal placement on testes and future fertility.	Provides opportunity to vent feelings and fears and secure information to reduce anxiety.
Communicate with parents (and child) and answer questions calmly and honestly; use pictures, models and drawings as aids where helpful in explanations.	Promotes calm and supportive trusting environment.
Give parents (and child) as much input in decisions about care and routines as possible.	Allows for more control over situation.
Provide as much privacy to the child as possible during assessments.	Promotes comfort and prevents embarrassment.
Inform parents that surgery is usually performed after the age of 1 but may be done during the preschool years by the age of 5 if testes have not spontaneously descended on their own.	Provides information about need for surgical correction before school age to prevent psychological and cosmetic embarrassment to the child and that exposure to the higher temperature in the abdomen may damage testes and predispose to formation of tumor and infertility.
Teach about procedure to the parents (and child).	Explains the surgical procedure to correct the deformity (orchiopexy).

INTERVENTIONS	RATIONALES
(Reassure child that his penis will remain in place and that the surgery will not affect the penis in any way.)	Alleviates any fear that the penis may be cut off.
Instruct parents and child in activity restrictions and play appropriate to age and trauma of surgery (as ordered, specify).	Provides information about return to normal activity without injury to operative area or disconnect the suture which may lead to testes again returning into inguinal canal.
(Demonstrate and teach self-examination of testes and allow for return demonstration; inform to report any change felt.)	Allows for early detection of a neoplasm.

NIC: *Anxiety Reduction*

Evaluation

(Date/time of evaluation of goal)

(Has goal been met? Not met? Partially met?)

(Did parents report decreased anxiety? Use quotes.)

(Revisions to care plan? D/C care plan? Continue care plan?)

RISK FOR INFECTION

Related to: Inadequate primary defenses (broken skin).

Defining Characteristics: (Specify: surgical incision proximity to urine and feces.)

Goal: Client will not experience infection by (date and time to evaluate).

Outcome Criteria

✔ Temperature remains <99° F.

✔ Incision is clean and dry without redness, edema, drainage, or odor.

NOC: *Risk Control*

INTERVENTIONS	RATIONALES
Assess wound for redness, warmth, swelling, discharge or odor (specify frequency).	Indicates infection at site.
Apply ice to wound postoperatively as ordered.	Reduces swelling.

(continues)

(continued)

INTERVENTIONS	RATIONALES
Carefully cleanse perineal area of any urine or stool as needed; teach parents.	Prevents contamination of wound and risk of infection.
Administer antibiotic therapy as ordered (specify).	Prevents or treats infection by preventing synthesis of cell wall of microorganisms.
Reinforce completion of course of antibiotic therapy.	Prevents recurrence of infection.
Teach child to wear clean undergarments or parents to change child's diaper frequently and not leave child in soiled diaper.	Maintains cleanliness of surgical area and prevents contamination.

NIC: *Infection Control*

Evaluation

(Date/time of evaluation of goal)

(Has goal been met? Not met? Partially met?)

(What is temperature? Describe wound assessment relative to outcome criteria.)

(Revisions to care plan? D/C care plan? Continue care plan?)

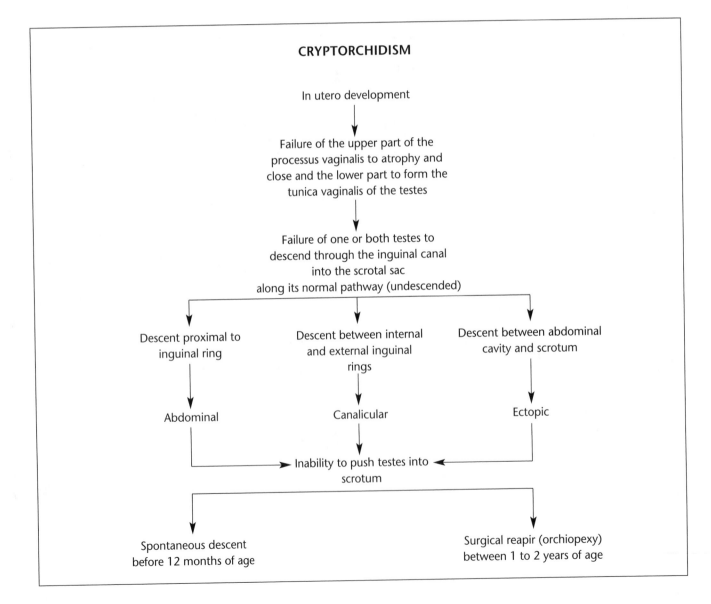

CRYPTORCHIDISM

In utero development

↓

Failure of the upper part of the processus vaginalis to atrophy and close and the lower part to form the tunica vaginalis of the testes

↓

Failure of one or both testes to descend through the inguinal canal into the scrotal sac along its normal pathway (undescended)

Descent proximal to inguinal ring → Abdominal

Descent between internal and external inguinal rings → Canalicular

Descent between abdominal cavity and scrotum → Ectopic

→ Inability to push testes into scrotum ←

Spontaneous descent before 12 months of age

Surgical reapir (orchiopexy) between 1 to 2 years of age

CHAPTER 5.7

URINARY TRACT INFECTION

Urinary tract infection (UTI) is defined as infection located in the lower tract (bladder or urethra) or in the upper tract (ureters or kidneys). The peak incidence of UTI observed in children occurs between 2 and 6 years of age, but can be observed at any age. The incidence of UTI in children also varies by gender: females have a 10% to 30% greater risk of developing a UTI; males have a 50% greater risk of developing a recurrent UTI; and during the newborn-age range only, male infants are at a greater risk of developing a UTI.

Etiologic factors associated with UTI in children include: 75% to 80% of bacterial infections are caused by Escherichia coli. Bacterial organisms occur more frequently than viral or fungal organisms which are more frequent in low-birth weight and preterm infants. The higher incidence in female children is attributed to the female child's anatomic differences from the male child (shorter urethra with an increased chance of contamination caused by the close proximity to the anus), other factors include: urinary stasis, poor hygiene practices, and external factors (i.e., Foley catheter, tight fitting diapers, exposure to bubble baths).

Diagnosis of UTI can be made by a urine culture from a clean-catch or a catheterized specimen. However, there is a high risk for contamination with clean-catch specimens. Lab result criteria for a UTI diagnosis: colony counts of 100,000 colonies in a clean-catch urine; and any urine culture greater than 5,000 colonies from urine obtained on a suprapubic puncture or catheterized specimen. Signs and symptoms of UTI in pediatric patients are age-related. For example, unique symptoms of UTI displayed by the infant: failure to thrive and fever; by the preschooler: anorexia and somnolence; by the school-ager: enuresis and personality changes; and those by the adolescent: fatigue and flank pain.

MEDICAL CARE

DIAGNOSTIC EVALUATION

Diagnosis Is Dependent Upon: age-related symptoms of UTI; an accurate and thorough history of UTI symptoms, patterns of voiding, health practices at home, recurrent treatment of UTI, physical growth and examination, and urine culture lab results.

Urine Culture and Sensitivity: the gold standard for the diagnosis of UTI, to determine the presence of bacteria in the urine and the drugs to which they are sensitive. UTI will have >100,000 colony formation units/ml (CFU/ml) in the first urine specimen in the morning. Evidence of a contaminated urine sample will reveal a report of fewer than 10,000 CFU/ml. Low colony formation may also occur because of very dilute or acidic urine, frequent voiding, chronic infection, or antibacterial therapy.

Urinalysis: may show elevated protein, leukocytes, casts, pus cells. The urinalysis may be normal, with a positive urine culture.

Radiographic Studies: (may be performed to identify any structural or functional renal abnormalities). These may include: renal ultrasound (RUS), voiding cystourethrogram (VCUG), intravenous pyelogram (IVP), and dimercaptosuccinic acid (DSMA).

Voiding Cystourethrogram (VCUG): reveals anatomic abnormality of bladder and urethra and reflux of urine into ureters which predisposes to recurrent infection.

Intravenous Pyelogram (IVP): reveals abnormalities in renal or bladder function caused by recurrent infections.

Renal Ultrasound (RUS): radiologic test to determine renal obstructions and structural abnormalities; renal size; renal calculit; and polycystic kidney.

MEDICAL MANAGEMENT

Is directed at early diagnosis, elimination of infection, identification of causative factors to prevent infection and preservation of renal function.

Anti-infectives: dependent on identification of the microorganism and sensitivity to specific anti-infectives.

Urine Culture: reveals colonization of bacteria and identification of specific organism and sensitivity to antimicrobials.

Follow-up Management: urine cultures should be repeated monthly for 3 months, every 3 months for 6 months, and annually thereafter to ensure early detection of any recurrent symptoms. The relapse rate of UTI is high in children and tends to occur within 1–2 months after termination of antibiotic therapy.

COMMON NURSING DIAGNOSES

See HYPERTHERMIA

Related to: Illness (urinary tract infections).

Defining Characteristics: (Specify: age-related symptoms of UTI in the pediatric patient, fever [temperature greater than 38.5° C], positive urine culture and sensitivity for bacteria in the urine.)

See RISK FOR DEFICIENT FLUID VOLUME

Related to: Abnormal loss of fluids and deviations affecting intake of fluids.

Defining Characteristics: (Specify: fever and chills; vomiting and diarrhea; anorexia, abdominal pain; reluctance of child to drink fluids; attempts to hold urine for long periods; enuresis; urgency and dysuria with voiding.)

ADDITIONAL NURSING DIAGNOSES

DEFICIENT KNOWLEDGE

Related to: UTI.

Defining Characteristics: (Specify: lacks accurate information related to diagnosis; treatment of current UTI and prevention or recurrent UTI; age-related signs and symptoms of UTI; home management and follow-up needs.)

Goal: Client will obtain information about UTIs by (date and time to evaluate).

Outcome Criteria

✔ Client verbalizes signs and symptoms of UTI and expected treatment regimen.

NOC: *Knowledge: Disease Process*

INTERVENTIONS	RATIONALES
Assess parents' knowledge of age-related signs and symptoms of UTI, associated anatomy effects related to UTI (girls vs. boys); assess history and past treatments for UTI, compliance of previous UTI management.	Provides information needed to develop plan of instruction to ensure compliance of medical regimen; UTI commonly occur in females and are prone to recurrent episodes; vesicoureteral reflux predisposes to UTI.
Teach parents about causes of the infection and predisposing factors; to be alert to dysuria, frequency, urgency, fever, foul odor to urine, cloudiness of urine, enuresis in the toilet trained child or flank pain, chills and fever, abdominal distention; and to report the presence of these signs and symptoms to physician.	Provides information that indicates lower or upper urinary tract infection.
Teach parents how to collect a mid-stream urine specimen for laboratory analysis before and after antibiotic therapy.	Reveals presence of infection and identifies organism responsible and if treatment is effective or needs changing.
Teach parents (and child) in antibiotic therapy and to take full course of medication.	Provides information about medication therapy for effective resolution of infection and prevention of relapse.
Teach parents and child to avoid bubble baths and tub baths and take showers; to wipe female from front to back and instruct child to do same after toileting.	Provides information about prevention of recurrence of infection and irritation to the urethra.
Instruct child to void frequently and increase daily fluids according to age (specify), include fluids that are acidic (citrus and cranberry juice).	Prevents retention and stasis of urine which predisposes to infection; fluids flush out bacteria and acidic fluids change pH of urine from alkaline to acid.
Teach parents and child to avoid wearing tight nonabsorbable undergarments.	Predisposes to harboring of bacteria, entry and ascending into urinary tract.

INTERVENTIONS	RATIONALES
If diagnostic tests are to be performed, provide information about type of procedure, reason for procedure to be done, what to expect during procedure, after care following procedure.	Prepares child and parents for procedures to diagnosis anatomic abnormalities that may be the source of UTI.
Instruct parents to obtain urine for analysis from the first morning void.	The first morning void is considered the most accurate for assessing growth of organisms; urine specimens will show a decline in colonization throughout the day from diuresis and frequent voiding.
Teach parents to avoid giving the child caffeine beverages and carbonated beverages.	Caffeine and carbonated beverages may cause irritation to the bladder mucosa.
Instruct sexually active adolescents to void immediately after sexual intercourse.	This measure is associated with decreasing the risk of exposure to UTI; it may also help prevent recurrence of UTI; this measure will aid in flushing out bacteria.

NIC: *Teaching: Disease Process*

Evaluation

(Date/time of evaluation of goal)

(Has goal been met? Not met? Partially met?)

(What did clients verbalize about the signs and symptoms and treatment of UTIs? Use quotes.)

(Revisions to care plan? D/C care plan? Continue care plan?)

URINARY TRACT INFECTION

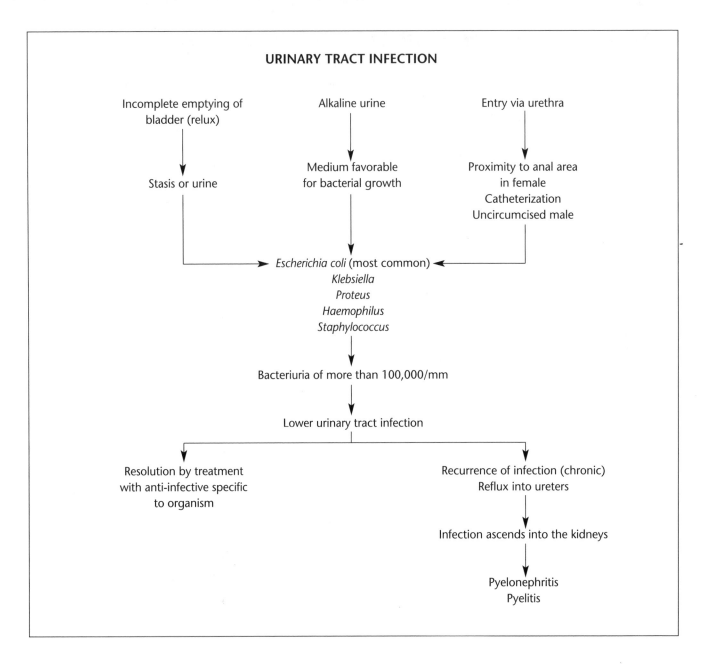

CHAPTER 5.8

VESICOURETERAL REFLUX

Vesicoureteral reflux is defined as a retrograde (or backflow) of urine into the ureters. The diagnosis for VUR rarely occurs after 5 years of age. The etiology of VUR is categorized into two types, primary and secondary reflux. Primary reflux is caused by an inadequate valvular mechanism at the ureterovesical junction and is not associated with any obstruction or neurogenic bladder. The inadequate valve in primary reflux is caused by the shortened submucosal tunnel that shortens bladder filling. Secondary reflux occurs secondary to obstruction (50% of cases in infants are caused by posterior urethral valves) or neurogenic bladder. Important risk factors associated with VUR include: age, urinary tract infection (UTI), and reflux.

The following effects of unrepaired reflux have been identified: urine concentration ability is inversely proportional to the grade of reflux; renal scarring; lower-weight percentiles (in physical growth); hypertension; proteinuria; and those with bilateral scarring and an increased risk of developing end stage renal failure (as high as 30%). In the majority of children, the problem will disappear spontaneously without surgical intervention if infection is controlled. Management of reflux includes antibacterial therapy for infection control.

MEDICAL CARE

DIAGNOSTIC EVALUATION

Ultrasound: to identify anatomic abnormalities and measure renal growth.

Voiding Cystourethrography (VCUG): visualizes bladder outline and urethra, reveals reflux of urine into ureters, and shows complications of bladder emptying.

Intravenous Pyelogram (IVP): provides information about the integrity of the kidneys, ureters and bladder. It is recommended after an abnormal ultrasound, especially if anatomy is poorly defined.

MEDICAL MANAGEMENT

Antibacterial Therapy: may be administered for short-term or long-term usage.

Ureteral Reimplantation Surgery: antireflux surgery, consists of reimplantation of ureters into the bladder.

Follow-up Evaluation: children with reflux should be evaluated at a clinic at 3-month intervals. VCUG: is recommended again, at 2 to 6 months postoperatively.

Analgesics: to control pain postoperatively.

Antispasmodics: flavoxate hydrochloride (Urispas), propantheline (Banlin), PO, belladonna and opium (BSO) suppository to relax smooth muscle of bladder and reduce discomfort caused by bladder irritation and spasms.

Urine Culture: reveals infectious agent and basis for antibacterial therapy or need for modification of therapy.

COMMON NURSING DIAGNOSES

See RISK FOR DEFICIENT FLUID VOLUME

Related to: Loss of fluid through abnormal routes, deviations affecting intake of fluid.

Defining Characteristics: (Specify: NPO status pre and postoperatively, urinary catheter [Foley or suprapubic], dry skin and mucous membranes, poor skin turgor, decreased urinary output via catheter or stents, temperature elevation.)

See RISK FOR IMPAIRED SKIN INTEGRITY

Related to: Surgical incision.

Defining Characteristics: (Specify: disruption of skin surface, catheter site irritation and discomfort.)

See HYPERTHERMIA

Related to: Illness.

Defining Characteristics: (Specify: increase in body temperature above normal range, evidence of infection at surgical or catheter site, or renal/urinary infection.)

ADDITIONAL NURSING DIAGNOSES

DEFICIENT KNOWLEDGE

Related to: Lack of exposure to information about disorder.

Defining Characteristics: (Specify: expressed need for information about continuous medical regimen to control renal/bladder infection and measures to prevent infection.

Goal: Clients will obtain information about child's illness and treatment by (date and time to evaluate).

Outcome Criteria

✔ Clients verbalize understanding of illness and treatment regimen.

NOC: *Knowledge: Disease Process*

INTERVENTIONS	RATIONALES
Assess parents' and child's understanding of vesicoureteral reflux. Provide necessary information and allow time for questions. Use teaching aids as needed (specify).	Provides basic understanding of the condition without repeating information the clients already know.
Instruct parents and child in antibacterial administration including information on action, dose, form, time, frequency, how to take, side effects to report (specify).	Promotes understanding of the medication regimen for long-term therapy to prevent recurrent or relapse of urinary infection.
Teach parents and child to develop strategies for administration of medications including the development of an organized plan using pill dispensers, alarms on a clock or watch, check-off list, reminder notes to prevent omissions (specify).	Empowers the parents and child to take control of medication administration on a long-term basis.

INTERVENTIONS	RATIONALES
Teach parents and child of need to obtain urine cultures by midstream and taking to a laboratory or use of dip-slide or strip to use at home (specify).	Reveals presence of urinary infection and assists to regulate antibacterial therapy.

NIC: *Teaching: Disease Process*

Evaluation

(Date/time of evaluation of goal)

(Has goal been met? Not met? Partially met?)

(What did clients verbalize about the illness and treatment regimen? Use quotes.)

(Revisions to care plan? D/C care plan? Continue care plan?)

ANXIETY

Related to: Change in health status, change in environment (hospitalization for surgery).

Defining Characteristics: (Specify: expressed apprehension and concern about surgery [ureteral reimplantation] and pre and postoperative procedures and care.)

Goal: Clients will experience decreased anxiety by (date and time to evaluate).

Outcome Criteria

✔ Clients verbalize decreased anxiety.

NOC: *Anxiety Control*

INTERVENTIONS	RATIONALES
Assess source and level of anxiety and need for information and interventions that will relieve it.	Provides information about anxiety level and need to relieve it; source for parent includes the procedure and care of child pre and postoperatively; source for child includes separation from parents, unfamiliar environment, and painful procedures.
Allow expression of concerns and time to ask questions about need of surgery, procedure to be done, procedures to prepare for surgery, procedures, care and recovery after surgery.	Provides opportunity to vent feelings and fears and to feel secure in the environment.

INTERVENTIONS	RATIONALES
Answer questions calmly and honestly, use pictures, drawings, models and therapeutic play.	Promotes trust and a calm and supportive environment.
Encourage parents to stay with child and assist in care.	Allows parents to care for and support child and continue parental role and increases child's comfort by having a familiar caretaker.
Allow as much input into decisions about care and usual routines as possible by parents.	Allows for more control over situations and maintains a familiar routine for care.
Orient and introduce child to the surgical unit preoperatively.	Reduces anxiety caused by fear of the unknown.
Teach parents and child about abnormal functioning ureter and reason for surgical repair, that the ureter will be reimplanted to prevent urine from backing up in the ureter and continuing problems with infections.	Provides information that will enhance understanding about surgery to reduce anxiety.
Teach about and prepare for preoperative procedures and tests necessary for visualization and diagnosis (specify).	Allays anxiety and provides accurate information of what to expect.
Teach parents and child that catheter and/or stent will be in place and where they will be placed, that they will be irrigated and receive special care, that urine output will be noted and measured for any abnormalities or complications, that a surgical dressing will be in place to protect the incision, and, in case of young child, restraints may be in place on arms and legs, and that medications will be given to control pain.	Provides information of what to expect following surgery.
Reassure parents and child that surgery and catheters will not affect sterility or sexual orientation.	Provides information that may cause anxiety.

NIC: *Anxiety Reduction*

Evaluation

(Date/time of evaluation of goal)

(Has goal been met? Not met? Partially met?)

(Did clients report decreased anxiety? Use quotes.)

(Revisions to care plan? D/C care plan? Continue care plan?)

 PAIN

Related to: Surgery.

Defining Characteristics: (Specify: communication of pain descriptors, crying, irritability, restlessness, withdrawal, flank pain, ureteral edema from surgery, bladder spasms.)

Goal: Client will experience decreased pain by (date and time to evaluate).

Outcome Criteria

✔ Client rates pain as less than (specify for child, indicate which pain scale is used).

NOC: *Comfort Level*

INTERVENTIONS	RATIONALES
Assess verbal and nonverbal behavior, type and location and severity of pain depending on age (specify pain scale and frequency).	Provides information about pain as a basis for analgesic therapy.
Administer analgesic based on pain assessment and before pain becomes severe (specify).	Reduces pain and promotes rest to reduce stimuli and restlessness (action of drug).
Place in a comfortable position; avoid unnecessary movement or manipulation of suprapubic catheter.	Promotes comfort and decreases bladder spasms that cause pain.
Administer antispasmodic as ordered (specify).	Reduces bladder spasms caused by irritation of suprapubic catheter.
Maintain catheter patency by ensuring placement, checking flow and presence of kinks or obstruction (specify when).	Reduces pain caused by distention as a result of catheter clogging or displacement.
Provide distractions and reassurance when spasms occur and stay with child when they occur to inform the child that the pain is temporary.	Reduces anxiety which tends to increase pain.
Inform parents and child that pain will subside 24 to 48 hours following surgery and teach measures taken to control pain.	Provides knowledge about duration of pain and causes of pain.

NIC: *Pain Management*

Evaluation

(Date/time of evaluation of goal)

(Has goal been met? Not met? Partially met?)

(What is pain rating? Specify scale used.)

(Revisions to care plan? D/C care plan? Continue care plan?)

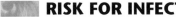 **RISK FOR INFECTION**

Related to: (Specify: urinary tract infection [acute, chronic or postoperative]; invasive postoperative drainage tubes (i.e., Silastic stents, urethral Foley or suprapubic tube].)

Defining Characteristics: (Specify: redness, abnormal drainage, and/or swelling at incision site; UTI symptoms [burning on voiding, cloudy and foul-smelling urine]; positive urine or wound culture; temperature elevation [38.5° C or higher].)

Goal: Client will not experience an infection by (date and time to evaluate).

Outcome Criteria

✔ Surgical incision remains clean and dry without redness, edema, odor, or drainage.

NOC: *Risk Control*

INTERVENTIONS	RATIONALES
Assess wound for redness, swelling, purulent drainage on dressing, healing.	Indicates presence of infectious process or poor healing.
Assess catheter site for redness, edema, irritation; urine collected in drainage system for cloudiness and foul odor.	Indicates infectious process at catheter site or in urinary bladder.
Collect urine for culture and sensitivities.	Reveals presence of urinary infection and sensitivity to specific antibacterial agent.
Administer antibacterial as ordered (specify).	Treats specific microorganism or prevents infection when catheter is in place.
Encourage increased fluid intake daily depending on age requirements when PO fluids are allowed (specify).	Promotes dilution of urine to prevent infection and encourage voiding after catheter is removed.

INTERVENTIONS	RATIONALES
Use sterile technique when changing dressings, giving catheter care or emptying drainage bag.	Prevents contamination of wound or urinary tract by the introduction of pathogens.
Maintain catheter and collection bag below level of bladder and maintain a closed, patent system free of kinks or obstructions.	Prevents backflow of urine into bladder or retention of urine which predisposes to infection.
Provide suprapubic catheter care by cleansing with peroxide solution after removing any meatal crusting, catheter care by washing perineum with mild soap and water, rinsing and applying antiseptic ointment.	Promotes comfort and prevents infection at suprapubic or meatal site.
Change dressings when soiled or wet 24 hours after surgery.	Promotes comfort and allows for wound assessment.
Instruct and demonstrate catheter care, irrigation, emptying of drainage system using sterile technique and allow for return demonstration.	Provides information and skill in caring for and maintaining catheter patency to prevent infection if child is to be discharged with catheter in place.
Inform parents of signs and symptoms of infection to report.	Allows for early intervention if infection is present.

NIC: *Infection Control*

Evaluation

(Date/time of evaluation of goal)

(Has goal been met? Not met? Partially met?)

(Describe incision)

(Revisions to care plan? D/C care plan? Continue care plan?)

RISK FOR INJURY

Related to: (Specify: catheter displacement; internal factor of complications of surgical trauma.)

Defining Characteristics: (Specify: catheter obstruction, postoperative bleeding catheter dislodgement, bladder distention, reduced urine output, dysuria, frequency, retention following removal of catheter.)

Goal: Client will not experience injury by (date and time to evaluate).

Outcome Criteria

✔ Urine is clear without blood or clots.

✔ Bladder is not distended.

✔ Client able to urinate after catheter is removed.

NOC: *Risk Control*

INTERVENTIONS	RATIONALES
Assess output via catheter and note characteristics of urine, passage of blood clots, color of urine and return to clear color; and if clots or return to red color occurs after a period of normal characteristics.	Provides information about possible complication of bleeding or obstruction.
Notify physician immediately if red color returns.	Allows for immediate interventions to treat hemorrhage.
Immobilize arms and legs with restraints, remove periodically; use bed cradle following surgery.	Prevents accidental dislodgement or removal of catheter.
Secure catheter to abdomen or leg with tape stents to catheter and avoid placing tension on the catheter when in place by gently holding it when performing care.	Prevents movement or manipulation of catheter that may cause displacement.
If catheter becomes displaced, notify physician for replacement (have a suprapubic catheter on hand at all times).	Ensures continued drainage of urine.
Measure I&O q h for an output of 1 ml/kg/hr and notify physician if less.	Provides information to ensure adequate output via catheters.
Note first voiding after catheter removed, time of voiding and amount, difficulty, presence of abdominal distention.	Provides information about return of urinary pattern, presence of retention.

INTERVENTIONS	RATIONALES
Support during first voiding (warm water over perineum, sitting or standing position) and privacy.	Prevents embarrassment and promotes voiding.
Encourage increase in fluid intake according to age requirements.	Promotes voiding.
Inform parents and child that physician should be notified if urinary pattern or characteristics change or if unable to void after catheter is removed.	Allows for early interventions if needed.
Teach parents about measures taken to ensure that catheters remain in place and patent (use of restraints, anchoring catheters, irrigations) and that this is a temporary situation.	Informs parents of need for measures to prevent displacement of catheter.
Teach child to void frequently after catheter removal.	Prevents stasis of urine leading to urinary infection.

NIC: *Surveillance*

Evaluation

(Date/time of evaluation of goal)

(Has goal been met? Not met? Partially met?)

(Describe urine. Is ladder distended?)

(Revisions to care plan? D/C care plan? Continue care plan?)

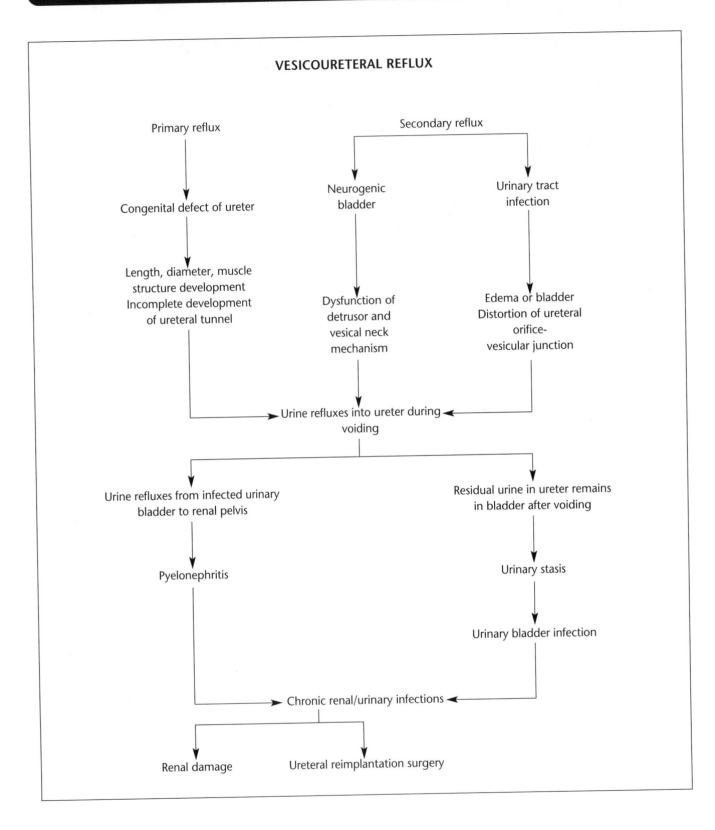

VESICOURETERAL REFLUX

CHAPTER 5.9

WILMS' TUMOR

Wilms' tumor (or nephroblastoma) is identified as the most common pediatric malignant renal tumor in children. Incidence of Wilms' tumor is slightly less frequent in boys than in girls. The average age at diagnosis with unilateral tumors is 41.5 months and with bilateral tumors is 29.5 months. Children with Wilms' tumor may have associated anomalies and chromosomal abnormalities, such as: aniridia (congenital absence of the iris); hypospadias; cryptorchidism; Beckwith-Wiedemann syndrome; Denys-Drash syndrome; Perlman and Sotos' syndrome. The appearance of the Wilms' tumor is usually referred to as the "pushing type" (or adjacent renal parenchyma, enclosed by a distinct intrarenal pseudocapsule).

The most frequent initial clinical presentation for most children with Wilms' tumor is abdominal swelling or the presence of an abdominal mass. This initial presentation is usually first noticed by a parent while bathing or dressing the child. Other frequent findings at diagnosis include: abdominal pain, gross hematuria, fever, and hypertension.

The most common sites of metastases of Wilms' tumor are the lungs, the regional lymph nodes, and the liver. Histology classifies the tumor into: (1) favorable or unfavorable histology; (2) 3 cell types: triphasic or biphasic; with blastemal, stromal, and epithelial elements; and (3) 10% have anaplastic or unfavorable histologic findings, including anaplastic Wilms' tumor, clear cell sarcoma of the kidney, rhabdoid tumor of the kidney. Other histologic patterns include: nephrogenic rests, congenital mesoblastic nephroma, and renal cell carcinoma. An unfavorable histology is associated with a poor prognosis and more extensive chemotherapy. Prognosis is determined by the pathologic staging of Wilms' tumor, defined by the National Wilms' Tumor Study Group. Both the histology classification and the pathologic staging of Wilms' tumor determine the type and length of time for administration of chemotherapy agents and radiation treatments.

MEDICAL CARE

Diagnostic Evaluation: complete peripheral blood count (including a differential white blood cell count platelet count); liver function test (SGOT, SGPT, bilirubin); urinalysis, renal functions tests (BUN, creatinine) and serum calcium determination. Elevated serum calcium is associated with a rhabdoid tumor of the kidney or congenital mesoblastic nephroma.

Abdominal Ultrasound Examination: can distinguish whether the abdominal mass is intrarenal or extrarenal; unilateral or bilateral; unifocal or multifocal; or solid or cystic.

Contrast-Enhanced Computed Tomography of the Abdomen: to evaluate the nature and extent of the mass; and whether the tumor has extended into adjacent structures such as the liver, spleen, or colon.

Supine X-ray Film of the Abdomen: is necessary for planning and review of radiation therapy.

Real-Time Ultrasonography: determines the patency of the inferior vena cava vessel (when the tumor is identified within this vessel, the proximal extent of the thrombus must be established before the operation).

Chest X-ray and Chest CT scan: to determine whether pulmonary metastases are present (are only performed if an unfavorable histology of the tumor is identified).

Radionuclide Bone Scan and X-ray Skeletal Survey: should be performed on all postoperative children with clear cell sarcoma of the kidney, presence of pulmonary or hepatic metastases.

Brain Imaging: should be obtained on all children with clear cell sarcoma of the kidney or with rhabdoid tumor of the kidney; both of these tumors are associated with intracranial metastases.

Bone Marrow Aspiration and Biopsy: usually not performed as bone marrow involvement is rare.

THERAPEUTIC MANAGEMENT

Chemotherapy and Radiation Therapy Protocol: Favorable Histology: vincristine and actinomycin-D (no radiation).

Unfavorable Histology: vincristine, actinomycin-D, cyclophosphamide, with radiation.

Renal Angiogram: reveals renal function and extent of involvement.

Scans of Kidney, Liver, Bone: reveals involvement of these organs if metastasis is present.

Inferior Venacavagram: reveals involvement adjacent to the vena cava if the tumor has grown to a large size.

Erythrocyte Sedimentation Rate (ESR): reveals increases as serum protein levels change.

Albumin: reveals decreases with renal involvement.

Enzymes: reveals increases in alanine aminotransferase (ALT), aspartate aminotransferase (AST), lactic dehydrogenase (LDH) with liver involvement; alkaline phosphatase (ALP) with bone involvement.

Complete Blood Count: reveals increases in RBC as tumor excretes more erythropoietin.

Urinalysis: reveals characteristics that indicate change in renal function caused by tumor, uric acid, erythropoietin increases.

COMMON NURSING DIAGNOSES

See IMBALANCED NUTRITION: LESS THAN BODY REQUIREMENTS

Related to: (Specify: inability to ingest and digest food, side effects from therapy.)

Defining Characteristics: (Specify: anorexia, nausea and vomiting from chemotherapy, obstruction postoperatively from chemotherapy causing adynamic ileus stomatitis [rare], abdominal cramping.)

See RISK FOR DEFICIENT FLUID VOLUME

Related to: (Specify: altered intake, excessive losses through normal routes, nausea and vomiting caused by chemotherapy and radiation therapy.)

Defining Characteristics: (Specify: diarrhea, vomiting from radiation.)

See DIARRHEA

Related to: Side effects.

Defining Characteristics: (Specify: increased frequency of bowel sounds and loose, liquid stools.)

See CONSTIPATION

Related to: (Specify: gastrointestinal obstructive lesions postoperatively, side effects.)

Defining Characteristics: (Specify: adynamicileus, decreased bowel sounds, abdominal distention, frequency less than usual pattern.)

See RISK FOR IMPAIRED SKIN INTEGRITY

Related to: (Specify: side effects and radiation therapy; secondary effects of chronic diarrhea.)

Defining Characteristics: (Specify: erythema or hyperpigmentation of previously irradiated skin; local phlebitis; transverse ridging of nails; redness and excoriation of perianal area from chronic diarrhea.)

ADDITIONAL NURSING DIAGNOSES

ANXIETY

Related to: (Specify: change in health status, threat of death, threat to self-concept.)

Defining Characteristics: (Specify: increased apprehension and fear of diagnosis, expressed concern and worry about preoperative procedures and preparation, postoperative care and effects of therapy, possible metastasis of disease.)

Goal: Clients will experience decreased anxiety by (date and time to evaluate).

Outcome Criteria

✔ Clients verbalize decreased anxiety.

NOC: *Anxiety Control*

INTERVENTIONS	RATIONALES
Assess source and level of anxiety and need for information and support that will relieve it.	Provides information about degree of anxiety and need for interventions and support; sources for parents may be guilt and uncertainty about surgery,

INTERVENTIONS	RATIONALES
	treatments and recovery, possible loss of child; sources for the child may be the multiple procedures of diagnosis and surgery and the effects of postoperative treatments.
Allow expression of concerns and inquiries about disease and possible consequences of surgery and prognosis.	Provides opportunity to vent feelings, secure information needed to reduce anxiety.
Encourage parents to stay with the child or open visitation, provide a telephone number to call for information about condition of child.	Promotes care and support of child by parents.
Provide continuing nurse assignment with the same personnel; encourage parents to participate in care.	Promotes trust and comfort and familiarity with staff giving care.
Orient child to the surgical and ICU unit, equipment, noises and staff.	Reduces anxiety caused by fear of unknown.
Teach parents and child about the disease process, surgical procedure, what to expect with procedures done preoperatively, and what will be experienced postoperatively including radiation and chemotherapy and its benefits and effects (alopecia, stomatitis, nausea, vomiting, diarrhea are possible but temporary).	Promotes knowledge and understanding of pre and postoperative treatments and effect on disease and self-image.
Explain all procedures and care in simple, direct, honest terms and repeat as often as necessary; reinforce physician information if needed and provide specific information as needed.	Prevents overwhelming child and parents with information in small amount of time as diagnosis and procedures usually carried out within a short period of time and anxiety will prevent ability to comprehend.
Teach parents and child the extent of surgery with the removal of a kidney and the staging process; discuss their understanding of the pathology report postoperatively and clarify information as needed.	Reduces anxiety when knowledge and support is given and child and parents will not feel betrayed by inadequate preparation of procedures and treatments.
Utilize therapeutic play, drawings, models for instruction of child.	Provides aids to assist child to understand what will be experienced and to express their feelings.

INTERVENTIONS	RATIONALES
Provide parents and child with information about community agencies and support groups.	Provides emotional support by those who have experiences with the effects of the disease.

NIC: *Anxiety Reduction*

Evaluation

(Date/time of evaluation of goal)

(Has goal been met? Not met? Partially met?)

(Did parents report decreased anxiety? Use quotes.)

(Revisions to care plan? D/C care plan? Continue care plan?)

RISK FOR INJURY

Related to: (Specify: side effects, complications.)

Defining Characteristics: Intestinal obstruction; edema; adhesion formation; stomatitis.

Goal: Child will not experience injury by (date and time to evaluate).

Outcome Criteria

✔ BP remains within (specify range for child).

✔ Tumor capsule remains intact.

✔ Surgical incision remains clean and dry without redness, edema, odor, or drainage.

NOC: *Risk Control*

INTERVENTIONS	RATIONALES
Assess blood pressure for increases pre and postoperatively q 2h, changes in pulse and respirations.	Provides information about vital signs caused by renal function abnormality preoperatively or by nephrectomy postoperatively, postoperative atelectasis.
Avoid any palpation of abdominal mass; post sign on bed stating not to palpate preoperatively.	Prevents trauma to tumor site and possible metastasis by dissemination of cancer cells.
Assess bowel activity postoperatively for elimination pattern, bowel sounds, bowel distention.	Provides information about possible adynamic ileus from chemotherapy causing bowel obstruction.

(continues)

(continued)

INTERVENTIONS	RATIONALES
Assess incision site for redness, swelling, drainage, intactness, and healing and change dressing when soiled or wet; assess oral and perineal area.	Indicates infectious process resulting from invasive procedure or inflammation resulting from immunosuppressive therapy for stomatitis or skin breakdown or inflammation; provides oral care and anal care after elimination; provides postoperative pulmonary care.
Assess urinary output for presence of cloudy, foul-smelling urine; collect specimen for culture analysis and report any change in renal function (hypertension, headache irritability, weight gain, behavior changes).	Indicates possible renal impairment and/or urinary bladder infection; renal involvement alters renin excretion which increases BP and immunosuppressive therapy leads to infection.
Maintain reverse isolation if leukopenia present or according to agency dictate.	Prevents transmission of infective agents to the immunosuppressed child.
Assess and document frequency of bowel movements; document a description of all bowel movements; measure abdominal girth.	To assess potential intestinal obstruction from vincristine-induced adynamic ileus.
Give stool softeners (as prescribed).	To prevent straining with bowel movements.
Teach parents and child about all assessments and procedures and reason for isolation precautions.	Promotes understanding and cooperation.
Teach parents to avoid exposing child to infectious agents; limit visitors.	Prevents exposure to possible pathogens in the immunosuppressed child.
Advise parents to dress child appropriate to weather conditions and to avoid rough activities or sports.	Prevents respiratory infections associated with exposure or trauma to the abdominal site preoperatively and surgical site postoperatively.
Instruct parents and child in mouth care (rinsing and swabbing with solutions, cleansing and drying after bowel elimination).	Prevents or treats skin and mucous membrane damage as a result of therapy.
Teach parents and child to report any changes in urinary pattern or characteristics or renal function promptly.	Allows for immediate attention to any genitourinary problems in remaining kidney.

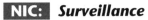 **NIC:** *Surveillance*

Evaluation

(Date/time of evaluation of goal)

(Has goal been met? Not met? Partially met?)

(What is BP? Is tumor capsule intact? Describe post-operative incision.)

(Revisions to care plan? D/C care plan? Continue care plan?)

IMPAIRED ORAL MUCOUS MEMBRANE

Related to: Chemotherapy.

Defining Characteristics: (Specify: stomatitis, oral ulcers, hyperemia, oral pain or discomfort, oral plaque.)

Goal: Child will be free of oral mucous membrane irritation by (date and time to evaluate).

Outcome Criteria

✔ No oral mucous membrane lesions present.

NOC: *Oral Health*

INTERVENTIONS	RATIONALES
Assess oral cavity for pain ulcers, lesions, gingivitis, mucositis or stomatitis and effect on ability to ingest food and fluids (specify frequency).	Provides information about effect of chemotherapy.
Administer medication (specify) before meals and offer bland, smooth foods that are not hot or spicy.	Permits eating with more comfort.
Administer an antiseptic mouth rinse 30 minutes before any food or fluid intake as ordered (specify).	Promotes comfort of oral mucosa and maintains integrity (action of drug).
Provide oral hygiene (30 minutes before or after meals): mouthwashes (specify); instruct patient not to eat or drink for 30 minutes after oral hygiene is completed.	To prevent oral mucositis.
Use soft-sponge toothbrush or sponge toothette or gauze to provide mouth rinse.	To avoid oral trauma.

INTERVENTIONS	RATIONALES
Administer local anesthetics to oral area as ordered; administer these before meals.	May be effective in temporary pain relief from oral lesions; permits eating with decreased oral pain.
Avoid oral temperatures.	To avoid oral trauma.
Avoid use of lemon glycerin swabs to oral lesions.	Lemon may increase irritation to oral lesions.
Offer moist, soft, bland foods.	To minimize irritation to oral ulcers; it may also be better tolerated by the child.
Avoid foods which are hot, spicy, or which include ascorbic acid.	To minimize irritation to oral ulcers; these foods may increase pain and irritation to oral areas.
Teach parents about effect of chemotherapy on oral mucosa and in treatments to decrease discomfort in oral cavity.	Promotes understanding of side effects that occur and temporary nature of the side effects.
Teach parents in mouth care.	Promotes effective care of oral cavity to relieve discomfort and prevent mucosa breakdown and increased inflammation.

NIC: Oral Health Maintenance

Evaluation

(Date/time of evaluation of goal)

(Has goal been met? Not met? Partially met?)

(Does child have any oral mucous membrane lesions?)

(Revisions to care plan? D/C care plan? Continue care plan?)

INEFFECTIVE PROTECTION

Related to: (Specify: drug therapy [antineoplastics]: abnormal blood profile [leukopenia, thrombocytopenia, anemia, coagulation]; treatments [radiation].)

Defining Characteristics: (Specify: altered clotting, bone marrow suppression, deficient immunity against infection, petechiae, bleeding from nose, gums, hematuria [25% of cases will display preoperatively], hemorrhagic cystitis [a common side effect of cyclophosphamide].)

Goal: Child will be protected from illness or injury by (date and time to evaluate).

Outcome Criteria

✔ Child does not experience bleeding.

✔ Temperature remains <100° F.

NOC: Infection Status

INTERVENTIONS	RATIONALES
Assess for bleeding from any site, WBC, platelet count, Hct, absolute neutrophil, count and febrile episodes (specify when).	Provides information about frank bleeding or blood profile abnormalities that predispose to bleeding caused by bone marrow suppression and immuno-suppression resulting from chemotherapy.
Administer blood transfusion as ordered for severe blood loss, monitor patency, vital signs, chills, fever, urticaria, rash, dyspnea, diaphoresis, headache throughout transfusion, and terminate if any of these changes occur.	Replaces blood loss when symptoms of anemia appear (dizziness, pallor, fatigue, increased pulse and respirations) or when Hct is less than 20% or platelet count less than 20,000/cu mm.
Pad sides of bed, avoid trauma with use of hard toothbrush or dental floss, apply pressure for 5 minutes after IV administration, discontinue taking rectal temperatures or performing unnecessary invasive procedures.	Prevents bleeding caused by trauma during chemotherapy administration which alters platelets and clotting factor.
Carry out handwashing technique before giving care, use mask and gown when appropriate, provide a private room, monitor for any signs and symptoms of infection.	Prevents transmission of pathogens to a compromised immune system during chemotherapy if the absolute neutrophil count is less than 1,000/cu mm.
Teach parents and child to avoid rough play or sports, straining at defecation, blowing nose hard.	Prevents trauma that causes bleeding.
Caution parents and child to avoid persons with upper respiratory infection or any illness.	Prevents risk for infection in the highly susceptible child.
Instruct parents to report any fever, behavior changes, headache, dizziness, fatigue, pallor, slow oozing of blood from any area, exposure to communicable diseases.	Indicates a complication associated with abnormal blood profile.

(continues)

(continued)

INTERVENTIONS	RATIONALES
Teach and allow for return demonstration of urine and stool testing for blood using dipstick and hematest.	Identifies presence of bleeding in gastrointestinal or urinary tract.

NIC: *Surveillance*

Evaluation

(Date/time of evaluation of goal)

(Has goal been met? Not met? Partially met?)

(Are there any indications of bleeding? What is child's temperature?)

(Revisions to care plan? D/C care plan? Continue care plan?)

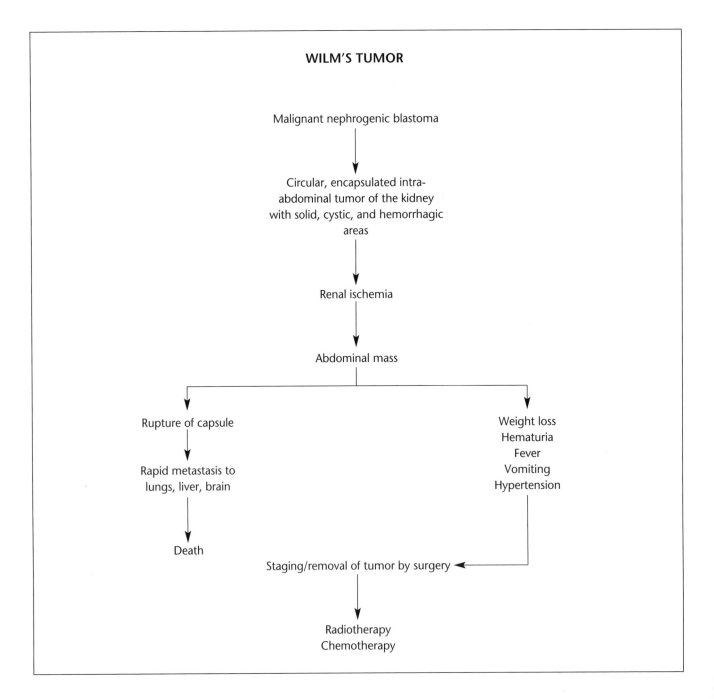

WILM'S TUMOR

Malignant nephrogenic blastoma

↓

Circular, encapsulated intra-abdominal tumor of the kidney with solid, cystic, and hemorrhagic areas

↓

Renal ischemia

↓

Abdominal mass

Rupture of capsule

↓

Rapid metastasis to lungs, liver, brain

↓

Death

Weight loss
Hematuria
Fever
Vomiting
Hypertension

↓

Staging/removal of tumor by surgery

↓

Radiotherapy
Chemotherapy

UNIT 6
MUSCULOSKELETAL SYSTEM

CHAPTER 6.0

MUSCULOSKELETAL SYSTEM: BASIC CARE PLAN

The musculoskeletal system includes components that are needed for the supportive and protective framework of the body. The system functions to provide the movement that is essential for interacting and adapting to the child's environment and is especially vulnerable to forces in the environment. The system includes bones which compose the skeletal system, muscles which compose the muscular system, joints which compose the articular system, tendons, and ligaments. Tendons and ligaments with muscle attach to the surfaces of bones and the combination of all of the components allows for ambulation, personal care, and play. The problems encountered in these systems are classified as traumatic (most common) and long-term disability (degenerative disease). Any problem or abnormality that affects this system commonly affects the function of one or more other organ systems. The functional disruption that occurs as a result of a musculoskeletal problem that requires immobilization leads to physical and emotional alterations in a child who is usually active and curious. With growth and development of the system structures and gross and fine motor development, the child progressively functions within adult parameters for movements and activities of daily living.

MUSCULOSKELETAL GROWTH AND DEVELOPMENT

BONE, MUSCLE, JOINT, TENDON, LIGAMENT STRUCTURE

- The spine in the newborn is rounded or has a convex curvature with the lumbar curve developed by 12 to 18 months of age; cervical spine is concave; thoracic spine is convex; and lumbar spine is concave after 18 months of age with the double S curve developed in the older child.

- Muscles are completely formed at birth with size increasing by hypertrophy and strength increasing with muscular functions of walking, climbing, running, and jumping which is well established by 3 years of age.

- Muscle development and bone growth continue to mature with skeletal lengthening and muscle strengthening increases throughout childhood.

- Bone ossification is continuous with 25 new ossification centers appearing during the second year and bones continue to ossify until maturity is reached.

- Bone growth occurs in the epiphysis at the end of long bones until it closes, at which time growth ceases.

- Height and rate of skeletal growth increases at a slower rate with age with the toddler increasing 3 to 5 inches/year.

- Feet of the infant and toddler appear flat and an arch develops with walking.

- Height averages vary with age and sex.

	Boys	Girls
6 mo	26¾ in	26 in
1 yr	30 in	29¼ in
2 yr	34¼ in	34¼ in
3 yr	37¼ in	37 in
4 yr	40½ in	40 in
6 yr	45¾ in	45 in
8 yr	50 in	49¾ in
10 yr	54¼ in	54½ in
12 yr	59 in	59¾ in

MUSCULOSKELETAL FUNCTION

- Development of gross and fine motor function and muscle strength and refinement continue in the preschool and school-age child.

- From the beginning of walking through toddler stage, legs are usually bowlegged until back and leg muscles develop and wide stance and waddle or toddling gait is apparent until 2 to 2½ years of age; by school-age the legs become closer together and walking and posture is sturdy and balanced.

■ Bones in the child resist pressure and muscle pull less than the adult, so injury by trauma is common.

■ Bones heal faster in children as the bones are still in the process of ossification and growth.

NURSING DIAGNOSES

IMPAIRED PHYSICAL MOBILITY

Related to: (Specify: intolerance to activity; decreased strength and endurance.)

Defining Characteristics: (Specify: inability to purposefully move within physical environment, including bed mobility, transfer and ambulation, limited range of motion, decreased muscle strength, control and/or mass, fatigue, bed rest.

Related to: Pain and discomfort.

Defining Characteristics: (Specify: reluctance to attempt movement, limited range of movement, painful and/or swollen joints, fracture, surgical procedure, infectious process.)

Related to: Neuromuscular impairment.

Defining Characteristics: (Specify: inability to purposefully move within physical environment, including bed mobility, transfer and ambulation, decreased muscle strength, control and/or mass, impaired coordination, paralysis [paraplegia or quadraplegia], progressive deterioration, inadequate gross and fine motor skills, diminished musculoskeletal responses.)

Related to: Musculoskeletal impairment.

Defining Characteristics: (Specify: inability to purposefully move within physical environment, including bed mobility, transfer and ambulation, reluctance to attempt movement, limited range of motion, decreased muscle strength, control and/or mass, imposed restrictions of movement including mechanical [cast, traction, splint, brace, or bed rest], contractures, fracture, joint disease and destruction inflammation, congenital disorders.)

Goal: Client will gain improved physical mobility by (date and time to evaluate).

Outcome Criteria

✔ (Specify, e.g., child will move self in bed with traction bar; walk the length of the hallway and back twice a day; etc.)

NOC: *Mobility Level*

INTERVENTIONS	RATIONALES
Assess muscle tone, strength, mass; joint mobility, pain, stiffness, swelling; ability to move and activity level in performing ADL (specify when).	Provides information about musculoskeletal condition and function.
Assess bed rest status, activity restrictions, imposed immobility by braces, casts, traction, splints.	Maintains rest during acute stages to promote healing and restoration of health.
Assess sensory (diminished sensation and numbness) and motor (gait and balance) function of extremities; presence of paralysis, fracture, surgical correction of musculoskeletal abnormalities.	Provides information about conditions or treatments that affect mobility.
Assess physical effects of immobilization on body systems; constipation, skin breakdown, urinary retention, hypercalcemia, loss of muscle strength, contractures, circulatory stasis, stasis of pulmonary secretions, anorexia, renal calculi, decreased metabolism and energy, loss of nerve innervation.	Prevents complications of immobility by monitoring and intervening when needed; mobility provides important contributions to development and physical health.
Assess psychologic effect of immobilization; reduced body image, inability to reduce stress, loss of stimuli, loss of independence and mastery, anxiety, regressive behavior, anger and aggression, passive and submissive behavior, crying, irritability, temper tantrums.	Provides information about behavior and deprivation resulting from immobilization that prevents children from dealing with feelings and expression of anxiety and tensions.
Avoid restriction in activities unless ordered; encourage and allow for as much movement as possible in performing daily activities; administer analgesic before activity.	Promotes mobility and activity synonymous with health and life; allows for autonomy and control for normal development.
Encourage all age-appropriate activities that facilitate mobility, allow infant to crawl (specify).	Promotes mobility according to limitations of illness and provides outlet for frustration of imposed immobility.

(continues)

(continued)

INTERVENTIONS	RATIONALES
Provide quiet play and progress in ambulation by scheduling dangling at bedside, standing with support, ambulation with support with increases daily and praise for all attempts regardless of progress.	Maintains large and small muscle strength as condition permits.
Transport/transfer infant/child by Hoyer lift, stroller, wheelchair, bed outside of room/hospital.	Provides stimulation by interacting in a different environment in absence of mobility.
Provide and apply brace, splint; use of aids including wheelchair, crutches, supportive reading, eating, and other aids for ADL as needed (specify).	Promotes independence and support in mobility and activities.
Maintain body alignment on bed rest, reposition q 2h or as needed; use a drawing for child to follow for position and where to lie in bed.	Prevents contractures and physical deformity and preserves joint function.
Coordinate rest with periods of mobility.	Prevents fatigue and conserves energy.
Perform muscle strengthening exercises, passive stretching exercises, joint mobilizing exercises if ordered or as appropriate (specify).	Preserves muscle strength or prepares for use of crutches or other mobility aids.
Apply special shoes, splint or appliance for day or night use (specify).	Maintains position at night and prevents deformity and allows for locomotion by increasing gait efficiency during day use.
Prepare for physical and/or occupational therapy during recuperative period as ordered (specify how).	Promotes and maintains optimal function and mobility of child.
Inform parents and child of hazards of immobility (specify).	Promotes compliance with program to maintain mobility and understanding of effects of immobility.

INTERVENTIONS	RATIONALES
Teach parents and child to use devices or aids for mobility and ADL (specify).	Promotes safe use of aids and apparatus and increased security.
Teach parents to provide clear pathways, remove rugs, make environmental modifications as needed.	Provides safe environment for mobility.
Teach parents and child about activities for large muscle strengthening (tricycle, swimming, running, skipping rope), and small muscle strengthening (games, puzzles, crayons, coloring books).	Promotes strengthening of muscles as condition improvement.
Encourage child with progress in ambulation and ADL.	Provides child with a goal to strive for and achieve.
Teach parents and child ROM, strengthening exercises as appropriate.	Maintains muscle and joint function.
Reinforce parents and child of importance of therapy and follow-up care, short- or long-term depending on need.	Promotes compliance with prescribed therapy especially if needed to ensure mobility or health maintenance in chronic disorders.

NIC: *Activity Therapy*

Evaluation

(Date/time of evaluation of goal)

(Has goal been met? Not met? Partially met?)

(What has been child's activity level? How does it compare with the outcome criteria?)

(Revisions to care plan? D/C care plan? Continue care plan?)

CHAPTER 6.1

FRACTURES

A fracture is a break in a bone which is usually caused by a fall or injury. Fractures are common in children because of their activity and continual changes and growth in gross motor function. Injury of this type in an infant or very small child is often the result of physical abuse. The most common type of fracture in children under 3 years of age is the greenstick which is an incomplete fracture and results in a compression of one side causing it to bend and the other side to fail. A bend fracture is the result of the bone bending and straightening on its own because of the flexibility of the bone at a young age. A buckle fracture is raised bulging of the bone resulting from compression of the bone near its most porous part. A complete fracture is a division in the bone with or without attachment of a periosteal hinge remaining. The most common sites of fractures in children are the femur, humerus, clavicle, ulna, radius, tibia, and fibula. Treatment includes reduction (open or closed), and immobilization by casting and/or traction depending on the type and severity of the fracture. Healing is faster in the child and takes place within 3 to 4 weeks. Remodeling is usually completed within 9 months depending on the type and site on the fracture, amount of fragmentation, and the age of the child.

MEDICAL CARE

Analgesics: for pain control depending on severity.

Bone X-ray: reveals trauma site, separation of the epiphysis in older child.

Enzymes: reveals increases in alkaline phosphatase (ALP), lactic dehydrogenase (LDH), creatine phosphokinase (CPK), aspartate aminotransferase (AST) with bone, and muscle damage.

Complete Blood Count (CBC): reveals increased WBC and neutrophils if infection present, decreased RBC, Hct, Hgb with destruction of RBC caused by muscle, bone and soft tissue injury.

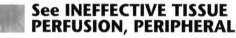

COMMON NURSING DIAGNOSES

See IMPAIRED PHYSICAL MOBILITY

Related to: Pain and discomfort, musculoskeletal impairment (fracture).

Defining Characteristics: (Specify: intolerance to activity, decreased strength and endurance, inability to purposefully move within physical environment including bed mobility, transfer and ambulation, reluctance to attempt movement, imposed restrictions of movement including mechanical medical protocol [cast, traction], inability to participate in activities and socializing.)

See INEFFECTIVE TISSUE PERFUSION, PERIPHERAL

Related to: Interruption in arterial and venous flow.

Defining Characteristics: (Specify: cold, pallor or blue color of extremity, decreased peripheral pulse, cast tightness.)

See RISK FOR IMPAIRED SKIN INTEGRITY

Related to: (Specify: external factor of physical immobilization, pressure of cast, traction apparatus, presence of surgical incision from open reduction; internal factors of altered circulation and sensation.)

Defining Characteristics: (Specify: disruption of skin surface, invasion of bony structures, redness, irritation of skin at cast edges or pressure areas, numbness or tingling of casted extremities.)

See CONSTIPATION

Related to: Inadequate physical activity or immobility.

Defining Characteristics: (Specify: frequency less than usual, hard formed stool, decreased bowel sounds, straining at defecation.)

ADDITIONAL NURSING DIAGNOSES

PAIN

Related to: Physical injuring agents (bone fracture); surgery to realign fracture.

Defining Characteristics: Communication of pain descriptors, guarding and protective behavior to injured part, crying, irritability, restlessness, swelling of part, muscle spasms.

Goal: Child will experience less pain by (date and time to evaluate).

Outcome Criteria

✔ Child rates pain as less than (specify desired level and pain scale used).

NOC: *Pain Level*

INTERVENTIONS	RATIONALES
Assess site for pain including type, severity, and duration using a pain scale if appropriate; pain as a result of surgical open reduction (specify frequency).	Provides information about pain as a basis for analgesic and muscle relaxant therapy.
Administer analgesic, muscle relaxant, or both as ordered and note response (specify drug, dose, etc.).	Reduces pain and promotes rest following injury or surgery (action of drug).
Apply ice to fracture if ordered.	Treats pain and edema by vasoconstriction.
Apply splint or Jones dressing (cotton wrapping over area covered by an Ace bandage).	Relieves pain and prevents further damage by protecting and immobilizing limb.
Elevate limb above heart level, maintain alignment of limb when positioning.	Promotes venous return to relieve edema which causes pain and prevents contractures.
Support limb above and below injured area when moving and positioning; use smooth movements and avoid abrupt movement of limb.	Prevents pain caused by movement.
Teach parents and child about pain medications and expected results and importance of reporting pain before it becomes too severe.	Provides information about expected effects of analgesic therapy during acute stages of pain and as pain subsides with healing.

INTERVENTIONS	RATIONALES
Show parents and child ways to move and position limb, maintaining immobilization of extremity, and to avoid weight-bearing exercise until advised by physician.	Prevents undue pain caused by movement of limb.

NIC: *Pain Management*

Evaluation

(Date/time of evaluation of goal)

(Has goal been met? Not met? Partially met?)

(What is pain rating? Specify scale used)

(Revisions to care plan? D/C care plan? Continue care plan?)

RISK FOR INJURY

Related to: (Specify: sensory dysfunction, tissue hypoxia, altered mobility resulting from cast application.)

Defining Characteristics: (Specify: change in color, temperature, edema, movement of fingers/toes; tingling or numbness of fingers/toes; drainage or musty odor from under cast; skin irritation at cast edges; moist, wet, or broken cast, foreign objects inserted between cast and skin.)

Goal: Child will not experience injury by (date and time to evaluate).

Outcome Criteria

✔ Affected area (specify remains pink and warm).
✔ Child reports sensation and is able to move affected area (specify).

NOC: *Risk Detection*

INTERVENTIONS	RATIONALES
Assess pulses in casted upper or lower extremity, swelling, coolness, inability to move digits, pallor or cyanosis, numbness of areas distal to the cast q 2h.	Provides information about the neurovascular status of an extremity following cast application as swelling continues causing the cast to become tight and compromise circulation; a bivalved cast treats excessive edema to prevent tissue damage.

INTERVENTIONS	RATIONALES
Allow cast to dry thoroughly using a fan, turning q 2h, support on pillows and use palm of hands to lift or handle cast exposing as much of the cast to the air as possible.	Prevents indentations in the cast that may cause pressure areas, allows cast to dry from inside out for 1/2 hour or more depending on substance used for cast and type of cast.
Do not use a heated fan or dryer.	Heat causes the cast to dry on the outside but stay wet underneath, or may cause burns from heat conduction through the cast.
Elevate casted part on pillow until completely dry and when at rest for a few days.	Promotes venous return to reduce swelling.
Provide quiet play for a few days and exercise muscle and joints above and below.	Maintains muscle and joint function.
Remove small articles or food that may be put into the cast.	Prevents pressure to injury and infection if skin is broken under the cast.
Clean plaster cast with vinegar and water; fiberglass casts are cleaned with mild soap and water.	Maintains cleanliness of the cast.
Petal cast if rough edges are present; massage skin near cast edges and note any reddened or abrasive areas.	Protects skin from irritation and breakdown.
Outline area of drainage on cast with pen; and include date and time.	Monitors increases in drainage under the cast.
Provide muscle strengthening exercises, ROM of unaffected parts, isometric exercises appropriate.	Prepares for crutch walking if appropriate and maintains joint and muscle mobility.
Teach parents and child about type of cast, type of fracture and how it heals.	Provides information about injury and type of immobilization to allow for healing process.
Reinforce to parents and child to restrict activities according to physician advice, to avoid placing articles, such as a coat hanger for scratching, into the cast.	Prevents damage to the cast and skin that may lead to infection or impair the desired effect of the cast.
Teach parents and child to avoid allowing limb to hang down and maintain elevation of the limb when sitting and support limb with a sling when standing; avoid standing for prolonged periods of time.	Maintains return venous flow and prevents fatigue from heavy cast.

INTERVENTIONS	RATIONALES
Instruct parents to note and report any pain, swelling, musty odor from cast; changes in neurovascular status in casted extremity, tightness or looseness of cast.	Indicates presence of infection or neurovascular compromise that may require a cast change.
Teach parents to massage skin at cast edges, avoid use of lotions and powder in these areas, and pad cast edges if needed.	Toughens skin to prevent breakdown and prevents infection by providing media for bacterial growth.
Instruct child in use of crutches or application of sling (specify).	Allows for mobility and participation in activities.
Teach parents and child about length of cast presence, need for physical therapy if appropriate, and method of maintaining clean cast (plaster or plastic).	Permits planning for continuing care if appropriate.

NIC: *Surveillance*

Evaluation

(Date/time of evaluation of goal)

(Has goal been met? Not met? Partially met?)

(Describe color, temperature, sensation, and movement of affected area. What does child say?)

(Revisions to care plan? D/C care plan? Continue care plan?)

RISK FOR INJURY

Related to: (Specify: sensory dysfunction, altered mobility resulting from skin or skeletal traction.)

Defining Characteristics: (Specify: redness, swelling, pain at pin site, change in neurovascular status of extremity, malfunction of traction apparatus, ineffective traction, contractures or weakness of joint and muscles.)

Goal: Child will not experience injury by (date and time to evaluate).

Outcome Criteria

✔ Traction is maintained.
✔ Child remains in correct body alignment. (Pin sites are not red or swollen.)

NOC: *Risk Control*

INTERVENTIONS	RATIONALES
Assess type and purpose of traction, extremity or body part involved (specify).	Provides information about use of traction to realign bone ends, provide immobilization of a part, reduce muscle spasms, correct a deformity, provide rest for an extremity; traction may be manual as in cast application, skin in which the pull is attached to the skin with bandages or straps, or skeletal in which the pull is attached to a pin, wire, or tongs inserted into the bone at a distal position to the fracture.
Assess functioning part of the traction apparatus including correct weight amount and hanging, ropes in tract with secure knots, pulleys in original site with movable wheels, position of frames, splints.	Provides information needed to ensure correct traction applied to body part.
Assess skin color, pulses, numbness, or changes in movement of body part; weakness or contractures of uninvolved muscles and joints: neurochecks q 2 to 4h.	Indicates neurovascular changes resulting from traction; muscular changes resulting from immobilization.
Assess pressure points noting any redness or breakdown and reposition if possible; massage uninjured skin areas.	Prevents prolonged pressure on skin that results in breakdown and decreased blood flow to area.
Maintain bed position as ordered with head or foot elevated.	Provides desired amount of pull and countertraction.
Maintain correct body alignment especially in hips, legs, arms, and shoulders; realign after the child has moved or changed position.	Promotes comfort and prevents deformity.
Perform ROM to unaffected joints, apply foot plate if appropriate.	Prevents contractures and foot drop.
Maintain nonadhesive straps or bandages used; do not remove or change unless permitted while someone maintains traction; note tightness or looseness that may cause ineffective traction.	Supplies attachment for pull in skin traction.

INTERVENTIONS	RATIONALES
Cleanse and dress pin site daily; apply antiseptic ointment if ordered; check skin for infection at site; examine screws within metal clamp for proper attachment of clamp to traction; do not remove traction.	Supplies attachment for pull in skeletal traction and treats pin site to prevent infection.
Assist child to perform ADL activities independently as much as possible; facilitate self-care with assistive aids.	Promotes independence in self-care within limitations of age and immobilization.
Suggest activities such as hobbies, TV, reading, games while in traction.	Allows for movement without disturbing traction.
Provide diversionary activities and encourage visits from family and friends, move bed to area of activity with peers.	Provides and promotes social interactions.
Teach parents and child as appropriate for age about reason for traction and length of time traction must be in place.	Provides information to assist with coping with immobility.
Teach child of amount and type of movement allowed while in traction.	Ensures that amount of activity is not exceeded and will not affect traction.
Reassure parents that traction will assist in the healing of fracture.	Promotes positive response to treatment.

NIC: *Surveillance*

Evaluation

(Date/time of evaluation of goal)

(Has goal been met? Not met? Partially met?)

(Has traction been maintained? Describe child's body alignment. Describe pin assessment.)

(Revision to care plan? D/C care plan? Continue care plan?)

FRACTURES

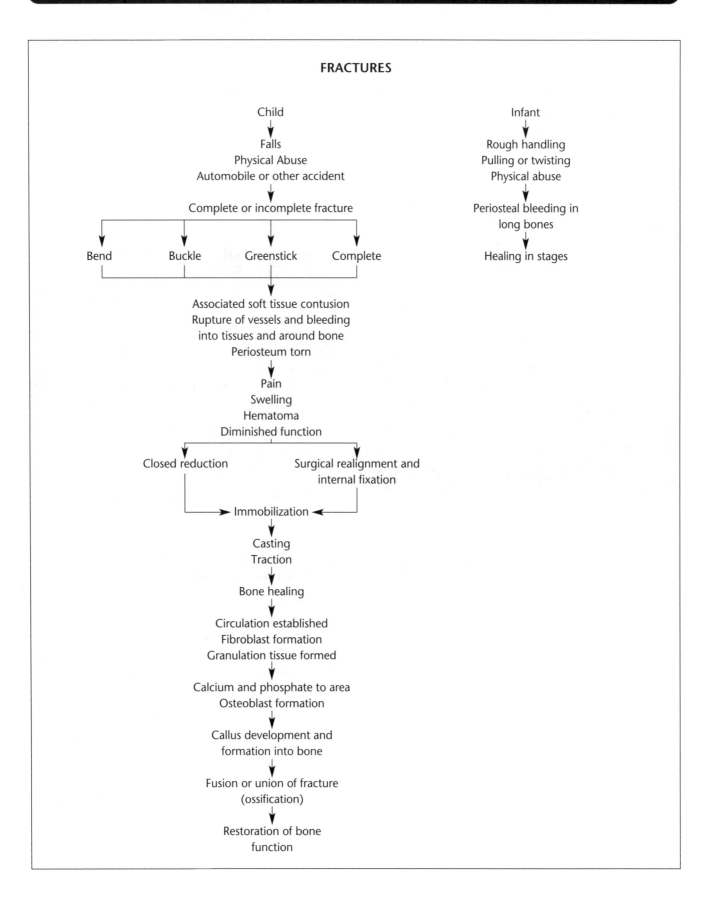

CHAPTER 6.2

CONGENITAL HIP DYSPLASIA

Congenital hip dysplasia is related to abnormal hip development. The abnormalities include hip instability, preluxation (shallow acetabulum), subluxation (incomplete dislocation of the hip), and dislocation (femoral head not in contact with the acetabulum). It usually involves one hip, but may involve both. It occurs 6 times more often in females than males. It is usually identified in the newborn period and responds to treatment best if initiated before 2 months of age. Therefore, it is important to examine every infant from birth to 12 months of age. Treatment is dependent on the age of the child and the degree of abnormality, and ranges from application of a reduction device, to traction and casting, to surgical open reduction. Casting and splinting with correction is usually impossible after 6 years of age.

MEDICAL CARE

Pelvic X-ray: reveals outward femoral displacement with upward slope of the roof of the acetabulum in infant/child over 4 months of age.

Ultrasound: reveals cartilaginous head displacement in infant under 1 to 4 months of age.

Ortolani Test: a maneuver abducting the infant's leg that, in the event of hip dysplasia, causes the femoral head to enter the acetabulum and is identified by a click as this occurs.

Barlow's Test: a maneuver adducting the infant's leg that, in the event of hip dysplasia, causes the femoral head to exit the acetabulum and is palpable by the examiner.

COMMON NURSING DIAGNOSES

See IMPAIRED PHYSICAL MOBILITY

Related to: Musculoskeletal impairment (hip defect).

Defining Characteristics: (Specify: imposed restriction of movement by harness, cast, traction, or splint;

inability to purposefully move within physical environment including bed mobility; ambulation.

See RISK FOR IMPAIRED SKIN INTEGRITY

Related to: External factor of physical immobilization; internal factor of altered circulation; sensation by pressure of device, cast, traction.

Defining Characteristics: Edema, tight appliance or cast, change in skin color and temperature proximal to spica cast or device or pin site, skin irritation at pin site or cast edges, numbness proximal to cast.

See CONSTIPATION

Related to: Musculoskeletal impairment, inadequate physical activity or immobility.

Defining Characteristics: Frequency less than usual, hard formed stool, decreased bowel sounds, straining at defecation.

See DELAYED GROWTH AND DEVELOPMENT

Related to: Effects of physical disability (immobilization).

Defining Characteristics: Environmental and stimulation deficiencies, inability to perform self-care activities appropriate for age, isolation with long-term immobilization.

ADDITIONAL NURSING DIAGNOSES

RISK FOR INJURY

Related to: (Specify: untreated or improper treatment for dislocation.)

Defining Characteristics: (Specify: late onset dislocation, absence of early recognition and intervention for correction, muscle contracture, muscle shortening, femoral and acetabulum deformity, tight spica cast, inappropriate traction or malfunctioning traction.)

Goal: Infant will not experience injury by (date and time to evaluate).

Outcome Criteria

✔ (Specify outcome criteria based on treatment mode, e.g., traction is maintained; Pavlik harness is applied properly; skin is free of irritation in spica cast.)

NOC: *Risk Detection*

INTERVENTIONS	RATIONALES
Assess infant up to 2 months of age for frank breech birth, cesarean birth, hip joint laxity or dislocation (Ortolani or Barlow test), degree of dysplasia or dislocation, shortened limb on the affected side (telescoping), broadened perineum, asymmetry of thigh and gluteal folds with increased number of folds and flattened buttocks.	Provides information about the presence and degree of dysplasia; may be preluxation, subluxation, or dislocation (luxation) and involve a laxity of the capsule or an abnormal acetabulum; identification of the presence of the deformity at this age results in the highest success rate in complete correction.
Assess child's shortened leg affected with telescoping; palpation of femur when thigh is extended and pushed toward the head and pulled in distal direction; delayed walking and a limp that causes lurching toward affected side; downward tilt of pelvis toward unaffected side if weight-bearing on affected side when standing (Trendelenberg sign); lordosis and waddling gait if both hips affected.	Provides information about the presence of deformity in one or both hips in the older infant or toddler and preschool age group; usually identified when the child begins to walk or stand, and limb is shortened and adductor and flexor muscle contracture has occurred; requires closed reduction (traction and cast) or open reduction (surgery, cast splint) to correct.
(Apply Pavlik harness splinting device to infant up to 6 months of age to be worn continuously for 3 to 6 months to ensure hip stability; apply double or triple diapers or Frejka pillow if this is treatment ordered.)	Maintains abducted, reduced position for maintaining the femur in the acetabulum; other methods to correct unstable hip may be used to stretch legs and maintain abducted position depending on degree of deformity.
(Maintain skin traction in presence of abduction contracture in the infant up to 6 months of age and spica cast if applied following the traction; maintain	Promotes hip abduction until stable; applies with a spica cast if unable to maintain stable reduction of the hip for 3 to 6 months; removal of the spica

INTERVENTIONS	RATIONALES
skin traction for gradual reduction of the hip adductor and flexor muscles with a spica cast application for immobilization in child 6 to 10 months of age.)	cast is followed by an abduction brace for protection.
(Provide traction care including correct alignment of extremity, correct amount of weights, free hang of weights, correctly functioning pulleys with secure knots, neurologic and circulatory checks q 4h for color, warmth, sensation.)	Maintains safe, effective traction to affected hip(s) with child's response to traction monitored.
(Provide spica cast care including support of cast when moving, removing crumbs and small articles that may get into cast, petal cast edges, avoiding insertion of anything into cast to scratch, clean cast when needed, allow to dry completely, protect cast from soiling and dampness from elimination or bathing; neurologic and circulatory checks q 4h for color, peripheral pulse, warmth, capillary refill, sensation; nausea and vomiting resulting from cast syndrome.)	Maintains safe, effective immobilization to ensure permanent stability of hip with child's response to cast monitored for cast syndrome caused by tight spica cast compressing the superior mesenteric artery of the duodenum.
(Provide diaper change frequently and as needed; use disposable diapers or plastic protection over diaper.)	Maintains clean harness brace, or cast.
(Teach parents about type and degree of deformity and cause and treatment plan for correction and prognosis by reinforcing physician information; inform of proposed operative reduction in older child or if obstruction of joint development by soft tissue is present in the young child.)	Provides information about abnormality, its classification, medical and/or surgical regimen that is determined by age and severity of the deformity.
(Teach parents to apply splint or harness correctly over the diaper and shirt, use disposable diapers or waterproof undergarment to protect appliance; on removal of harness for bathing if allowed or sponge bathing child with harness in place, padding shoulder straps, changing position q 2h; to avoid adjusting the harness.)	Promotes and maintains reduction of hip to correct deformity.

(continues)

(continued)

INTERVENTIONS	RATIONALES
(Teach parents about traction care including reason and purpose for traction, amount of movement that the child is allowed, performing neurovascular assessment and what to report, correct weight for amount and hanging with pulleys and knots if present, maintaining body alignment.)	Ensures correct traction for gradual reduction of the hip and/or preoperative if surgery anticipated.
(Teach parents in spica cast care including reason and purpose; support of the cast during movement; maintaining clean, dry cast and protecting it from stool and urine with waterproof tape or plastic cover; padding cast edges; avoid lifting by crossbar; disallowing small objects or crumbs to enter cast; cast signatures without leaving white space between writing; instruct in diapering or bedpan/toilet use; use of a diaper tucked into the perineal opening on cast; feeding infant in supine position [head elevated propped with pillows or while being held in upright position on lap or in a car seat]; inform parents that specially made car seats for infants with casts/harness are available and must be used if the child rides in a car; refer to social worker if cost prevents access to the seats.)	Ensures correct cast care for immobilization of hip following reduction of the hip; traction or surgical correction may be used for reduction or reconstruction of the acetabulum.
Refer parents to crippled children or other community agencies available.	Provides information and support services to the child and family.

NIC: *Surveillance*

Evaluation

(Date/time of evaluation of goal)

(Has goal been met? Not met? Partially met?)

(Provide data related to outcome criteria, e.g., Has traction been maintained? Is Pavlik harness correctly applied? Describe skin around spica cast.)

(Revisions to care plan? D/C care plan? Continue care plan?)

IMPAIRED SOCIAL INTERACTION

Related to: Limited physical mobility.

Defining Characteristics: (Specify: change in pattern of interaction, lengthy treatment and immobilization, boredom, inability to engage in usual activities for age group, environment that lacks diversion.)

Goal: Infant will experience adequate social interaction by (date and time to evaluate).

Outcome Criteria

✔ Parent stays with infant and provides social interaction.

✔ Infant responds positively to parental interaction.

✔ Infant is included in family activities.

NOC: *Social Involvement*

INTERVENTIONS	RATIONALES
Assess infant's social interaction with parents.	Provides information about infant stimulation.
Provide age appropriate toys to be used in bed while in a prone or sitting position depending on type of treatment and degree of immobilization.	Promotes social and developmental activities and reduces boredom during long-term treatment.
Provide exposure to other children by moving bed near areas of activity or near a window; wheel on a stretcher, wheelchair, or stroller; allow to walk with cast or brace if permitted.	Provides environmental stimulation and social interaction; promotes social interaction with others during long-term treatment and reduces boredom.
Encourage family and friends to visit or stay with child.	Promotes social interaction with others during long-term treatment and reduces boredom.
Place toys and other articles within reach.	Provides access to diversion activities when needed.
Teach parents to include infant/child in family activities.	Promotes feeling of acceptance and well-being as part of the family.
Assist parents with devices available or methods of converting aids used for mobility to fill needs of child with a cast or appliance.	Promotes exposure to a variety of activities and changes of environmental stimuli.

INTERVENTIONS	RATIONALES
Encourage parents to allow as much independence if self-care by child as possible.	Promotes independence and allows some control over the situation.

NIC: *Socialization Enhancement*

Evaluation

(Date/time of evaluation of goal)

(Has goal been met? Not met? Partially met?)

(Do parents provide social interaction for infant? Does infant respond positively? Is infant included in family activities?)

(Revisions to care plan? D/C care plan? Continue care plan?)

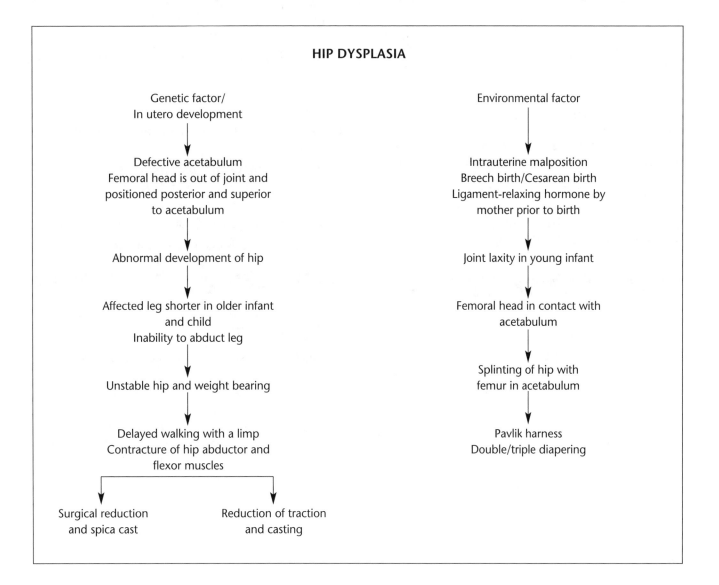

CHAPTER 6.3

LUPUS ERYTHEMATOSUS

Lupus erythematosus is a chronic systemic inflammatory disease of the collagen or supporting tissues and affects any organ in the body. It is classified into a transient type affecting neonates and a type with an onset after infancy that is the same as systemic lupus erythematosus affecting adults. The disease is characterized by remissions and exacerbations and may appear in children as young as 6 years of age but is most commonly seen in those 10 years of age and older. Disease manifestations include lesions or rash on face, neck, trunk and extremities; pleurisy; pericarditis; kidney failure; arthritis; anemia; gastrointestinal abnormalities; and enlarged lymph nodes. Prognosis is dependent on the response to the medical regimen and prevention of exacerbations and severe complications of the renal system.

MEDICAL CARE

Anti-inflammatories (Nonsteroidal): aspirin given to relieve joint pain by decreasing inflammation.

Anti-inflammatories (Steroidal): prednisone given to relieve severe manifestations of the disease; oral dose is tapered to lowest effective amount to control symptoms.

Immunosuppressants: azathioprine (Imuran) given in combination with an anti-inflammatory to reduce amount of steroids.

Antimalarials: hydroxychloroquine sulfate, chloroquine given as second line therapy to relieve symptoms caused by skin, joint, and renal complications and to reduce amounts of steroids needed.

Antibiotics: given specific to identified microorganisms and sensitivity to tested antibiotics.

Anticonvulsants: phenytoin given to control or prevent seizure activity if central nervous system affected.

Antihypertensives: given with a diuretic to lower blood pressure if needed.

Diuretics: given to promote diuresis and elimination of sodium by preventing reabsorption if renal function affected or if blood pressure elevated.

Electrocardiogram: reveals changes and arrhythmias if cardiac output decreased.

Blood Urea Nitrogen (BUN): reveals increases in impaired renal function.

Creatinine: reveals increases in impaired renal function.

Complete Blood Count: reveals increased WBC in presence of infection, decreased Hgb, and platelet and RBC decreases.

Urinalysis: reveals protein, RBC with renal impairment.

Guaiac Test: reveals occult blood in stool.

COMMON NURSING DIAGNOSES

See RISK FOR IMPAIRED SKIN INTEGRITY

Related to: (Specify: altered pigmentation, circulation, immunologic.)

Defining Characteristics: (Specify: disruption in skin surface; scaly erythematmous blush or patchy area over nose and cheeks in the shape of a butterfly; sensitivity to cold in hands and feet with or without cyanosis; dry, cracked skin; alopecia.)

See IMPAIRED PHYSICAL MOBILITY

Related to: (Specify: intolerance to activity, decreased strength and endurance, pain and discomfort.)

Defining Characteristics: (Specify: generalized weakness; joint swelling, stiffness, and pain; limited range of motion; generalized aching; arthralgia; fatigue.)

See HYPERTHERMIA

Related to: Inflammation.

Defining Characteristics: (Specify: increase in body temperature above normal range, low grade elevation.)

See DISTURBED THOUGHT PROCESSES

Related to: Physiologic changes.

Defining Characteristics: (Specify: forgetfulness, changes in consciousness, excitability, seizures, psychosis, irritability, nystagmus, diplopia, disorientation.)

See RISK FOR DEFICIENT FLUID VOLUME

Related to: Renal failure.

Defining Characteristics: (Specify: increased urine output, altered intake, weight loss or gain, edema, dry skin and mucous membranes, thirst, hypotension, increased pulse rate, proteinuria.)

See DECREASED CARDIAC OUTPUT

Related to: (Specify: alteration in preload, electrical factor of altered conduction.)

Defining Characteristics: (Specify: variations in hemodynamic readings, arrhythmias, ECG changes, cyanosis, skin and mucous membrane pallor, decreased peripheral pulses, rales, dyspnea, orthopnea, restlessness.)

See IMBALANCED NUTRITION: LESS THAN BODY REQUIREMENTS

Related to: Inability to ingest, digest, and absorb nutrients.

Defining Characteristics: Anorexia, nausea, vomiting, diarrhea, abdominal discomfort.

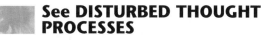
ADDITIONAL NURSING DIAGNOSES

DISTURBED BODY IMAGE

Related to: Biophysical and psychosocial factors.

Defining Characteristics: (Specify: verbal and nonverbal responses to change in body appearance [alopecia, skin rashes, steroid side effects], negative feelings about body, multiple stressors and change in daily living limitations and social relationships.)

Goal: Child will gain improved body image by (date and time to evaluate).

Outcome Criteria

✔ Child verbalizes positive feelings about self.
✔ Participates in social gatherings.

NOC: *Body Image*

INTERVENTIONS	RATIONALES
Assess child for feelings about multiple restrictions in lifestyle, chronic illness, difficulty in school and social situations, inability to keep up with peers and participate in activities.	Provides information about status of self-concept and body image that require special attention.
Encourage expression of feelings and concerns and support communications with parents, teachers, and peers.	Provides opportunity to vent feelings and reduce negative feelings about changes in appearance.
Avoid negative comments and stress positive activities and accomplishments.	Enhances body image and confidence.
Note withdrawal behavior and signs of depression.	Reveals responses to body image changes and possible poor adjustment to changes.
Note hair loss, skin rashes or changes, weight gain and shift in body fat distribution, hirsutism, edema and effect on child.	Reveals side effects of steroid therapy and disease manifestations that affect body image.
Show support and acceptance of changes in appearance of child; provide privacy as needed.	Promotes trust and demonstrates respect for child.
Teach parents to maintain support for child.	Encourages acceptance of the child with special needs (long-term steroid therapy and side effects, risk for infection and bleeding tendency, lifelong activity restrictions).
Suggest use of wig, scarf, makeup, clothing selection as indicated.	Supports child during body image changes involving skin, hair, edema, weight gain, hirsutism.
Encourage parents to be flexible in care of child and to integrate care and routines so child may participate in peer activity.	Promotes well-being of child and sense of belonging and control of life events.

(continues)

(continued)

INTERVENTIONS	RATIONALES
Assist parents and child to deal with peer and school perceptions of appearance and to tell others about change in appearance.	Prevents stigmatization of child by those who are not apprised of the child's disease; attitudes of others will affect child's body image.

NIC: *Socialization Enhancement*

Evaluation

(Date/time of evaluation of goal)

(Has goal been met? Not met? Partially met?)

(What did child say about self? Use quotes. Does child participate in social gatherings? Specify.)

(Revisions to care plan? D/C care plan? Continue care plan?)

PAIN

Related to: Inflammatory process.

Defining Characteristics: (Specify: communication of pain descriptors, joint pain, achiness, joint swelling and stiffness.)

Goal: Child will experience decreased pain by (date and time to evaluate).

Outcome Criteria

✔ Child rates pain as less than (specify expected level and pain scale used).

NOC: *Pain Level*

INTERVENTIONS	RATIONALES
Assess severity of joint pain, location, duration, remissions, and exacerbations and what precipitates pain such as weight gain, activity; affect on mobility and participation in ADL; presence of joint deformity.	Provides information symptomatic of the effect of the disease on the musculoskeletal system; allows for analgesic selection and better management of activity involvement.
Administer analgesic (specify) and anti-inflammatories (specify) and assess effect of medications in relieving pain.	(Action of drugs.)
Apply warm compresses or packs to painful areas.	Promotes circulation to the area by vasodilation to relieve pain.

INTERVENTIONS	RATIONALES
Provide 1 to 2 rest periods during day and quiet environment for sleep.	Decreases stimulation that increases pain, and promotes rest.
Encourage to assume position of comfort.	Promotes comfort and rest for joints to reduce pain.
Provide toys, TV, books, games, for quiet play during painful episodes.	Promotes diversionary activity to detract from pain.
Explain cause of pain to child and measures that should be taken to relieve pain (specify).	Provides reasons for treatments and medications.
Inform child of factors that exacerbate pain episodes and to express or report presence of pain at the onset.	Promotes opportunity to avoid those situations or activities that contribute to pain and to provide for immediate relief.

NIC: *Pain Management*

Evaluation

(Date/time of evaluation of goal)

(Has goal been met? Not met? Partially met?)

(What is pain rating? Specify scale used.)

(Revisions to care plan? D/C care plan? Continue care plan?)

DEFICIENT KNOWLEDGE

Related to: Lack of information about chronic illness.

Defining Characteristics: (Specify: request for information about disease and the special needs associated with the disease; prevention of exacerbation and complications of the disease; risk of noncompliance with multiple preventive precautions.)

Goal: Clients will gain knowledge about lupus erythematosus by (date and time to evaluate).

Outcome Criteria

✔ Clients verbalize how lupus affect each body system.

✔ Clients identify 3 ways to avoid exacerbations of the condition.

✔ Clients verbalize understanding of treatment regimen.

NOC: *Knowledge: Disease Process*

INTERVENTIONS	RATIONALES
Assess knowledge of disease, type of treatments, effect on all systems, and medical regimen.	Provides information needed to understand this complex disease and adjust long-term treatment and restrictions.
Teach parents and child about the disease process, effect on connective tissue and all systems, and treatment regimen needed to maintain remission.	Provides information about known facts related to the disease to enhance knowledge of potential for exacerbations that may lead to early death.
Teach parents and child about the administration and side effects of anti-inflammatories and immunosuppressant drugs (specify), not to decrease or skip the dose if side effects appear, and the need to adjust dosage during stressful situations.	Promotes understanding of long-term medication regimen even when affected by undesirable side effects; an abrupt withdrawal of the medication may cause a serious physiologic complication.
Teach parents and child about activity restrictions or moderate activities allowed and to weigh one activity against another as appropriate for the child.	Prevents exacerbation of the symptoms while considering the long-term difficulty the child faces when activities are restricted.
Teach child to avoid sun exposure directly, through clouds, or reflected from water or snow; to use special sun screen or brimmed or visored hat to protect face.	Prevents skin eruptions/reactions common to this disease when exposed to the sun.
Teach clients about child's need to take naps and have 8 hours of sleep/night; avoid fatigue or stressful situations; avoid medications such as sulfonamides, tetracyclines, anticonvulsants, and others that cause an exacerbation.	Prevents exacerbations of the disease symptoms.
Teach parents and child to report bruising, petechiae, elevated temperature, blood in urine or stool, increased irritability, vomiting, inability or remission in taking medications, respiratory or urinary changes.	Provides for early interventions if complications occur.
Refer to community agencies or American Lupus Society for contact and support.	Provides information and support for families and children to assist in adjusting to the disease and its lifelong limitation.

NIC: *Teaching: Disease Process*

Evaluation

(Date/time of evaluation of goal)

(Has goal been met? Not met? Partially met?)

(What did clients verbalize about lupus? What 3 ways to avoid problems did clients identify? What did clients verbalize about treatment regimen? Use quotes.)

(Revisions to care plan? D/C care plan? Continue care plan?)

INEFFECTIVE COPING

Related to: (Specify: multiple life changes, personal vulnerability.)

Defining Characteristics: (Specify: alteration in social participation, inappropriate use of defense mechanisms [denial, regression, projection], withdrawal, intolerance of new experiences, lifelong hardships of medical regimen and limitations.)

Goal: Child will cope effectively with illness by (date and time to evaluate).

Outcome Criteria

✔ Child expresses feelings about chronic illness.
✔ Child identifies 3 effective coping mechanisms to use.

NOC: *Coping*

INTERVENTIONS	RATIONALES
Assess coping behaviors of child and factors that induce use of defense mechanisms, response to stressful situations (avoidance behavior, cooperation or resistance, aggression, regression, delaying tactics, inappropriate humor).	Provides information about child's coping mechanisms and pattern and use of coping strategies.
Allow child to express feeling and provide outlet for release of feeling in an accepting environment.	Promotes independence and control over a situation.
Provide therapeutic play including throwing ball or balloons, pounding board, hand painting, water play.	Provides expression of feelings and outlet to release aggression.
Involve child in care decisions and encourage independence in as much of the care as possible.	Promotes active participation in care with assistance as needed.

(continues)

(continued)

INTERVENTIONS	RATIONALES
Assist child to identify at least 3 coping mechanisms to use during play, social interactions, painful procedures, restrictions, and bed rest.	Allows for experiences which gives the child an opportunity to practice successful coping behaviors that enhance development of one's self-esteem.
Encourage parents to participate in child's care and support.	Increases feelings of security when the child must deal with new situations.
Assist child to identify behaviors that are positive and negative and discuss the factors that influence coping pattern (age, development, past experiences, ability to adapt, support, perception of what is happening, inner resources).	Promotes understanding of coping pattern and reasons for behavior.
Teach child about any procedures well before scheduling and that support will be given to assist through the event.	Promotes coping with new and painful experiences.

INTERVENTIONS	RATIONALES
Suggest psychological consultation if appropriate.	Assists child to deal constructively with frustration and compliance with medical regimen for lifelong illness.

NIC: *Self-Esteem Enhancement*

Evaluation

(Date/time of evaluation of goal)

(Has goal been met? Not met? Partially met?)

(What feelings about chronic illness did child verbalize? What 3 ways to cope did child identify? Use quotes.)

(Revisions to care plan? D/C care plan? Continue care plan?)

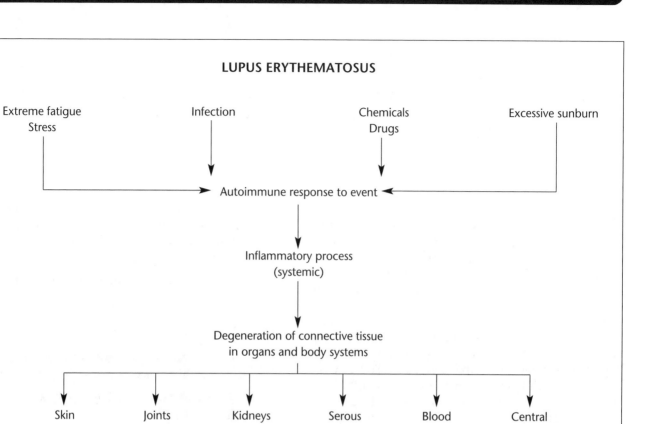

CHAPTER 6.4

LEGG-CALVÉ-PERTHES DISEASE

Legg-Calvé-Perthes disease (osteochondritis deformans), is a disease of the femoral head occurring in children between 3 to 12 years of age. Its cause is unknown but the disease is characterized by a necrosis of the femoral head which results from an impaired circulation of the femoral epiphysis extending to the acetabulum. Joint dysfunction with hip pain or ache and a limp that is continuous or intermittent are common signs and symptoms of the condition. Early treatment to maintain the femoral head in the acetabulum determines the prognosis. The disease progression and resolution is classified into four stages: stage I is the necrosis and degeneration of the femoral head (avascular); stage II is the bone absorption and vascularization (revascularization); stage III is the new bone formation with ossification (reparative); and stage IV is the reformation of the femoral head to a sphere (regenerative).

MEDICAL CARE

X-ray: reveals changes in the femoral head and hip from a flattened appearance (stage I) to a mottled appearance and progressing to increased bone density and normalization of the rounded appearance of the femoral head (stage IV).

Magnetic Resonance Imaging (MRI): useful early in the disease to detect changes as radiographic changes are not present for several months after onset. MRIs are useful later in assessing containment of the femoral head in the acetabulum.

Abduction Traction: used to increase the range of motion in a child who has developed limited hip motion from pain and spasm. Abduction traction is gradually increased on a daily basis to a point comfortably tolerated by the child. Traction may be used prior to surgical intervention and may be used in a home-based program.

Serial Casting: casting of the hips in an abducted position with weekly cast changes using a progres-

sively longer bar until full range of abduction is achieved. Casting also contains the femoral head in the acetabulum. The cast may be bivalved later and used as a splint.

Osteotomy: surgical realignment of the femur so that the head of the femur is securely contained within the acetabulum. Requires 6 to 8 weeks of a hip spica cast after surgery and may be preceded by traction.

COMMON NURSING DIAGNOSES

See IMPAIRED PHYSICAL MOBILITY

Related to: Musculoskeletal impairment (femoral head).

Defining Characteristics: (Specify: imposed restrictions of movement by medical protocol of corrective device [cast, brace, traction], reluctance to attempt movement, restriction in weight-bearing, limited ROM, bed rest.)

See RISK FOR IMPAIRED SKIN INTEGRITY

Related to: (Specify: physical immobilization, pressure of cast or appliance and altered circulation, sensation.)

Defining Characteristics: (Specify: change in skin color and temperature proximately to cast, skin irritation at cast edges, numbness or tingling distal to cast, redness on skin from prolonged pressure, break in skin from surgical correction.)

See DELAYED GROWTH AND DEVELOPMENT

Related to: Effects of immobilization.

Defining Characteristics: (Specify: environmental and stimulation deficiencies, inability to perform self-care activities appropriate for age, inability to participate in school and social activities.)

ADDITIONAL NURSING DIAGNOSES

▨ DEFICIENT KNOWLEDGE

Related to: Lack of information about the disease.

Defining Characteristics: (Specify: request for information about initial and long-term treatment, management of the therapy, and modification of activities.)

Goal: Clients will obtain knowledge about the illness by (date and time to evaluate).

Outcome Criteria

✔ Parents verbalize understanding of the four stages of the disease.

✔ Parents and child (if applicable) verbalize understanding of treatment plan (specify).

NOC: *Knowledge: Disease Process*

INTERVENTIONS	RATIONALES
Assess knowledge of pathology of the disease and its four stages, treatment and prognosis, signs and symptoms. Provide information as needed.	Provides information needed to develop a plan of instruction to ensure compliance of the medical regimen for correction; usually lasts 1 to 4 years and affects children 3 to 12 years of age with each stage lasting approximately 9 to 12 months; the younger the child at the time of diagnosis, the more positive the results and prognosis.
Teach parents and child that hip pain or stiffness that is constant or intermittent with involvement of the knee or thigh, limited ROM of the hip joint, a limp on the affected side may indicate aseptic necrosis of the femoral capital epiphysis with degenerative changes in the femoral head.	Reveals signs and symptoms of the disease usually noted in the second stage.
Teach parents and child about use and purpose of traction if used.	Applied to stretch adductor muscles before abduction cast is used, or before surgery.
(If home traction is used, refer parents to a home health agency.)	Home traction allows child to be in comfortable, familiar surroundings while maintaining therapeutic regimen; visits from home nurse allow evaluation of treatment and provision of family support and education.

INTERVENTIONS	RATIONALES
(For surgical correction, inform parents that child will need prophylactic antibiotics, will receive IV narcotics for pain for 2 to 3 days after surgery, will have a hip spica cast applied, and will be discharged to home 4 to 5 days after surgery.)	Decreases anxiety about the surgical procedure through knowledge of postoperative care.
(Teach parents about purpose and application of an abduction splint; after ROM achieved, demonstrate and allow for return demonstration of application.)	Provides containment of the position of the femur while allowing for supported weight-bearing during healing, and is removable for bathing.
Teach child to avoid weight-bearing on the affected limb (except as prescribed by physician) and to be relatively inactive; advise activities suitable to stage of condition such as hobbies, crafts, games, museums, events of interest.	Prevents degeneration of the hip joint caused by femoral damage resulting from weight-bearing activities; prolonged bed rest is no longer required.
Encourage parents to advise school of activities that are allowed for learning and peer interactions.	Provides special needs of child in order to continue school attendance and activities that may be adapted to appliance to promote feeling of acceptance.
Teach parents about care of cast or splint including cleaning, tightness, and alignment with joints.	Promotes proper function of appliance used and prevents complications associated with its use.
Instruct parents and child in use and care of crutches if used including swing through gait; monitor for repair needs as presence of loose screws and worn tips.	Promotes safe use of crutches for mobility.
Encourage parents to maintain pathways clear of clutter or toys in home.	Prevents falls and injury.
Suggest to parents to prepare for attendance at special activities by calling in advance for special transportation, use of wheelchairs or other aids.	Provides for participation in outside activities to enhance growth and development needs in long-term therapy.

NIC: *Teaching: Disease Process*

Evaluation

(Date/time of evaluation of goal)

(Has goal been met? Not met? Partially met?)

(What did clients verbalize about the four stages of Legg-Calvé-Perthes disease? What did clients verbalize about treatment regimen? Use quotes.)

(Revisions to care plan? D/C care plan? Continue care plan?)

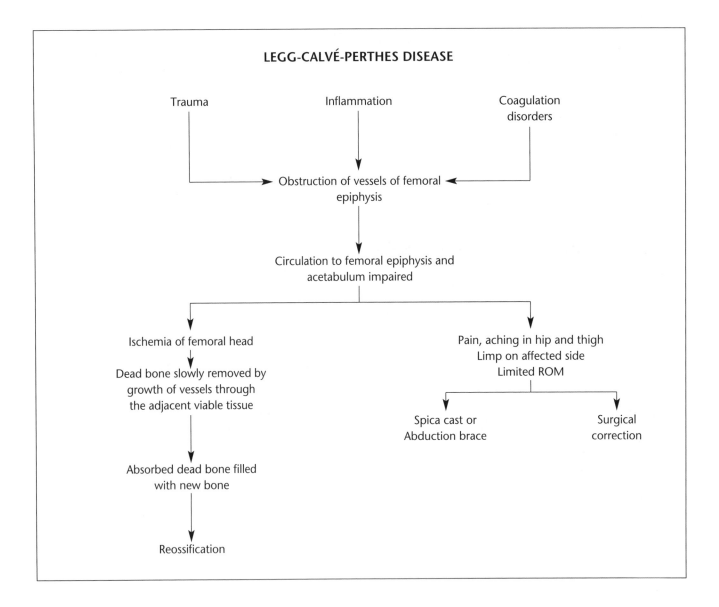

LEGG-CALVÉ-PERTHES DISEASE

Trauma   Inflammation   Coagulation disorders

Obstruction of vessels of femoral epiphysis

Circulation to femoral epiphysis and acetabulum impaired

Ischemia of femoral head

Dead bone slowly removed by growth of vessels through the adjacent viable tissue

Absorbed dead bone filled with new bone

Reossification

Pain, aching in hip and thigh
Limp on affected side
Limited ROM

Spica cast or Abduction brace

Surgical correction

CHAPTER 6.5

OSTEOGENIC SARCOMA

Osteogenic sarcoma is a primary malignancy of the bone with the metaphysics of the long bones most commonly affected. These include the femur, humerus, and tibia. Metastasis most commonly affects the lungs but may involve other organs. The disease most commonly occurs in children over 10 years of age. Treatment consists of amputation of the limb with chemotherapy before and/or following surgery, or a bone and joint replacement in selected children to salvage the limb with chemotherapy before the surgery.

MEDICAL CARE

Analgesics: to control postoperative pain.

Chemotherapy Protocol: methotrexate with leucovorin calcium, doxorubicin, dactinomycin cyclophosphamide, cisplatin.

Antigout Agent: allopurinol to reduce the severity of hyperuricemia caused by chemotherapy which promotes nucleic acid degradation causing increased plasma uric acid levels.

Bone X-ray: reveals bone lesion, fracture caused by tumor invasion.

Bone Scan: reveals presence of bone lesions and size.

Bone Biopsy: reveals presence of malignant tumor.

Computerized Tomography (CT): reveals metastasis of bone and other organs.

Enzymes: alkaline phosphatase (ALP): reveals increased level caused by abnormal osteoblastic activity or bone cell production; also reveals presence of isoenzymes (ALP2) of bone origin.

COMMON NURSING DIAGNOSES

 See IMBALANCED NUTRITION: LESS THAN BODY REQUIREMENTS

Related to: (Specify: inability to ingest and digest food, chemotherapy.)

Defining Characteristics: (Specify: anorexia, nausea, vomiting from chemotherapy, anxiety, grieving, weight loss, NPO status before and after surgery.)

 See RISK FOR DEFICIENT FLUID VOLUME

Related to: (Specify: altered intake; excessive losses through normal routes.)

Defining Characteristics: (Specify: diarrhea, vomiting from chemotherapy, NPO status before and after surgery.)

See RISK FOR IMPAIRED SKIN INTEGRITY

Related to: (Specify: chemotherapy, IV, surgical site, and use of prosthesis.)

Defining Characteristics: (Specify: disruption of skin surfaces, destruction of skin surfaces, redness, edema, excoriation of stump site, improper fit or application of prosthesis, extravasation of IV site with swelling skin, redness, and tissue necrosis.)

See IMPAIRED PHYSICAL MOBILITY

Related to: Amputation.

Defining Characteristics: (Specify: inability to move within physical environment, reluctance to attempt movement, imposed restrictions of movement with loss of limb, inability to adapt to prosthesis or brace, use of crutches or wheelchair.)

See DIARRHEA

Related to: Chemotherapy.

Defining Characteristics: (Specify: increased frequency of bowel sounds and loose, liquid stools.)

ADDITIONAL NURSING DIAGNOSES

ANXIETY

Related to: Change in health status, threat of death, threat to self-concept.

Defining Characteristics: (Specify: increased apprehension and fear of diagnosis; expressed concern and worry about preoperative procedures and preparation, postoperative effects of therapy on physical and emotional status, possible metastasis of disease, loss of limb and use of prosthesis.)

Goal: Clients will experience decreased anxiety by (date and time to evaluate).

Outcome Criteria

✔ Parents and child express feelings about illness.
✔ Clients verbalize feeling less anxious.

NOC: *Anxiety Control*

INTERVENTIONS	RATIONALES
Assess level of anxiety of parents and child and how it is manifested; the need for information that will relieve anxiety.	Provides information about source and level of anxiety and need for interventions to relieve it; sources for the child may be procedures, fear of mutilation or death, unfamiliar environment of hospital and may be manifested by restlessness, inability to play, sleep, or eat.
Assess possible need for special counseling services for child.	Reduces anxiety and supports child dealing with illness and promotes adjustment to lifestyle changes.
Allow open expression of concerns about illness, procedures, treatments, and possible consequences of surgery.	Provides opportunity to vent feelings and fears to reduce anxiety.
Communicate with child at appropriate age level and answer questions calmly and honestly; use pictures, models, and drawings for explanations.	Promotes understanding and trust.
Provide child with as much input in decisions about care and routines as possible.	Allows for more control and independence in situations.
Encourage parents to stay with child; provide a telephone number to call for information.	Promotes care and support by parents.

INTERVENTIONS	RATIONALES
Provide continuing nurse assignment with the same personnel.	Promotes trust and comfort and familiarity with staff giving care.
Orient child to surgical and ICU unit, equipment, noises, and staff.	Reduces anxiety caused by fear of unknown.
Teach parents and child about the disease process, surgical procedure, what to expect preoperatively and postoperatively including chemotherapy and its benefits and side effects (nausea, vomiting, diarrhea, stomatitis, alopecia, and others are possibilities but are temporary; phantom pain).	Provides information to promote understanding that will relieve fear and anxiety; understanding of preoperative and postoperative treatments and effect on body image.
Explain all procedures and care in simple, direct, honest terms and repeat as often as necessary; reinforce physician information if needed and provide specific information as requested.	Supplies information about all diagnostic procedures and tests such as CBC, platelets with chemotherapy and scans, and X-rays for diagnosis.
Inform parents and child of the extent of surgery planned with the removal of a limb (that a temporary prosthesis will be fitted immediately following surgery, and a permanent one will be fitted in 6 to 8 weeks; that recreational and physical therapy will be undertaken following amputation).	Reduces anxiety when knowledge and support is given, and child and parents will not feel betrayed by inadequate preparation of procedures and treatments.
Introduce child to another who has same disease and amputation.	Provides information and support from a peer with the same condition and who would have empathy.
Refer to American Cancer Society.	Provide resource for information and support groups.

NIC: *Anxiety Reduction*

Evaluation

(Date/time of evaluation of goal)

(Has goal been met? Not met? Partially met?)

(Did parents and child express feelings about the illness? Did clients verbalize decreased anxiety? Use quotes.)

(Revisions to care plan? D/C care plan? Continue care plan?)

IMPAIRED ORAL MUCOUS MEMBRANE

Related to: Chemotherapy.

Defining Characteristics: (Specify: stomatitis, oral ulcers, hyperemia, oral pain or discomfort, oral plaque.)

Goal: Child will be free of oral mucous membrane irritation by (date and time to evaluate).

Outcome Criteria

✔ No oral mucous membrane lesions present.

NOC: *Oral Health*

INTERVENTIONS	RATIONALES
Assess oral cavity for pain ulcers, lesions, gingivitis, mucositis or stomatitis and effect on ability to ingest food and fluids.	Provides information about effect of chemotherapy.
Provide mouth rinses, cleansing with swabs or soft toothbrush.	Provides mouth care without irritating oral mucosa.
Administer medication topically as ordered (specify) before meals and offer bland, smooth foods that are not hot or spicy.	Permits eating with more comfort (action of drug).
Administer an antiseptic mouth rinse (specify) 30 minutes before any food or fluid intake, as ordered.	Promotes comfort of oral mucosa and maintains integrity.
Encourage child to select foods they prefer from list.	Allows for independence and control over situation to reduce helplessness and increase nutrition.
Teach parents about the effect of chemotherapy on oral mucosa and in treatment to decrease discomfort in oral cavity.	Promotes understanding of side effects that occur and temporary nature of the side effects.
Teach parents about mouth rinses and topical application of medications.	Promotes effective care of oral cavity to relieve discomfort and prevent mucosa breakdown and increased inflammation.
Instruct to use soft brush or swabs to clean mouth.	Prevents trauma to mucosa.

NIC: *Oral Health Maintenance*

Evaluation

(Date/time of evaluation of goal)
(Has goal been met? Not met? Partially met?)

(Does child have any oral mucous membrane lesions?)
(Revisions to care plan? D/C care plan? Continue care plan?)

INEFFECTIVE PROTECTION

Related to: (Specify: drug therapy [antineoplastics]: abnormal blood profile [leukopenia, thrombocytopenia, anemia, coagulation].)

Defining Characteristics: (Specify: altered clotting, bone marrow suppression, deficient immunity against infection, hematoma, petechiae, bleeding from nose or gums, hematemesis, blood in stool.)

Goal: Child will be protected by (date and time to evaluate).

Outcome Criteria

✔ Child does not experience bleeding.
✔ Temperature remains <100° F.
✔ Breath sounds clear bilaterally.

NOC: *Infection Status*

INTERVENTIONS	RATIONALES
Assess for bleeding from any site, WBC, platelet count, Hct, absolute neutrophil count, and febrile episodes.	Provides information about frank bleeding or blood profile abnormalities that predispose to bleeding caused by bone marrow suppression and immuno-suppression resulting from chemotherapy.
Avoid trauma by use of hard toothbrush or dental floss, taking rectal temperatures, performing unnecessary invasive procedures.	Prevents bleeding caused by trauma during chemotherapy which alters platelet and clotting factors.
Carry out handwashing technique before giving care, use mask and gown when appropriate, provide a private room, monitor for any signs and symptoms of infections, especially pulmonary.	Prevents transmission of pathogens to a compromised immune system during chemotherapy if neutrophil count is less than 1,000/cu mm.
Teach parents and child to avoid rough play or sports, straining at defecation, forcefully blowing nose.	Prevents trauma that causes bleeding.
Teach parents and child to avoid people with upper respiratory infection or any illness.	Prevents risk for infection in the highly susceptible child.

(continues)

(continued)

INTERVENTIONS	RATIONALES
Teach parents to report any fever, behavior changes, headache, dizziness, fatigue, pallor, slow oozing of blood from any area, exposure to a communicable disease.	Indicates a complication associated with an abnormal blood profile.
Instruct and allow for return demonstration of urine and stool testing for blood using dipstick and hematest.	Identifies presence of bleeding in gastrointestinal or urinary tract.

NIC: *Surveillance*

Evaluation

(Date/time of evaluation of goal)

(Has goal been met? Not met? Partially met?)

(Is there any sign of bleeding? What has been looked for? What is temperature? Describe breath sounds.)

(Revisions to care plan? D/C care plan? Continue care plan?)

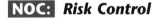 **RISK FOR INJURY**

Related to: (Specify: broken skin and altered mobility; prosthesis use.)

Defining Characteristics: (Specify: amputation of a limb, changes in stump incision [redness, irritation, swelling, drainage], improper fit of prosthesis and failure to adapt to it, improper positioning and alignment of the stump, psychosocial maladaption to prosthesis.)

Goal: Child will not experience injury by (date and time to evaluate).

Outcome Criteria

✔ Stump is clean and dry without redness, odor, or drainage.

✔ Child and parents begin to care for stump (specify).

NOC: *Risk Control*

INTERVENTIONS	RATIONALES
Assess child for type of surgery and condition and healing of the stump, type of bandaging or cast, presence of drains, type of prosthetic device and fit.	Provides information about amputation needed to provide specific care of stump and rehabilitation.
Assess dressing for bleeding, redness, pain, drainage at stump area q 2 to 4h; maintain dressing (pressure) or wrapping of stump as ordered; change dressing only if ordered.	Indicates infection or risk of hemorrhage at amputation.
Maintain Trendelenburg and prone position as ordered; avoid elevation (with pillow), external rotation, or abduction of stump.	Prevents deformities and contractures caused by hip flexion.
Perform ROM daily and exercises recommended by physical therapist.	Promotes mobility and healing of the stump and prevents contractures.
Cleanse stump and socket daily with mild soap and warm water, rinse and pat dry.	Promotes adaptation to device and prevents infection caused by pathogens transmitted via the prosthetic device.
Support expressions about loss of lifestyle and permanent disability adjustment difficulties (age appropriate).	Promotes venting of feelings and assists to cope with change in body image.
Instruct parents and child in stump care, toughening exercises, application of stocking and prosthesis, care of device.	Promotes adaptation to loss and correct care of stump and prosthesis.
Instruct child in stump positioning and exercising, ROM of muscles and joints.	Prevents muscle or joint complications and enhances mobility.
Inform child of importance of daily activities to perform and those to avoid and explain reasons for restrictions.	Promotes mobility and return to former activities within limitation imposed by amputation and use of prosthetic device.
Teach parents and child to continue chemotherapy and rehabilitation therapy.	Promotes healing.
Discuss modification of clothing and instruct in crutch walking and how to get around in room, at home, and at school.	Enhances body image and return to limited activities.
Reassure child that feelings of anger, denial, and hostility are normal following such a loss.	Promotes acceptance of child while grieving for loss.

NIC: *Surveillance*

Evaluation

(Date/time of evaluation of goal)

(Has goal been met? Not met? Partially met?)

(Describe stump. Describe stump care provided by parents and child.)

(Revisions to care plan? D/C care plan? Continue care plan?)

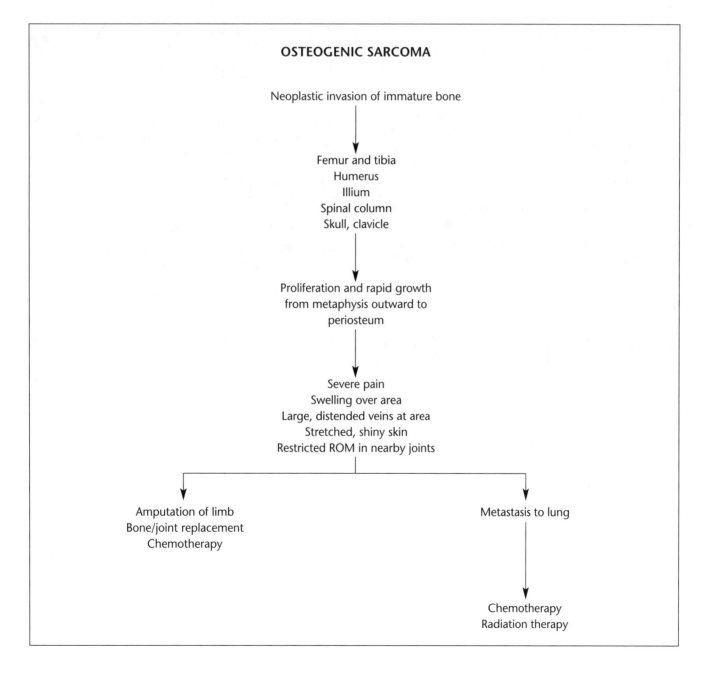

CHAPTER 6.6

OSTEOMYELITIS

Osteomyelitis is an infection of the bone caused by any infectious agent, but most commonly by *Staphylococcus aureus*, hemolytic streptococci, *E. coli*, or *Haemophilus influenzae*. In children, the metaphyses of long bones (tibia, femur) are the sites most frequently involved. The infectious agent usually enters the bone through the blood (hematogenous) after trauma or an upper respiratory infection. Less commonly, the infection can spread to the bone secondary to a contiguous focus of infection. The disease can be acute, with a rapidly destructive pyogenic infection of the bone and marrow and signs of systemic infection as well as local pain, swelling, and redness of the involved area. In subacute osteomyelitis, the disease is insidious in onset and the child has pain and dysfunction without systemic infection. The subacute form may be caused by children receiving antibiotics during a presymptomatic period. Osteomyelitis most commonly occurs in children 5 to 14 years of age. The disease can usually be treated with antibiotics, but may require surgical drainage as well.

MEDICAL CARE

Analgesics/Antipyretics: acetaminophen for pain and to reduce fever.

Antibiotics: dependent on identification of infective agent and sensitivity to the antibiotic.

Bone X-ray: shows changes in the involved area after the first 2 weeks.

Computerized Tomography (CT): reveals bone changes early in the disease.

Bone Scan: reveals infectious process in bone by increased uptake of radionucleotides.

Erythrocyte Sedimentation Rate (ESR): reveals increases in acute stage.

Complete Blood Count (CBC): reveals increased WBC during infectious process.

Blood/Wound Cultures: reveals organisms responsible for infection by culture of site.

COMMON NURSING DIAGNOSES

 ### See HYPERTHERMIA

Related to: Infection.

Defining Characteristics: (Specify: increase in body temperature above normal range, warm to touch, increased respiratory and pulse rate.)

See RISK FOR DEFICIENT FLUID VOLUME

Related to: Excessive losses.

Defining Characteristics: (Specify: elevated temperature, diaphoresis, thirst, altered intake, insensitive losses.)

See IMPAIRED PHYSICAL MOBILITY

Related to: Pain and discomfort, musculoskeletal impairment.

Defining Characteristics: (Specify: reluctance to attempt movement, imposed restrictions of movement by immobilization of part by cast and/or bed rest, restriction in weight-bearing.)

See IMBALANCED NUTRITION: LESS THAN BODY REQUIREMENTS

Related to: Inability to ingest food.

Defining Characteristics: (Specify: anorexia, irritability, restlessness, weight loss, inadequate food intake.)

See RISK FOR IMPAIRED SKIN INTEGRITY

Related to: (Specify: physical immobilization, pressure of cast and altered circulation, sensation.)

Defining Characteristics: (Specify: change in color and temperature of skin proximal to cast or device, skin irritation at cast edges, numbness distal cast, prolonged pressure on an area with redness present, break in skin from surgical wound.)

ADDITIONAL NURSING DIAGNOSES

ANXIETY

Related to: Change in health status, change in environment (hospitalization).

Defining Characteristics: (Specify: expressed apprehension and concern about prolonged hospitalization resulting from spread of infection, possible surgical drainage of infected area.)

Goal: Clients will experience decreased anxiety by (date and time to evaluate).

Outcome Criteria

✔ Clients identify source of anxiety.
✔ Clients verbalize decreased anxiety.

NOC: *Anxiety Control*

INTERVENTIONS	RATIONALES
Assess source and level of anxiety and need for information that will relieve anxiety.	Provides information about anxiety, its effect and need to relieve it; sources may include prolonged immobilization and hospitalization, long-term IV antibiotic therapy, possible surgical drainage and antibiotic instillation into wound, risk of complications from disease and high-dose medication therapy.
Encourage expression of concerns and time to ask questions about condition, procedures, prognosis, recovery time by parents or child.	Provides opportunity to vent feelings and fears to reduce anxiety.
Answer questions calmly and honestly; use pictures, drawings, and models for information about demonstrations.	Promotes trust and secure, supportive environment.
Encourage parents to stay with child during hospitalization, and to assist in care; encourage visits from friends and relatives.	Allows parents to care for and support child, continue parental role and promote security for the child.

INTERVENTIONS	RATIONALES
Give parents and child as much input into decisions about care and usual routines as possible.	Allows for more control over situation and maintains familiar routines for care.
Teach parents and child about cause and course of the disease, extent of the infectious process, and treatment modalities.	Provides information that will enhance understanding of the disease to relieve anxiety.
Inform parents and child of tests and procedures to be done and the reasons for them; include surgical procedure if planned.	Provides rationale for diagnostic procedures and surgery to prepare for these experiences and reduce fear of unknown that increases anxiety.
Teach parents and child of reason for antibiotic therapy.	Provides rationale for long-term therapy to control infectious process and prevent its spread to reduce anxiety.
Teach parents and child about treatment to expect following surgery including presence of cast on the affected extremity, antibiotic therapy instillation into the wound, and continuous removal of drainage from the wound by low suction.	Provides information about postoperative care to reduce anxiety.
Teach parents and child that although weight-bearing will be disallowed until healing is well established, appetite, quiet activity, and improved sense of well-being will be increased as acuity of the disease is reduced.	Promotes comfort and positive attitude and reduces anxiety level when expectations are known.
(Inform parents that physical therapy may be prescribed after infection subsides, acute healing assured.)	Permits optimal function of affected extremity and allows for feeling of positive outcome.

NIC: *Anxiety Reduction*

Evaluation

(Date/time of evaluation of goal)

(Has goal been met? Not met? Partially met?)

(Did parents and child identify source of anxiety? Did clients verbalize decreased anxiety? Use quotes.)

(Revisions to care plan? D/C care plan? Continue care plan?)

PAIN

Related to: Inflammation/infection.

Defining Characteristics: (Specify: communication of pain descriptors, crying, irritability, restlessness, withdrawal, reluctance to use or move affected limb, tenderness.)

Goal: Child will experience decreased pain by (date and time to evaluate).

Outcome Criteria

✔ Child rates pain as a (specify using a pain scale. Identify scale used).

NOC: *Pain Level*

INTERVENTIONS	RATIONALES
Assess site for pain on movement of extremity; resistance of muscles to passive movement, holding extremity in semi-flexion; severity, type, and duration of pain using a pain scale if appropriate.	Provides information about pain as a basis for analgesic therapy.
Administer analgesic and sedative as ordered (specify drug, dose, route) and note response.	Reduces pain and promotes rest to reduce stimuli that cause pain (action of drug).
Place extremity in position of comfort and support with pillows at 30 degrees elevation.	Promotes comfort and reduces or prevents pain by reducing edema when venous return is enhanced.
Move extremity with smoothness and care.	Prevents pain caused by careless handling or abrupt movement of affected part.
Provide diversionary activities and quiet play during acute stage (specify).	Diverts attention from the pain.
Teach parents and child about analgesic medications and expected results.	Provides information about effects expected from analgesic therapy to relieve pain until acute stage subsides or healing is underway.
Suggest to parents and child ways to move, position extremity; importance of maintaining immobilization of the extremity and avoiding any weight-bearing activity until advised.	Prevents undue pain caused by movement of affected area.

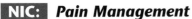 **NIC:** *Pain Management*

Evaluation

(Date/time of evaluation of goal)

(Has goal been met? Not met? Partially met?)

(What is pain rating? Specify scale used)

(Revisions to care plan? D/C care plan? Continue care plan?)

▨ **RISK FOR INJURY**

Related to: (Specify: infection spread, immobilization, effects of cast application.)

Defining Characteristics: (Specify: changes in color and temperature, tactile perception of casted extremity, increased body temperature, purulent drainage, edema, erythematic infection site, musty odor under cast, increased WBC, positive wound culture.)

Goal: Child will not experience injury by (date and time to evaluate).

Outcome Criteria

✔ Child denies increased pain. WBC levels remain < (specify).

NOC: *Risk Control*

INTERVENTIONS	RATIONALES
Assess presence of localized pain, swelling, and warmth over the affected bone; purulent drainage with a musty odor from open wound, under cast, or over the infected area that is left open for observation.	Provides information about site of infection(s) which may be open wound, bone, or surgical drainage wound; inadequate treatment may result in chronic osteomyelitis or persistence and spread of infection.
Administer antibiotics based on physician orders (specify).	(Action of drug.)
Administer antibiotic solution (specify) into the wound, as ordered, via an IV administration set at a regulated rate; provide wound drainage by connecting tubes from wound to low suction.	Treats open wound infections and ensures continuous wound drainage.
Place child in isolation and maintain body fluid precautions (wound and skin) if wound is open and draining.	Prevents wound contamination or spread of infection; agency policy dictates measures for precautions.
Maintain sterile technique for all procedures and dressing changes; cleanse, pack wound as ordered.	Prevents introduction of infectious organisms.

INTERVENTIONS	RATIONALES
Measure limb circumference when assessing infectious process.	Reveals changes caused by edema.
Monitor WBC, ESR, and antibiotic levels as appropriate.	Increases in WBC and ESR found in infections and antibiotic levels reveal if therapeutic levels are maintained for effective treatment.
Provide immobilization of limb by maintaining cast, splint, and bed rest status; monitor color, temperature, sensation, and motion of digits.	Maintains limb alignment, limits spread of infection, and prevents possible fraction or complications resulting from neurovascular problems.
Teach parents and child about proper technique for hand-washing, wound care and handling contaminated articles/supplies.	Prevents transmission of microorganisms to or from child.
Instruct parents about antibiotic administration including action, dose, time, frequency, side effects, and expected results; length of time that antibiotic therapy may last.	Promotes long-term therapy to ensure effective results.
Teach parents and child about measures to maintain immobility and reason for isolation precautions.	Prevents further spread of infection and possible damage to affected area and surrounding tissue.
Teach parents to care for cast or splint including petaling edges, maintaining dry and clean cast or splint, preventing small particles or objects from entering cast or splint.	Ensures effective immobilization and prevents complications caused by whole or bivalve cast or splint.
Inform parents and child that physical therapy may follow healing and resolution of infection.	Ensures optimal functioning of affected limb.

NIC: *Surveillance*

Evaluation

(Date/time of evaluation of goal)

(Has goal been met? Not met? Partially met?)

(Does child complain of increased pain? What is WBC level—include date and time of test.)

(Revisions to care plan? D/C care plan? Continue care plan?)

IMPAIRED SOCIAL INTERACTION

Related to: (Specify: limited physical mobility, therapeutic isolation.)

Defining Characteristics: (Specify: change in pattern of interaction, lengthy treatment and immobilization, boredom, inability to engage in usual activities for age group, environment that lacks diversion.)

Goal: Child will increase social interaction by (date and time to evaluate).

Outcome Criteria

✔ Child participates in family activities.
✔ Child socializes with friends.

NOC: *Social Involvement*

INTERVENTIONS	RATIONALES
Provide age-appropriate toys that can be used in bed while in a prone or sitting position depending on type of treatment and degree of immobilization.	Promotes social and developmental activities and reduces boredom during long-term treatment.
Provide exposure to other children by moving bed near areas of activity or near a window; wheel on a stretcher or in a wheelchair or stroller, allow to walk with cast or splint when permitted.	Provides environmental stimulation and social interaction.
Encourage family and friends to visit, call, or stay with child; if in isolation provide frequent interactions or someone to stay with child.	Promotes social interaction with others during long-term treatment and reduces boredom.
Place toys and other articles within reach.	Provides access to diversion activities when needed.
Inform parents to include infant/child in family activities.	Promotes feeling of acceptance and well-being as part of the family.
Inform of devices available or methods used for mobility to fit needs of child with a cast or splint.	Promotes exposure to various activities and changes of environmental stimuli.
Encourage parents to allow as much independence in self-care by child as possible.	Promotes independence and allows some control over the situation.

NIC: *Socialization Enhancement*

Evaluation

(Date/time of evaluation of goal)

(Has goal been met? Not met? Partially met?)

(Does child participate in family activities? Does child socialize with friends? Specify.)

(Revisions to care plan? D/C care plan? Continue care plan?)

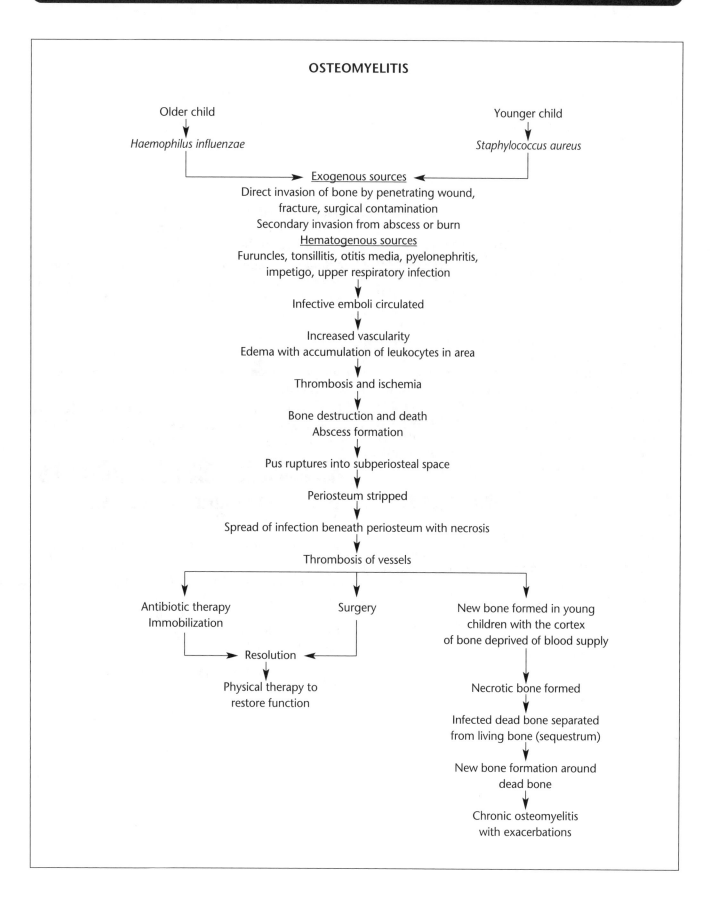

OSTEOMYELITIS

Older child   Younger child

Haemophilus influenzae   *Staphylococcus aureus*

Exogenous sources
Direct invasion of bone by penetrating wound,
fracture, surgical contamination
Secondary invasion from abscess or burn
Hematogenous sources
Furuncles, tonsillitis, otitis media, pyelonephritis,
impetigo, upper respiratory infection

Infective emboli circulated

Increased vascularity
Edema with accumulation of leukocytes in area

Thrombosis and ischemia

Bone destruction and death
Abscess formation

Pus ruptures into subperiosteal space

Periosteum stripped

Spread of infection beneath periosteum with necrosis

Thrombosis of vessels

Antibiotic therapy   Surgery   New bone formed in young
Immobilization   children with the cortex
                                                 of bone deprived of blood supply

Resolution

Physical therapy to   Necrotic bone formed
restore function
                                                 Infected dead bone separated
                                                 from living bone (sequestrum)

                                                 New bone formation around
                                                 dead bone

                                                 Chronic osteomyelitis
                                                 with exacerbations

CHAPTER 6.7

JUVENILE RHEUMATOID ARTHRITIS

Juvenile rheumatoid arthritis (JRA) is a chronic inflammatory disease that involves the synovium of the joints resulting in effusion and eventual erosion and destruction of the joint cartilage. It is classified into different types and characterized by remissions and exacerbations with the onset most common between 2 to 5 and 9 to 12 years of age. Pauciarticular arthritis involves only a few joints, usually under five; polyarticular arthritis involves many joints, usually more than four. Systemic arthritis involves the presence of arthritis and associated high temperature, rash, and effects on other organs such as the heart, lungs, eyes, and those located in the abdominal cavity. Prognosis is based on the severity of the disease, type of arthritis, and response to treatment with the most severe complications of permanent deformity, hip disease, and iridocyclitis with visual loss.

MEDICAL CARE

Anti-inflammatories (Nonsteroidal): for analgesia, antipyretic action as well as anti-inflammatory and antirheumatic effects; may be used in combination with steroids and gold salts; action thought to be the inhibition of prostaglandin synthesis.

Anti-inflammatories (Steroidal): prednisone (Deltasone) given PO to suppress inflammatory responses and reactions, also reduces antibody titers and inhibits phagocytosis and release of allergic substances.

Antirheumatics (Slow acting): to inhibit collagen formation or alter immune responses and inhibit prostaglandin synthesis in the treatment of rheumatic diseases.

Cytotoxics: to treat rheumatoid arthritis when response to other anti-inflammatory drugs are not effective if the disease is severe and debilitating; usually used in combination with other drugs.

Joint X-ray: reveals widened joint spaces with later joint destruction and fusion, evidence of osteoporosis and inflammation at affected joint sites.

Erythrocyte Sedimentation Rate (ESR): reveals increases in systemic type but may be increased or decreased depending on the degree of inflammation.

Antinuclear Antibodies: reveals presence in 75% of rheumatoid factor with a positive result in 25%; positive or negative result depending on type of arthritis.

Rheumatoid Factor: reveals presence in those with later onset type with a positive result in pauciarticular type.

Complete Blood Count: reveals increased WBC in early stages.

Synovial Fluid Culture: reveals absence of infectious process and confirms absence of other conditions by joint aspiration of fluid for examination.

COMMON NURSING DIAGNOSES

See IMPAIRED PHYSICAL MOBILITY

Related to: Musculoskeletal impairment, pain, and discomfort.

Defining Characteristics: (Specify: reluctance to attempt movement, limited range of motion, imposed restrictions of movement by medical protocol, resting or immobilization of joint(s) by splinting and positioning, fatigue, malaise.)

See RISK FOR IMPAIRED SKIN INTEGRITY

Related to: (Specify: external factor or physical immobilization.)

Defining Characteristics: (Specify: skin irritation under splint(s), redness from prolonged pressure, break in skin from surgery if done, macular rash on extremities and trunk areas.)

See DELAYED GROWTH AND DEVELOPMENT

Related to: Effects of physical disability.

Defining Characteristics: (Specify: environmental and stimulation deficiencies, inability to perform self-care activities appropriate for age, growth retardation during active disease, reduced peer relationships.)

 See HYPERTHERMIA

Related to: Illness of inflammation.

Defining Characteristics: (Specify: increase in body temperature above normal range, chills, low-grade temperatures or high elevation late in day or twice a day.)

See IMBALANCED NUTRITION: LESS THAN BODY REQUIREMENTS

Related to: Inability to ingest food.

Defining Characteristics: (Specify: anorexia, weight loss or poor gain, weakness, fatigue, irritability.)

ADDITIONAL NURSING DIAGNOSES

CHRONIC PAIN

Related to: Chronic physical disability.

Defining Characteristics: Verbalization or observed evidence of pain experienced for more than 6 months, guarded movement, fear of reinjury, altered ability to continue activities, physical and social withdrawal. Single or multiple joint involvement, joint stiffness, loss of motion, edema, and warmth in joint(s) and painful to touch.

Goal: Child will experience decreased chronic pain by (date and time to evaluate).

Outcome Criteria

✔ Child rates pain as less than (specify using a scale. Specify scale.).

NOC: *Comfort Level*

INTERVENTIONS	RATIONALES
Assess severity of joint pain, location, duration, remissions and exacerbations, stiffness and	Provides information symptomatic of the effect of the disease on the musculoskeletal system:
what precipitates pain such as weight gain, activity, fatigue; effect on mobility and participation in ADL; presence of joint deformity.	allows for analgesic/ anti-inflammatories selection and better management of activity involvement; inflammatory process cause pain with the edema resulting from joint effusion and synovial thickening and limited motion resulting from muscle spasms; joint deformity results from joint destruction.
Administer medications (specify) as ordered and assess effect of medications in relieving pain.	(Action of drugs: relieves pain and the inflammatory process associated with the pain; drugs may be administered alone or in combination including the nonsteroidal anti-inflammatory drugs that act as analgesic, antipyretic and anti-inflammatory; slower acting antirheumatic drugs which may be added for optimal effect if NSAIDs are ineffective; corticosteroid drugs in lowest effective dose for short period of time especially in the presence of a life-threatening situation.)
Apply warm compresses, packs, or soaks to painful areas; paraffin baths and whirlpool as ordered.	Promotes circulation to the area by vasodilation to relieve pain; moist heat relieves painful, stiff areas.
Provide 1 to 2 rest periods during day and quiet environment for sleep.	Decreases stimulation that increases pain, and it promotes rest, especially during acute episodes.
Encourage child to assume position of comfort; elevate and support painful joints when changing position.	Promotes diversionary activity to detract from pain.
Apply splints if ordered for night use.	Provides immobilization of joints to ease pain during movement.
Explain cause of pain to child and measures that should be taken to relieve pain.	Provides reasons for treatments and medications.
Teach child and parents about factors (stress, climate movement) that exacerbate pain episodes, and to express or report presence of pain at the onset.	Promotes opportunity to avoid those situations or activities that contribute to exacerbations of pain and to provide for immediate relief.

(continues)

(continued)

INTERVENTIONS	RATIONALES
Instruct parents and child in accurate administration of medications including side effects and importance of compliance with regimen whether taken qid, h.s., or bid and side effects to report (specify).	Promotes compliance with medical regimen to control pain and inflammation.
Teach parents to give warm bath daily for 10 minutes or warm wet packs with a towel bath to painful areas.	Supplies heat to affected joints to relieve pain and stiffness.
Instruct parents and child to avoid overactivity or movement of affected joints.	Prevents injury to affected joints during the acute episode when immobilization is important.
Teach child relaxation techniques, music therapy and diversionary activities such as TV, reading, games.	Provides nonpharmacologic interventions to relieve pain.

NIC: *Pain Management*

Evaluation

(Date/time of evaluation of goal)

(Has goal been met? Not met? Partially met?)

(What is pain rating? Specify scale used.)

(Revisions to care plan? D/C care plan? Continue care plan?)

DISTURBED BODY IMAGE

Related to: Biophysical and psychosocial factors.

Defining Characteristics: (Specify: verbal and nonverbal responses to change in body appearance [joint deformity, steroid side effects], negative feelings about body, multiple stressors and change in daily living limitations and social relationships.)

Goal: Child will experience improved body image by (date and time to evaluate).

Outcome Criteria

✔ Child expresses feelings about illness.

✔ Child identifies at least 1 positive thing about his or her body.

NOC: *Body Image*

INTERVENTIONS	RATIONALES
Assess child for feelings about multiple restrictions in lifestyle, chronic illness, difficulty in school and social situations, inability to keep up with peers and participate in activities.	Provides information about status of self-concept and body image that require special attention.
Encourage expression of feelings and concerns, and support communications with parents, teachers, and peers.	Provides opportunity to vent feelings and reduce negative feelings about changes in appearance.
Avoid negative comments and stress positive activities and accomplishments.	Enhances body image and confidence.
Note withdrawal behavior and signs of depression.	Reveals responses to body image changes and possible poor adjustment to changes.
Note presence of joint deformities, need to use splints, weight gain, shift in fat distribution, edema and effect on child.	Reveals side effects of steroid therapy and disease manifestations that affect body image.
Show support and acceptance of changes in appearance of child; provide privacy as needed.	Promotes trust and demonstrates respect for child.
Teach parents about maintaining support for child.	Encourages acceptance of the child with special needs (long-term steroid therapy and side effects, lifelong activity restrictions).
Discuss with parents and child the impact of the disease on body systems and risk for deformity and disabilities; correct misinformation and inform of ways to cope with body changes.	Provides correct information to assist in dealing with negative feelings about body.
Encourage parents to be flexible in care of child and to integrate care and routines into family activities; to allow child to participate in peer activity.	Promotes well-being of child and sense of belonging and control of life events by participating in normal activities for age and enhancing developmental task achievement.
Discuss with parents and child how to deal with peer perceptions of appearance and how to tell others about change in appearance.	Prevents stigmatization of child by those who are not apprised of the child's disease; attitude of others will affect child's body image.
Suggest psychological counseling or child life worker and inform of functions performed by these professionals.	Assists to improve self-esteem and to learn coping and problem solving skills.

INTERVENTIONS	RATIONALES
Refer to Juvenile Arthritis Foundation.	Promotes support from others and how they handle the changes.

NIC: *Self-Esteem Enhancement*

Evaluation

(Date/time of evaluation of goal)

(Has goal been met? Not met? Partially met?)

(What feelings about chronic illness did child verbalize? What positive thing about their body did child identify? Use quotes.)

(Revisions to care plan? D/C care plan? Continue care plan?)

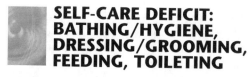

SELF-CARE DEFICIT: BATHING/HYGIENE, DRESSING/GROOMING, FEEDING, TOILETING

Related to: Pain, discomfort, and musculoskeletal impairment.

Defining Characteristics: (Specify: impaired ability in performance of ADL and maintenance of complete physical care; pain and weakness of joints and intolerance to activity; immobility status; joint deformity and/or contractures.)

Goal: Child will perform self care within limits of illness by (date and time to evaluate).

Outcome Criteria

✔ (Specify several self-care activities the child is capable of.)

NOC: *Self-Care: Bathing/Hygiene, Dressing/Grooming, Feeding, Toileting*

INTERVENTIONS	RATIONALES
Assess abilities and level of care and assistance.	Provides information about child's ability to perform self-care and to monitor progress.
Allow as much independence in ADL as possible but assist when needed.	Promotes independence and control over daily personal care needs without damage to joints.

INTERVENTIONS	RATIONALES
Encourage to perform own care and praise all accomplishments.	Promotes sense of accomplishment and independence; motivates to continue progress in ADL.
Position articles needed for care within reach; provide physical aids/devices to assist in performance of ADL (crutches, wheelchair, utensils that are easy to handle, hand bars, handles that are easy to open, clothing that is easy to put on and take off with zippers, Velcro, etc.).	Promotes independence and allows child access to aids to enhance independence.
Assist parents and child to develop plan and goals for daily ADL and suggest inclusions of actions taught by physical and occupational therapist.	Promotes independence and compliance in self-care.
Teach parents and child about application and use of aids and devices to accommodate self-care activities.	Promotes independence in ADL and self-confidence.
Discuss possible changes or adjustments in home and school environment to accommodate child's independence in meeting physical needs (pathways, furniture, doors).	Allows for safe participation in activities that are usually carried out by child on a daily basis.

NIC: *Self-Care Assistance*

Evaluation

(Date/time of evaluation of goal)

(Has goal been met? Not met? Partially met?)

(What self-care activities did the child perform relative to the outcome criteria?)

(Revisions to care plan? D/C care plan? Continue care plan?)

COMPROMISED FAMILY COPING

Related to: (Specify: inadequate or incorrect information or understanding, prolonged disease or disability progression that exhausts the physical and emotional supportive capacity of caretakers.)

Defining Characteristics: (Specify: expression and/or confirmation of concern and inadequate knowledge about long-term care needs, problems and complications, anxiety and guilt, overprotection of child.)

Goal: Family will cope more effectively by (date and time to evaluate).

Outcome Criteria

✔ Clients express feelings about child's chronic illness.

✔ Clients identify 3 positive coping mechanisms to implement.

NOC: *Family Coping*

INTERVENTIONS	RATIONALES
Assist family to assess coping methods used and effectiveness, family interactions and expectations related to long-term care, developmental level of family, response of siblings, knowledge and use of support systems and resources, presence of guilt and anxiety, overprotection and/or overindulgence behaviors.	Provides information identifying coping methods that work and the need to develop new coping skills and behaviors, family attitudes; child with special long-term needs may strengthen or strain family relationships and an undue degree of overprotection may be detrimental to child's growth and development (disallow school attendance and peer activities, avoiding discipline of child, and allowing child to assume responsibilities for ADL).
Encourage family members to express problem areas and explore solutions responsibly.	Reduces anxiety and enhances understanding; provides family an opportunity to identify problems and develop problem solving strategies.
Assist family to establish short- and long-term goals for child and to integrate child into family activities, include participation of all family members in care routines.	Promotes involvement and control over situations and maintains role of family members and parents.
Refer to assistance of social worker, counselor, clergy, or other as needed.	Provides support to the family faced with long-term care of child with a chronic illness.
Refer to community agencies and contact with the Arthritis Foundation or other families with a child with arthritis.	Provides information and support to child and family.

INTERVENTIONS	RATIONALES
Assist family members to express feelings, how they deal with the chronic needs of family member and coping patterns that help or hinder adjustment to the problems.	Allows for venting of feelings to determine need for information and support, and to relieve guilt and anxiety.
Inform family that overprotective behavior may hinder growth and development, and to treat child as normally as possible.	Promotes understanding of importance of making child one of the family and the adverse affects of overprotection of the child.
Teach family about remissions and exacerbations of the disease and that an exacerbation may last for long periods of time (over a period of months); that exacerbations may be precipitated by overactivity, stress, presence of other illnesses, climate changes.	Provides a realistic view of the chronic nature of the disease.
Inform parents and child of suggestions of unorthodox cures for the disease by friends, and the harmful effects caused by some of them.	Prevents injury as well as disappointment when cures do not measure up to expectations.
Assist family to identify positive coping mechanisms they may use (e.g., discussing feelings and issues openly, hiring a baby-sitter once a week, family movie nights, etc.).	Promotes ownership of solutions to coping difficulty.

NIC: *Family Involvement*

Evaluation

(Date/time of evaluation of goal)

(Has goal been met? Not met? Partially met?)

(Did clients discuss feelings about child's chronic illness? Provide quotes. List 3 positive coping mechanisms the family plans to implement.)

(Revisions to care plan? D/C care plan? Continue care plan?)

JUVENILE RHEUMATOID ARTHRITIS

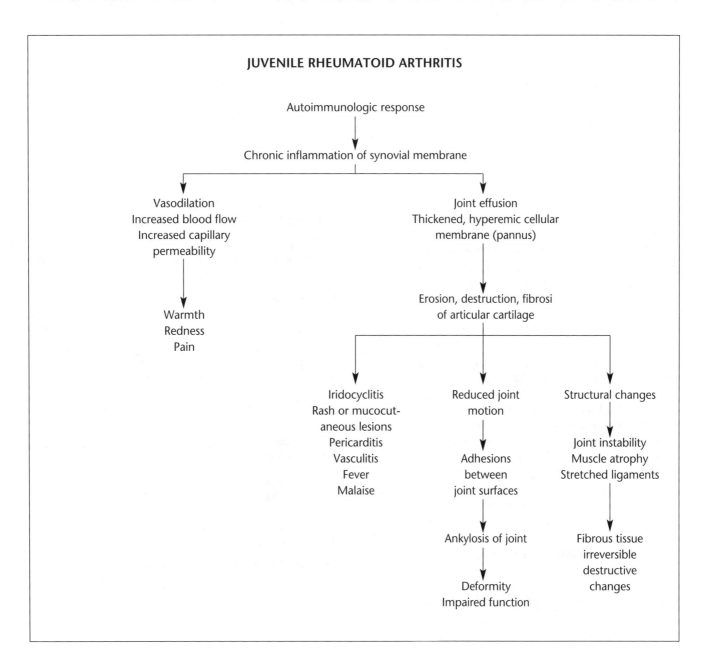

Autoimmunologic response

↓

Chronic inflammation of synovial membrane

Vasodilation
Increased blood flow
Increased capillary
permeability

↓

Warmth
Redness
Pain

Joint effusion
Thickened, hyperemic cellular
membrane (pannus)

↓

Erosion, destruction, fibrosi
of articular cartilage

Iridocyclitis
Rash or mucocut-
aneous lesions
Pericarditis
Vasculitis
Fever
Malaise

Reduced joint
motion

↓

Adhesions
between
joint surfaces

↓

Ankylosis of joint

↓

Deformity
Impaired function

Structural changes

↓

Joint instability
Muscle atrophy
Stretched ligaments

↓

Fibrous tissue
irreversible
destructive
changes

CHAPTER 6.8

SCOLIOSIS

Scoliosis is a lateral curvature of the spine with the thoracic area being the most commonly affected. It can be classified as functional or structural. Functional scoliosis is the result of another deformity and is corrected by treating the underlying problem. Structural scoliosis is most often idiopathic although it may be congenital or secondary to another disorder. There is a growing body of evidence that idiopathic scoliosis is probably genetic but the etiology is not completely understood. Structural scoliosis is more progressive and causes changes in supporting structures, such as the ribs. Management includes observation, bracing, and surgical fusion. Patients with idiopathic curves of less than 25 degrees are observed for progress until they have reached skeletal maturity. Bracing is recommended for adolescents with curves between 30 and 45 degrees, while curves greater than 45 degrees usually require surgery. The deformity may occur at any age, from infancy through adolescence, but the best prognosis belongs to those who are almost fully grown and whose curvature is of a mild degree. Idiopathic scoliosis most commonly occurs in adolescent girls.

MEDICAL CARE

Analgesics: to control postoperative pain depending on severity.

Spinal X-ray: reveals curvature of the spine via different views (A, P, and lateral) with head and hips unaligned.

Myelogram: reveals presence of neurologic abnormalities of muscle function.

Scoliometer: reveals deformity of back when in a forward bending position.

Thoracolumbosacral brace (TLSO): an underarm brace of molded plastic fitting from below the rib cage to the lower pelvis to correct thoracolumbar and lumbar curves. This brace is also worn 23 hours per day until skeletal maturity.

Boston brace: a type of corset with metal stays that is a more comfortable type of brace for scoliosis than molded plastic.

Surgical Fusion: includes the use of instrumentation and bone grafts to maintain internal fixation to correct severe deformities (greater than 45 degrees). The newer instruments no longer require postoperative casting, but immobility after surgery is maintained through bracing. The instruments include:

Harrington rods: metal rods connected by wires to the vertebrae.

Luque rods: flexible L-shaped metal rods fixed by wires to the bases of the spinous processes.

Dwyer instrumentation: a titanium cable fixed by screws to the vertebrae.

Cotrel-Dubousset (CD) procedure: bilateral segmental fixation using 2 rods and multiple hooks.

Electrical Stimulation: an electrical pulse transmitted to muscles on the convex side of the curve causing muscles to contract to straighten the spine. May be used for mild to moderate curves, but the effectiveness of this treatment is not well documented.

COMMON NURSING DIAGNOSES

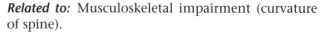 ### See IMPAIRED PHYSICAL MOBILITY

Related to: Musculoskeletal impairment (curvature of spine).

Defining Characteristics: (Specify: imposed restrictions of movement by medical protocol of corrective device [brace, traction], bed rest and inability to purposefully move within the physical environment following surgery or with halo traction.)

See RISK FOR IMPAIRED SKIN INTEGRITY

Related to: (Specify: physical immobilization, traction, or brace and altered sensation and circulation, surface electrical stimulation.)

Defining Characteristics: (Specify: change in skin color and temperature, skin irritation at stimulation, brace, redness on areas from prolonged pressure, break in skin from surgical correction or implantation of stimulators.)

See DELAYED GROWTH AND DEVELOPMENT

Related to: Effects of immobilization and restricted movement from spinal curvature.

Defining Characteristics: (Specify: environmental and stimulation deficiencies, difficulty participating in self-care and social activities with long-term continuous brace use.)

ADDITIONAL NURSING DIAGNOSES

DEFICIENT KNOWLEDGE

Related to: Lack of information about correction of functional or structural scoliosis.

Defining Characteristics: (Specify: request for information about treatments for scoliosis, application of brace and surgical procedure to correct scoliosis.)

Goal: Clients will obtain information about scoliosis by (date and time to evaluate).

Outcome Criteria

✔ Clients verbalize understanding of scoliosis and the treatment plan.

NOC: *Knowledge: Disease Process*

INTERVENTIONS	RATIONALES
Assess knowledge of deformity, cause and treatments.	Provides information about teaching needs.
Teach parents and child about functional or structural defect and methods of treatment modalities specific to age of child and severity of the deformity.	Promotes understanding of type of defect and treatment protocol to relieve anxiety; functional scoliosis is corrected by treating the underlying problem, and

INTERVENTIONS	RATIONALES
	structural scoliosis is treated with long-term bracing and exercising or surgical fixation to straighten and realign spine.
Teach parents and child about application, care, and removal of brace or orthoplast jacket, and inform that appliance must be worn for 23 hours/day and may be removed for bathing and exercise.	Provides nonoperative bracing to prevent progressive curvatures; higher curves are treated with the Milwaukee brace and lower curves with the TLSO brace and both are worn until growth is complete.
Teach child exercises to be performed in and out of the brace or other appliance and to perform them daily.	Prevents atrophy of muscle of spine and abdomen.
Teach child to maintain proper posture, use shoe lifts, exercises, and other prescribed treatments for functional scoliosis.	Corrects functional scoliosis which is usually caused by poor posture or unequal length of legs.
(Teach parents and child to use electrical stimulation, application of electrodes, skin protection, connection of leads, operation of machine to be used at night.)	Provides stimulation to the muscles to prevent progression of curvature.
(Teach parents and child of operative procedure planned and preoperative preparation required; reinforce physician information and use pictures, models and drawings to aid in teaching.)	Provides information about option for internal surgical instrumentation of curves over 45 degrees or those which are rapidly progressing to 45 degrees.
(Prepare parents and child for postoperative care, especially activity restrictions, log rolling, progression to ambulation, use of pillows for proper support, maintaining flat position, and possible use of special bed such as Stryker frame.)	Provides information about what to expect following surgery depending on the type of procedure.
(Teach parents and child of use of safety belt and walker when ambulating; instruct in safety precautions to take for child wearing brace [clear pathways, handrails, performing ADL using aids].)	Prevents trauma caused by fall from postoperative weakness, unassisted ambulation, or wearing of brace causing awkwardness in ambulation and ADL performance.
(Reassure parents and child that physical and occupational therapy will be prescribed after surgery.)	Provides information and support services.

(continues)

(continued)

INTERVENTIONS	RATIONALES
Refer to agencies for assistance such as National Scoliosis Foundation, community support groups.	Promotes optimal physical activity.

NIC: *Teaching: Disease Process*

Evaluation

(Date/time of evaluation of goal)

(Has goal been met? Not met? Partially met?)

(What did clients verbalize about scoliosis and the treatment plan? Use quotes.)

(Revisions to care plan? D/C care plan? Continue care plan?)

DISTURBED BODY IMAGE

Related to: Biophysical and psychosocial factors of spinal deformity

Defining Characteristics: (Specify: verbal response to actual change in structure of spine, negative feelings about body, dependence on long-term use of brace, feeling of rejection by peers, inability to participate in some activities.)

Goal: Child will experience improved body image by (date and time to evaluate).

Outcome Criteria

✔ Child expresses feelings about scoliosis and long-term treatment.

✔ Child identifies at least 1 positive thing about his or her body.

NOC: *Self-Esteem*

INTERVENTIONS	RATIONALES
Assess child for feelings about wearing brace, long-term treatments, restrictions in lifestyle, inability to keep up with peers and participate in activities.	Provides information about status of self-concept and changes in appearance.
Encourage expression of feelings and concerns and support child's communications with parents, peers and teachers.	Provides opportunity to vent and reduce negative feelings about changes in appearance and continuing wearing of an appliance.

INTERVENTIONS	RATIONALES
Maintain positive environment and promote activities that are allowed (sports, play, games).	Enhances body image and confidence, and promotes trust and respect of child.
Assist with plan for independence in ADL, application and removal of appliance, selection of shoes and clothing to wear such as T-shirt.	Promotes independence and adjustment to appliance.
Assist child to adjust to self-perception of short leg, use of appliance and effect on appearance.	Promotes positive self-image and realistic view of appearance.
Suggest open communication with school nurse and teacher.	Promotes adaptation to school within activity limitations.
Reassure parents and child that most activities are allowed with use of appliance.	Promotes positive feelings about treatment and restrictions imposed by the deformity.
Assist child to type of clothing to cover appliance that is stylish and has peer acceptance.	Enhances appearance and body image.
Help child find ways to inform others about wearing appliance.	Assist child in dealing with questions and curiosity of others about differences caused by deformity.
Teach child of activity restrictions that include progression from quiet activities to involvement in those to avoid: contact sports, bike riding, driving, skating, or those that may result in a fall if surgery has been done.	Prevents injury following surgical correction of the deformity.

NIC: *Self-Esteem Enhancement*

Evaluation

(Date/time of evaluation of goal)

(Has goal been met? Not met? Partially met?)

(What feelings about scoliosis and treatment did child verbalize? What positive thing about body did child identify? Use quotes.)

(Revisions to care plan? D/C care plan? Continue care plan?)

SCOLIOSIS

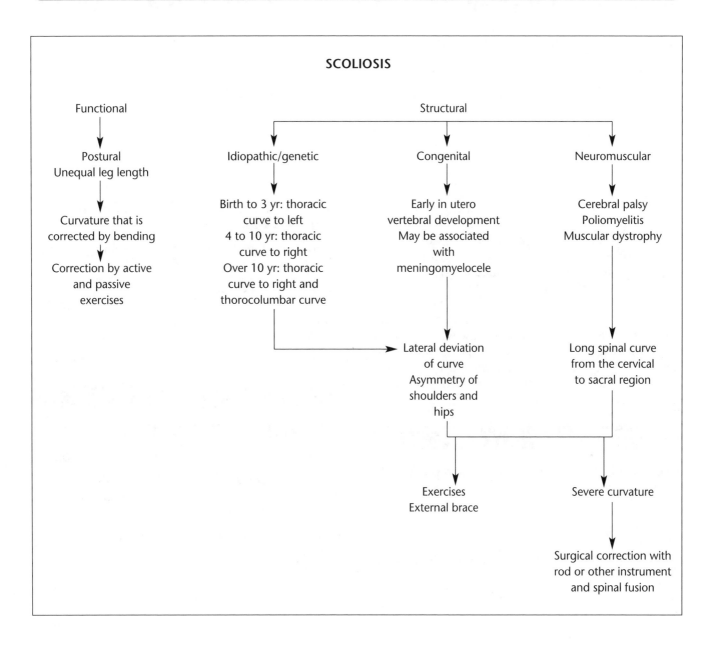

Functional

Structural

Postural
Unequal leg length

Idiopathic/genetic

Congenital

Neuromuscular

Curvature that is
corrected by bending

Birth to 3 yr: thoracic
curve to left
4 to 10 yr: thoracic
curve to right
Over 10 yr: thoracic
curve to right and
thorocolumbar curve

Early in utero
vertebral development
May be associated
with
meningomyelocele

Cerebral palsy
Poliomyelitis
Muscular dystrophy

Correction by active
and passive
exercises

Lateral deviation
of curve
Asymmetry of
shoulders and
hips

Long spinal curve
from the cervical
to sacral region

Exercises
External brace

Severe curvature

Surgical correction with
rod or other instrument
and spinal fusion

CHAPTER 6.9

TALIPES

Talipes (club foot) is a congenital disorder of the foot usually with ankle involvement characterized by a twisting out of a normal position that is unable to be manipulated into a different position. The deformity is typed and named according to the position of the foot and includes talipes varus (foot inversion), talipes valgus (foot eversion), talipes equinus (plantar flexion), and talipes calcaneus (dorsiflexion). Most are a combination of these with the most common deformity known as talipes equinovarus (inversion and plantar flexion of the foot). The defect may occur alone or in association with other congenital syndromes or defects.

MEDICAL CARE

Foot/Ankle X-ray: reveals abnormal bone deformity or distortion.

Casting
Surgical Correction

COMMON NURSING DIAGNOSES

See IMPAIRED PHYSICAL MOBILITY

Related to: Musculoskeletal impairment (talipes deformity).

Defining Characteristics: (Specify: imposed restrictions of movement by medical protocol of corrective device, serial cast application.)

See RISK FOR IMPAIRED SKIN INTEGRITY

Related to: (Specify: physical immobilization by cast(s), internal factors of altered circulation, sensation by cast pressure.)

Defining Characteristics: (Specify: edema, rapid growth rate, tight cast or appliance, color change and cool skin proximal to cast.)

See DELAYED GROWTH AND DEVELOPMENT

Related to: Effects of physical disability (immobilization).

Defining Characteristics: (Specify: delay in performing motor skills typical of age group during cast applications, lack of stimulation while cast is present.)

ADDITIONAL DIAGNOSES

DEFICIENT KNOWLEDGE

Related to: Lack of information about condition.

Defining Characteristics: (Specify: request for information about disorder, its cause and treatment for correction, follow-up care.)

Goal: Parents will gain information about talipes by (date and time to evaluate).

Outcome Criteria

✔ Parents verbalize understanding of condition of infant.
✔ Parents state the planned corrective treatment.

NOC: *Knowledge: Treatment Procedures*

INTERVENTIONS	RATIONALES
Assess knowledge of disorder, type of deformity, and if one or both feet are involved; type of immobilization and application and/or care; presence of associated congenital disorders or syndromes.	Provides information needed to develop plan of instruction to ensure compliance to medical regimen for correction; usually begins in infancy and lasts for 3 to 5 months, and most commonly occurs in males.

INTERVENTIONS	RATIONALES
Teach parents about type of talipes deformity and describe the position of the foot and ankle and the stages of corrective treatment.	Provides information about how the correction is accomplished, maintained, and re-evaluated to ensure the correction and prevent recurrence of the deformity.
Instruct parents in manipulation of feet in one smooth motion, demonstrate and allow for return demonstration.	Ensures correct positioning of the feet in preparation for immobilization.
Teach parents about casting procedure and type of cast applied (midthigh long led) and that new successive casts will be applied q 2 to 3 days for 1 to 2 weeks and then q 1 to 2 weeks with the final cast remaining in place for 4 to 8 weeks.	Ensures correction by the most reliable method of manipulation and serial casting to stretch tight structures and contract lax structures; frequent castings allow for rapid growth in infant.
Teach parents to monitor extremities for color, peripheral pulses, and coolness, and report changes in these circulatory parameters.	Prevents circulation and neurologic impairment from tight casts.

INTERVENTIONS	RATIONALES
Teach parents that if conservative treatment fails or child is older, surgery may be needed to correct deformity by releasing ligaments, lengthening tendons, or correcting bone deformity with casting following immobilization of the feet.	Prepares parents for possibility of surgical correction if manipulation is ineffective after 5 months of treatment.
Encourage parents to plan for follow-up physician evaluations and cast changes.	Ensures compliance over long-term correction of deformity by casting or appliance.

NIC: *Teaching: Disease Process*

Evaluation

(Date/time of evaluation of goal)

(Has goal been met? Not met? Partially met?)

(What did clients verbalize about infant's condition and the treatment plan? Use quotes.)

(Revisions to care plan? D/C care plan? Continue care plan?)

TALIPES

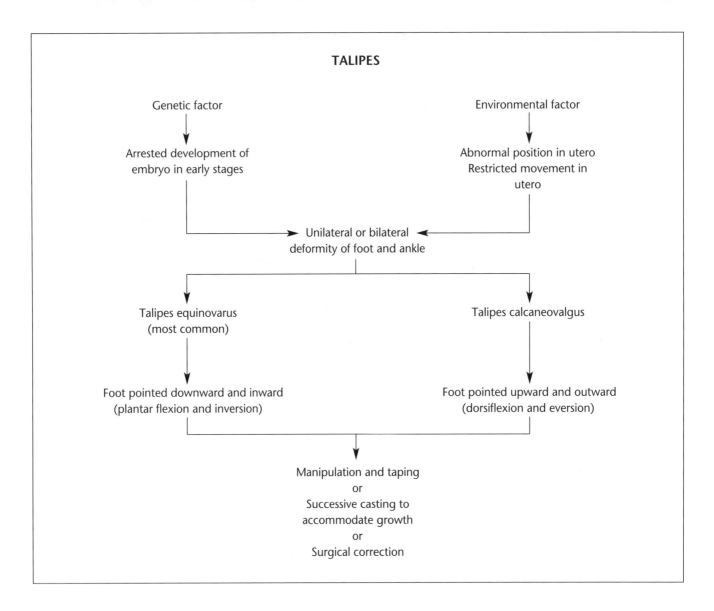

Genetic factor

↓

Arrested development of
embryo in early stages

Environmental factor

↓

Abnormal position in utero
Restricted movement in
utero

→ Unilateral or bilateral ←
deformity of foot and ankle

Talipes equinovarus
(most common)

↓

Foot pointed downward and inward
(plantar flexion and inversion)

Talipes calcaneovalgus

↓

Foot pointed upward and outward
(dorsiflexion and eversion)

↓

Manipulation and taping
or
Successive casting to
accommodate growth
or
Surgical correction

UNIT 7

NEUROLOGIC SYSTEM

CHAPTER 7.0

NEUROLOGIC SYSTEM: BASIC CARE PLAN

The neurologic system includes the central nervous system (CNS) consisting of the cerebrum, cerebellum, brain stem, and the spinal cord; the peripheral nervous system consisting of the motor (efferent) and sensory (afferent) nerves; and the autonomic nervous system (ANS) consisting of the sympathetic and parasympathetic systems that provide control of vital body functions. Alterations in the neurologic system affect the process of receiving, integrating, and responding to stimuli that enter the system. This results in disturbances with signs and symptoms dependent on the type and site of the impairment and the normal functioning of the system. The disturbances may be manifested by alterations in consciousness, sensation, or muscle function. Changes in the system also occur as the child develops neurologically and completes the growth and development requirements for adulthood; this system is one of the last to complete development after birth.

NEUROLOGIC GROWTH AND DEVELOPMENT

BRAIN AND SPINAL CORD STRUCTURE

- Skull structure is expansible during infancy and young childhood and becomes rigid with growth in older child.

- Head circumference at birth is 13 to 14 inches in size, increases to 17 inches at 6 months of age, and 18 inches at 12 months.

- Cranial sutures close during infancy (by 6 months), posterior fontanel at 6 to 8 weeks, and anterior fontanel at 12 to 18 months.

- Increases in brain size and cell numbers occur between birth and 1 year of age; growth continues with increases primarily in size from 1 year of age until maturity. Weight of the brain at birth is approximately 350 g or 12% of total body weight,

doubles by 1 year of age, and is approximately 1,000 g or 2/3 of adult size by 2 years of age, a continual slower pace until adulthood follows with a final size of 2% of total body weight.

- Cortex is 1/2 the thickness of the adult brain at birth and continues to develop and mature with growth.

- Myelinization of nerves and fiber tracts develops rapidly after birth with sensory pathways before motor pathways; continue to develop with growth of the child until reaching completion in late adolescence.

- Myelinization of nerve tracts follows a cephalocaudal and proximodistal sequence that allows for progressive neuromotor function; begins with cranial nerve fibers and spinal cord nerve fibers and then proceeds to brain stem and corticospinal nerve tracts.

- At birth, spinal nerves are attached to the cord in a horizontal position in relation to the vertebral column; with growth, lower nerves are directed more downward, and sacral and coccygeal nerves are directed in a vertical direction while cervical nerves remain in a horizontal position.

SENSORY AND MOTOR FUNCTION

- As the neurologic system develops, integrated functions of consciousness, mentation, language, motor function, sensory function, and bowel and bladder function develop to completion.

- Infant has reflexive responses and learns to bring responses under conscious control with growth and development of cortex—areas of cerebral development correspond to the development of intellect, control of attention span, and responses to stimuli.

- Neuromuscular maturity and myelinization of spinal cord promote walking by the age of 2 with skills perfected through preschool years.

- Gross and fine motor development and coordination develop by age 3 for most activities and continue with growth; physical strength and endurance continue to develop throughout school age.

- At birth, response to sound is present with ability to locate and identify sounds as myelinization of auditory pathways beyond the midbrain occurs; curvature of the external equal develops to adult position by 3 years of age.

- Hearing fully developed by 5 months of age; child proceeds to listen and react to sounds and understand words by 1 year of age.

- Sense of taste, smell, and touch are present at birth; responses to strong odors, sour solutions, pin prick apparent.

- In the infant, ciliary muscles are immature, which limits accommodation and the ability of the eye to fixate on an object for a period of time.

- Macula and muscles develop with growth.

- Response to color by 1 to 2 months, color vision at 6 months.

- Eye movement coordination by 3 months, function matures at 6 months.

- Binocular vision by 4 months, tear glands function by 4 months.

- Depth perception by 6 to 9 months, detail perception by 8 months.

- Peripheral vision by 1 year of age.

- Permanent iris color by 18 months of age.

- Visual acuity matures at 6 years of age.

Infant:	20/100 to 20/400 (technique dependent)
2 years:	20/40
4 years:	20/30
School-age:	20/20

- Body temperature regulation unstable at birth with decrements and improved regulation taking place with maturity

Infant:	99.4 to 99.5 degrees F
Toddler:	99.7 to 99 degrees F
Preschool:	99 to 98.6 degrees F
School-age:	98.6 to 97.8 degrees F

- Length of sleep time decreases from infancy throughout childhood; amount of REM sleep is 20% compared to 50% in infancy, non-REM sleep increases with age; length of the sleep cycle increases from 50 minutes in the infant to 90 minutes in later childhood, number of hours decrease with age.

NURSING DIAGNOSES

HYPERTHERMIA

Related to: Illness or trauma.

Defining Characteristics: (Specify: increase in body temperature above normal range, flushed skin, warm to touch, increased respiratory rate, tachycardia, seizures/convulsions.)

Related to: Dehydration.

Defining Characteristics: (Specify: increase in body temperature above normal range, flushed, dry skin, warm to touch, increased respirations, pulse, oliguria, poor skin turgor, sunken eyeballs.)

Goal: Child's temperature will be decreased by (date and time to evaluate).

Outcome Criteria

✔ Return of body temperature to (specify).

✔ Child's temperature will remain < (specify for child).

NOC: *Thermoregulation*

INTERVENTIONS	RATIONALES
Assess temperature via axillary method in infants and children to age 5 years, oral in children 5 to 6 years and older, depending on the individual child's ability to safely and accurately keep the thermometer in their mouth; check for malaise or lethargy and compare to normal ranges for age or low grade or high elevations associated with specific microorganisms or diseases.	Provides information about temperature changes caused by high susceptibility to fluctuations in infants and young children as their regulatory function is unstable (regulated in the hypothalamus); temperature in infant and young child responds to infection with higher and more rapid elevations and may become overheated as environmental temperatures change or from activity, crying and emotional upsets since regulating mechanism immature until age 8.
Assess temperature q 1 to 2h for sudden increase in presence of any temperature elevation or illness.	Sudden temperature elevation may induce a seizure.

(continues)

(continued)

INTERVENTIONS	RATIONALES
Teach parents that the main reason for treating a fever is discomfort; two antipyretic drugs of choice: Acetaminophen and nonsteroidal anti-inflammatory drugs such as Ibuprofen; administer as ordered in the form (liquid, tablet) that is appropriate for the age of the child and illness severity.	Reduces temperature; (lowers set point); prevents possible toxicity caused by accumulation if given too often, may be administered by tablet, liquid, chewable, suppository (action of drugs).
Teach that cooling measures such as lightweight clothing, skin exposure, decreasing room temperature and cool, wet compresses to skin are only effective if given one hour after antipyretic.	Antipyretics lower the set point, enabling cooling measures to be effective.
Instruct that sponging/tepid baths are not recommended for children with fever.	Utilized only for child with hyperthermia caused by elevated set point; hyperthermia is a condition where body temperature exceeds set point—more heat created than eliminated caused by internal factors such as hyperthyroidism, cerebral dysfunction, "malignant hyperthermia" (a reaction to anesthesia), or external factors (heat stroke).
Encourage parents to provide additional fluid.	Maintains hydration when fluids are lost through fever or hyperthermia.
Treat shivering by warming the body with clothing (especially extremities), increasing room temperature, and warm baths.	Shivering increases metabolic demands that produce more heat; it is the body's natural mechanism to maintain the higher set point by producing more heat.
Promote rest and provide a stress-free environment, hold and rock infant/child if needed.	Decreases metabolic requirements.
For hyperthermia only: cooling measures such as cooling blankets/mattresses and tepid tub baths are utilized; water temperature should be 1 to 2 degrees less than the child's temperature; recheck temperature 30 minutes after intervention; discontinue if shivering occurs.	Cooling measures are effective because of normal set point in hyperthermia; antipyretics are not effective.

INTERVENTIONS	RATIONALES
Teach parents to take oral and axillary temperature and allow for return demonstration; instruct in use of digital thermometers and plastic strips.	Allows parents to monitor temperature for elevation when child feels warm.
Teach parents of the difference between fever and hyperthermia and use of antipyretics to reduce fever and cooling baths to treat hyperthermia; instruct in safe use of antipyretics including type, dosage, frequency, form and limitations in 24-hour administration and sponging without use of cold water or alcohol.	Antipyretics given to control fever which is an elevation in set point, and cooling measures given to control hyperthermia which is a temperature that exceeds the set point.
Teach parents to report to physician immediately if: child is less than 2 months old with any fever; fever greater than 40.5° C. (105° F); presence of excessive crying; decreased level of consciousness; seizures; stiff neck; difficulty breathing; or if child has underlying illness.	Prevents severe complications from elevated temperature that persists and is not relieved by medications; physician intervention to initiate or change treatment may be necessary.
Inform parents that temperature may become elevated without the presence of a serious illness.	Reduces parental anxiety if unduly concerned about fever.

NIC: *Surveillance*

Evaluation

(Date/time of evaluation of goal)

(Has goal been met? Not met? Partially met?)

(What is child's temperature?)

(Revisions to care plan? D/C care plan? Continue care plan?)

DISTURBED SLEEP PATTERN

Related to: Illness.

Defining Characteristics: (Specify: interrupted sleep, temperature elevation, irritability, restlessness, listlessness, fatigue, weakness, nightmares.)

Related to: Environmental changes.

Defining Characteristics: (Specify: hospitalization, interrupted sleep, separation anxiety, stimuli overload, lack of privacy, breaks in bedtime rituals or routines.)

Goal: Client will be able to sleep without interruption by (date and time to evaluate).

Outcome Criteria

✔ Client goes to bed without difficulty.

✔ Client sleeps (specify number of hours) without waking.

✔ Client appears rested.

NOC: *Sleep*

INTERVENTIONS	RATIONALES
Assess sleep patterns and changes, nap times and frequency, sleep problems, pattern of awakenings and reason.	Provides information about fulfillment of sleep needs related to age requirements: infants need 10 to 20 hours/24 hours with a routine and sleep through the night by 5 months of age; toddlers need 12 hours/night and 2 naps which gradually changes to 10 hours/night and 1 nap; preschoolers need 10 hours/night with or without a nap; school-age children need 10 hours/night; wakenings may be caused by anxiety; nightmares and the absence of good sleep habits may create sleep problems.
Assess presence of temperature elevation, restlessness caused by pain, dyspnea, other signs and symptoms of an illness.	Provides possible reasons for restlessness, wakenings, and sleep/rest deficit.
Assess for fatigue, irritability, weakness, lability, yawning.	Results of sleep deficit or deprivation, overactivity.
Place infant (0–6 months) on back or side-lying position for sleep, utilizing positioning aids such as rolled blankets to maintain desired position; infants with gastroesophageal reflux, premature infants, and infants with specific upper airway problems may sleep in prone position; premature infants benefit developmentally from the prone position as it often facilitates flexion, and is soothing.	Recent research has led the American Academy of Pediatrics to recommend these positions which have shown to decrease the incidence of SIDS (sudden infant death syndrome).

INTERVENTIONS	RATIONALES
Avoid waking/interrupting sleep for feedings or caregiving.	Provides comfort for sleep without interruptions.
Offer snack and preferred toy at bedtime for child, follow home routines for time, night light, reading a story at bedtime, playing, tapes of music.	Promotes comfort and familiar bedtime pattern.
Allow time for quiet play before bedtime.	Avoids overstimulation before bedtime.
Provide soothing comfort if child has a nightmare and explain bad dream, stay until child returns to sleep.	Provides security and explanation to encourage child to sleep without fear.
Promote naps during day if such a routine has been established.	Follows usual age dependent nap/rest pattern.
Provide environment that is quiet, calm and warm; proper clothing, covers, and diaper change as needed.	Promotes sleep and/or rest periods.
Try to avoid painful procedures prior to bedtime when possible.	Decreases stimuli that prevent rest and sleep.
Encourage parent to stay with child at night if possible or hold, rock, or stroke child "until" asleep.	Promotes sleep and relaxation with a familiar person giving care.
Discuss with parents the amount of sleep needed by infant/child.	Promotes parental understanding of sleep needs which are age dependent.
Teach parents: Infant: feed, change diaper, dress appropriately, place in side-lying or supine position. Toddler: remind of bedtime or nap in advance, offer snack, allow preferred toy in bed, can assist to prepare for bed. Preschool: provide own sleeping area, night light, story or music. School-age: provide time before sleep for talk, review activities of day.	Provides suggestions that may assist to establish bedtime rituals.
Teach parents to maintain same sleep schedule, set limits, reinforce appropriate behaviors.	Promotes sleep pattern and avoids sleep problems.
Teach child relaxation techniques such as tensing each part of the body and slowly relaxing each part, taking deep breaths, repeating a word that the child associates with relaxation (specify).	Promotes rest and induces sleep.

(continues)

INTERVENTIONS	RATIONALES
Assist parents to solve chronic sleep problems after acute illness is resolved and child is at home; suggestions may include: a bedtime ritual; a consistent bedtime and location; use of a favorite blanket or toy to increase feelings of security; avoid use of bed as punishment; avoid feedings/drinks at night; if child consistently awakens at night, implement strategies which promote gradual change such as: entering room without picking up the child, then leaving for progressively longer periods of time until the child falls asleep by him/herself.	Routines greatly promote the child's sleep quality and quantity; promote the child's feelings of security; improve the quality of the parent-child relationship; promote the child's own natural body defenses.

NIC: *Sleep Enhancement*

Evaluation

(Date/time of evaluation of goal)

(Has goal been met? Not met? Partially met?)

(Did child go to bed without problems? How long did client sleep? Does client appear rested? Describe.)

(Revisions to care plan? D/C care plan? Continue care plan?)

DISTURBED THOUGHT PROCESSES

Related to: Physiologic changes.

Defining Characteristics: (Specify: altered attention span, disorientation to time, place, person, circumstances and events, changes in consciousness, hallucination, cognitive dissonance, inappropriate affect, memory deficit.

Goal: Client will experience improved thought processes by (date and time to evaluate).

Outcome Criteria

✔ (Specify for client, e.g., will have decreased ICP; will be alert and oriented × 3; will deny hallucinations, etc.)

NOC: *Cognitive Orientation*

INTERVENTIONS	RATIONALES
Assess history for neurologic conditions or infection, cognitive functioning.	Provides information about reason for mentation changes.
Assess for increased ICP and effects on orientation mentation, intellectual function, motor function.	Provides information about increased ICP which results from brain edema, shift or distortion and brain hypoxia.
Perform neurologic checks q 2h including PERL, orientation, grip and grasp and pain response, presence of irritability, confusion, memory loss; include cranial nerve function if indicated.	Provides data about changes in thought processes that indicate serious pathology.
Elevate head of bed 30 degrees and maintain proper head and neck alignment.	Promotes blood flow to brain and prevents hypoxia.
Provide toys and stimulation that are age-appropriate and modified for illness.	Promotes developmental level within prescribed limitations to improve orientation and attention span.
Limit sensory and motor expectations if unable to maintain thought processes and independence in activities.	Prevents frustration and insecure feelings.
(Inform parents of reason for loss of thought processes and temporary nature of this condition.)	Relieves doubts and anxiety about mental status of infant/child.
Encourage parents to expose infant/child to stimulation, toys, and play activities and praise desired behaviors indicating orientation.	Promotes developmental task achievement.

NIC: *Surveillance*

Evaluation

(Date/time of evaluation of goal)

(Has goal been met? Not met? Partially met?)

(Provide information related to the outcome criteria chosen, e.g., what is ICP? Describe level of alertness and orientation, etc.)

(Revisions to care plan? D/C care plan? Continue care plan?)

CHAPTER 7.1

HYDROCEPHALUS

Hydrocephalus is the enlargement of the intracranial cavity caused by the accumulation of cerebrospinal fluid in the ventricular system. This results from an imbalance in the production and absorption of the fluid which causes an increase in intracranial pressure as the fluid builds up. Fluid may accumulate as a result of blockage of the flow (noncommunicating hydrocephalus) or impaired absorption (communicating hydrocephalus). As the head enlarges to an abnormal size, the infant experiences lethargy, changes in level of consciousness, lower extremity spasticity and opisthotonos and, if the hydrocephalus is allowed to progress, the infant experiences difficulty in sucking and feeding, emesis, seizures, sunset eyes, and cardiopulmonary complications as lower brain stem and cortical function are disrupted or destroyed. In the child, increased intracranial pressure (ICP) focal manifestations are experienced related to space-occupying focal lesions and include headache, emesis, ataxia, irritability, lethargy, and confusion. Treatment may include surgery to provide shunting for drainage of the excess fluid from the ventricles to an extracranial space such as the peritoneum or right atrium (in older children) or management with medications to reduce IC if progression is slow or surgery is contraindicated.

MEDICAL CARE

Anticonvulsants: to interfere with impulse transmission of cerebral cortex and prevent seizures.

Antibiotics: culture and sensitivity dependent for shunt infections such as septicemia, meningitis, ventriculitis or given as prophylactic treatment.

Skull X-ray: reveals increasing head enlargement, widening of suture lines and fontanelles.

Magnetic Resonance Imaging: reveals presence of hydrocephalus.

Echoencephalogram: reveals comparison of ratio of ventricle to cortex.

Ventriculogram: reveals size of ventricles and patency of a shunt if present.

Surgical Management: therapy of choice in almost all cases. Includes use of ventriculo-peritoneal shunt (VP), ventriculo-atrial shunt (VA), temporary ventriculostomy.

Electrolyte Panel: reveals changes indicating dehydration or losses from diuretic therapy.

Complete Blood Count: reveals increased WBC if infection, presence of dehydration.

COMMON NURSING DIAGNOSES

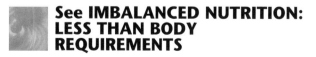

See EXCESS FLUID VOLUME

Related to: Compromised regulatory mechanism shunt placement—ventriculoatrial or VP.

Defining Characteristics: (Specify: decreased cardiac output, change in respiratory pattern, tachycardia, tachypnea, dyspnea, weight gain, chest pain, cardiac arrhythmias, pulmonary congestion.)

See RISK FOR DEFICIENT FLUID VOLUME

Related to: Excessive losses.

Defining Characteristics: (Specify: postoperative vomiting or diarrhea, use of diuretics, altered intake, thirst, dry skin and mucous membranes.)

See IMBALANCED NUTRITION: LESS THAN BODY REQUIREMENTS

Related to: Inability to ingest food/feedings.

Defining Characteristics: (Specify: advanced stage of hydrocephalus, postoperative vomiting, NPO status.)

See RISK FOR IMPAIRED SKIN INTEGRITY

Related to: Physical immobilization.

Defining Characteristics: (Specify: decreased movement of head, disruption of skin surface by surgical procedure [shunt insertion] or diagnostic procedure.)

See HYPERTHERMIA

Related to: Illness (infection).

Defining Characteristics: (Specify: increase in body temperature above normal range.)

See DELAYED GROWTH AND DEVELOPMENT

Related to: Effects of disorder or disability.

Defining Characteristics: (Specify: altered physical growth, mental retardation, delay or difficulty in performing motor, social skills typical of age, dependence.)

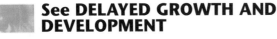

ANXIETY

Related to: (Specify: threat to or change in health status; threat to or change in environment [hospitalization].)

Defining Characteristics: (Specify: increased apprehension that condition of infant might worsen or condition may develop in child as a complication, expressed concern and worry about preoperative preparation and the surgical procedure, possible or actual physical, neurologic and mental deficits.)

Goal: Client will experience decreased anxiety by (date and time to evaluate).

Outcome Criteria

✔ Clients verbalize feeling better.

✔ Anxiety is decreased.

NOC: *Anxiety Control*

INTERVENTIONS	RATIONALES
Assess source and level of anxiety and need for information and support about condition and impending surgery.	Provides information about severity of anxiety and need for interventions and support; allows for identification of fear and uncertainty about condition and/or surgery and treatments and recovery; guilt about condition, possible loss of infant/child or of parental responsibility.
Allow expressions of concern and opportunity to ask questions about condition and recovery of ill infant/child.	Provides opportunity to vent feelings, secure information needed to reduce anxiety.
Communicate therapeutically with parents and answer questions calmly and honestly.	Promotes calm and supportive environment.
Encourage parents to remain involved in care and decision-making regarding infant/child.	Promotes constant monitoring of infant/child for improvement or worsening of symptoms.
Encourage parents to stay with infant/child or visit when able if hospitalized, assist in care (hold, feed, diaper) and make suggestions for routines and methods of treatment.	Allows parents to care for and support child instead of becoming increasingly anxious because of absence from child and wondering about infant/child's condition.
When surgery is planned, answer all questions from parents and child with honesty; refer to physician for answers and explanations if needed.	Promotes supportive environment and reduces anxiety caused by fear of unknown.
Prepare child/parents for diagnostic tests and potential surgical procedures.	Promotes reduction in anxiety if they have knowledge of expectations.
Explain reason for and what to expect for each procedure or type of therapy; use drawings and pictures, video tapes for child.	Reduces fear which causes anxiety.
Teach parents and child (age dependent) about reason for and type of surgery to be done, site and dressings, time of surgery and length of time of procedure, preoperative care and treatments.	Provides information about surgery and desired effects as well as possible residual effects.
Clarify any misinformation and answer all questions honestly and in simple understandable language.	Prevents unnecessary anxiety resulting from inaccurate information or beliefs.

INTERVENTIONS	RATIONALES
Teach about shunt placement and reason; possible future revision of shunt placement, signs and symptoms of shunt complication or malfunction.	Shunt is placed to by-pass an obstruction or remove excess cerebrospinal fluid that predisposes to increased ICP; a shunt revision may be done to treat shunt complication such as infection or obstruction or as a result of child growth.

NIC: *Anxiety Reduction*

Evaluation

(Date/time of evaluation of goal)

(Has goal been met? Not met? Partially met?)

(Did parents and child verbalize feeling better? Did clients verbalize decreased anxiety? Use quotes.)

(Revisions to care plan? D/C care plan? Continue care plan?)

RISK FOR INJURY

Related to: (Specify: sensory, integrative and effector dysfunction preoperatively.)

Defining Characteristics: (Specify: neuromuscular changes, neurosensory changes, behavioral changes, increased ICP, CSF accumulation, vital signs changes, seizure activity.)

Goal: Client will not experience any injury by (date and time to evaluate).

Outcome Criteria

✔ Head circumference remains (specify cm).

✔ Client will not demonstrate (specify several signs of increased ICP to observe for, e.g., irritability, bulging fontanels, sunset sign, vomiting, headache, seizures).

NOC: *Risk Detection*

INTERVENTIONS	RATIONALES
Assess for rapidly increased circumference of head, tense, bulging fontanels, widening suture lines, irritability, lethargy, "cracked pot" sound percussion,	Indicates increasing ICP in infant/small child.

INTERVENTIONS	RATIONALES
sunset sign, opisthotonos, spasticity of lower extremities, seizures, high-pitched cry, distended scalp veins, changes in normal feeding patterns.	
Assess for early signs including: headache, nausea, vomiting, diplopia, blurred vision, seizures, irritability, restlessness, decrease in school performance, decreased motor performance, sleep loss, weight loss, memory loss progressing to lethargy and drowsiness. Late signs: decreased level of consciousness, decreased motor response to commands, decreased response to pain, change in pupils, posturing, papilledema.	Indicates increasing ICP in children with symptoms related to cause of hydrocephalus.
Perform neurologic and vital sign assessment q 4h or as needed (specify).	Provides data indicating an increasing ICP causing decreased respirations, increased blood pressure and pulse.
Position with head elevated 30 degrees and support head when handling or changing position; monitor skin integrity with position change.	Promotes drainage of CSF and reduces accumulation of CSF; infant may not be able to lift and move head.
Carry out seizure precautions including padding of crib/bed, remove toys and objects from bed, maintain suction and oxygen at bedside, note and report characteristics of seizure.	Prevents injury to self during seizure activity caused by increased ICP and to treat apnea during seizure activity.
Support an enlarged head by cradling it in an arm when holding, place infant on a pillow when moving, move head and body of infant at the same time.	Protects infant's head from trauma and neck from strain.
Teach parents signs and symptoms of increased ICP and changes to report to physician (specify).	Promotes knowledge of risk of developing increased ICP and encourages preventive measures.
Inform parents that condition is life-long and monitoring and follow-up care on a regular basis is required.	Provides realistic and honest information that promotes optimal health and function for the infant/child.

NIC: *Surveillance*

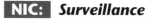

Evaluation

(Date/time of evaluation of goal)

(Has goal been met? Not met? Partially met?)

(Provide information related to the outcome criteria chosen, e.g., is child irritable? Are fontanels of infant bulging? Does child exhibit sunset sign? Complain of headache? Has there been any vomiting or seizure activity?)

(Revisions to care plan? D/C care plan? Continue care plan?)

RISK FOR INJURY

Related to: (Specify: shunt placement and potential complications of shunt functioning.)

Defining Characteristics: (Specify: increased ICP, kinking or plugging of shunt tubing, separation of tubing, changing of position of tubing, obstruction of shunt, displacement with growth.)

Goal: Client will not experience any injury by (date and time to evaluate).

Outcome Criteria

✔ Client will remain alert without signs of increased ICP.

NOC: *Risk Control*

INTERVENTIONS	RATIONALES
Assess for signs and symptoms of increased ICP, swelling along shunt tract; note presence/severity of headache and neck pain; behavior changes (lethargy, irritability), physical changes (full fontanel, nausea, vomiting, edematous eyes, tender, swollen abdomen).	Provides data that indicates shunt malfunction.
Note vomiting, drowsiness, irritability, swelling at pump site, redness, exudate and temperature of child.	Indicates shunt blockage.
Position carefully on nonoperative side postoperatively; maintain bed position and activity level as ordered depending on shunt dynamics.	Prevents trauma to surgical site; maintain shunt patency.

INTERVENTIONS	RATIONALES
Instruct parent on hydrocephalus and shunt placement; teaching should include: definition of hydrocephalus (brain anatomy), causes, diagnostic tests, treatments, signs of shunt malfunction and infection, interventions and proper notification of health professionals, and documentation; supplemental written materials are important; emphasize the importance of early identification of infection/malfunction and prompt notification.	Promotes understanding of illness/treatments which may decrease anxiety; knowledge of prompt treatment of complications often life-saving.
Teach parents about need for bowel elimination at least every 2 days and steps to take to ensure bowel movement.	Prevents complications associated with ventriculo-peritoneal shunt.
Inform parents of agencies for guidance and support such as National Hydrocephalus Foundation.	Provides assistance with management of child with hydrocephalus.
Discuss and encourage parents to treat child as member of family and instruct in activities to be avoided such as rough contact sports.	Promotes growth and development and feeling of belonging.

NIC: *Surveillance*

Evaluation

(Date/time of evaluation of goal)

(Has goal been met? Not met? Partially met?)

(Provide information related to the outcome criteria chosen, e.g., is child irritable? Are fontanels of infant bulging? Does child exhibit sunset sign? Complain of headache? Has there been any vomiting or seizure activity?)

(Revisions to care plan? D/C care plan? Continue care plan?)

RISK FOR INFECTION

Related to: Invasive procedure of shunt insertion.

Defining Characteristics: (Specify: elevated temperature, swelling, redness at shunt tract or operative site, nausea, vomiting, lethargy, excessive drainage on dressing, poor feeding.)

Goal: Client will not experience any infection by (date and time to evaluate).

Outcome Criteria

✔ Temperature remains <99° F.
✔ WBC levels (specify maximum for age).

NOC: *Risk Detection*

INTERVENTIONS	RATIONALES
Assess site for inflammatory process, temperature for elevation, WBC for increases, characteristics of drainage on dressings.	Provides data indicating presence or potential for infection which affects shunt function.
Follow principles of asepsis when performing procedures such as dressing changes.	Prevents transmission of microorganisms to shunt site.
Monitor temperature q 4h.	Elevation of temperature indicates infection.
Avoid positioning head of valve site for at least 2 days postoperatively.	Alleviates the risk of infection.

INTERVENTIONS	RATIONALES
Teach about signs and symptoms of infection of site and shunt tract and to notify physician if noted.	Promotes early detection of infection that may occur for up to 1 to 2 months after shunt insertion.
Teach parents about wound care and dressing change, emphasize importance of good handwashing techniques.	Provides clean, sterile dressings when soiled or wet.

NIC: *Surveillance*

Evaluation

(Date/time of evaluation of goal)

(Has goal been met? Not met? Partially met?)

(What is temperature? What is WBC level—include date and time of test.)

(Revisions to care plan? D/C care plan? Continue care plan?)

HYDROCEPHALUS

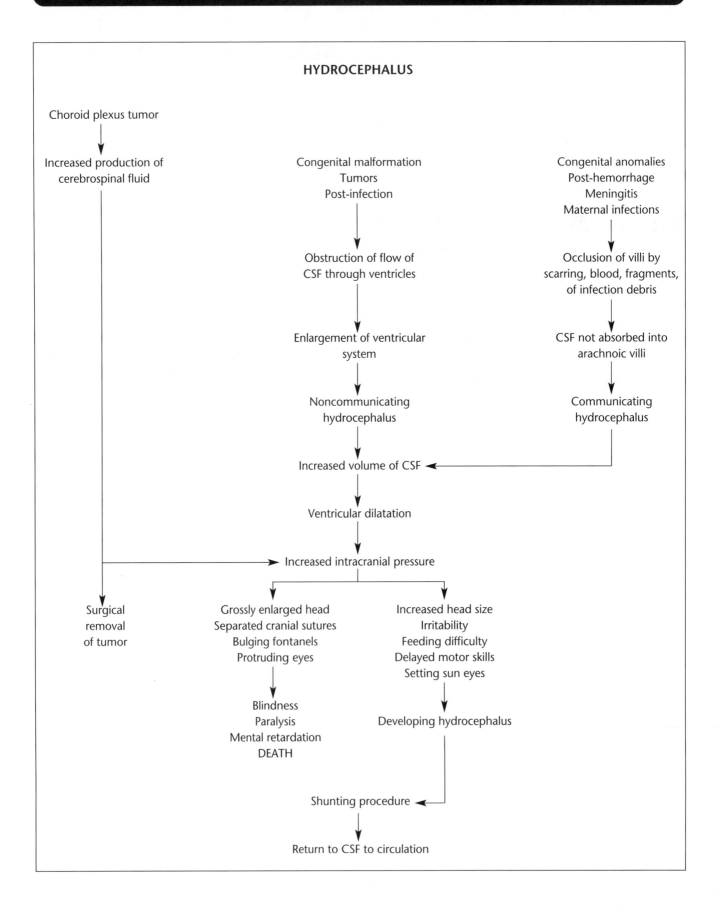

CHAPTER 7.2

BRAIN TUMOR

A brain tumor is a solid tumor that may be benign, malignant, or a metastatic growth from a tumor in another part of the body. Most central nervous system tumors occur in the cerebellum or brain stem and cause increased intracranial pressure and the symptoms associated with it. Other tumors occur in the cerebrum. A malignant brain tumor is the second most common type of cancer in children and has a poor prognosis as the tumor usually enlarges and becomes advanced before signs and symptoms appear or are detected as they are easily missed. Signs and symptoms are site and size dependent. Brain tumors are most prevalent in children 3 to 7 years of age. Treatment includes surgery, although total removal is not usually possible, chemotherapy, and radiation, which may be done to decrease the size of the tumor before surgery. One or a combination of these procedures may be done with each resulting in possible residual neurologic deficits.

MEDICAL CARE

Analgesics/Antipyretics: for headache to reduce fever and to decrease pain.

Diuretics (Osmotic): mannitol to induce diuresis with a hypertonic solution to prevent reabsorption of water by the glomeruli and decrease cerebral edema.

Antibiotics: specific to microorganisms identified by culture and sensitivities to treat infection or given to prevent infection.

Anti-inflammatories: cortisone to reduce the inflammation process in brain.

Saline Solution: given as eye drops or eye irrigation to prevent corneal ulceration.

Stool Softeners: for easier elimination to prevent constipation and Valsalva's maneuver which increase intracranial pressure.

Computerized Tomography Scan (CT): reveals changes in position of brain parenchyma, ventricles, and subarachnoid space caused by tumor growth.

Stereotactic Surgery: use of CT/MRI to reconstruct brain tumor three-dimensionally to accurately remove it surgically.

Laser Therapy: vaporization of tumor tissue.

Radiotherapy: use of radiation to shrink tumor size.

Chemotherapy: used to treat malignant tumors.

Cerebral Angiogram: reveals vascularity and blood supply to the tumor before surgery.

Magnetic Resonance Imaging (MRI): reveals tumor growth and size before, during, and after treatment.

Electrolyte Panel: reveals changes indicating dehydration or losses from diuretic therapy.

Complete Blood Count: reveals increased WBC if infection present.

Urinalysis: reveals increased sp.gr. in presence of dehydration.

COMMON NURSING DIAGNOSES

See HYPERTHERMIA

Related to: Illness.

Defining Characteristics: (Specify: increase in body temperature above normal range, presence of infection [meningitis or upper respiratory], surgical procedure [anesthesia, brain stem or hypothalamus area].)

See DISTURBED SLEEP PATTERN

Related to: Sensory alternations.

Defining Characteristics: (Specify: lethargy, restlessness, irritability, disorientation, coma, frequent napping.)

See RISK FOR DEFICIENT FLUID VOLUME

Related to: Excessive losses.

Defining Characteristics: (Specify: vomiting, altered intake, diuresis with use of diuretic, diabetes insipidus development, thirst, dry skin and mucous membranes.)

 See IMBALANCED NUTRITION: LESS THAN BODY REQUIREMENTS

Related to: Inability to ingest food.

Defining Characteristics: (Specify: vomiting, nausea, choking and possible aspiration with facial paralysis or edema, refusal to eat or drink, gavage feedings, depressed gag reflex.)

See IMPAIRED PHYSICAL MOBILITY

Related to: Neuromuscular impairment.

Defining Characteristics: (Specify: inability to purposefully move within physical environment, impaired coordination, loss of balance, decreased muscle strength and control spasticity, hypo or hyperreflexia, paralysis, general weakness, ataxia following surgery.)

See DELAYED GROWTH AND DEVELOPMENT

Related to: Effects of disorder following surgery/other.

Defining Characteristics: (Specify: delay or difficulty in performing skills typical of age group [motor, social or expressive], inability to perform self-control activities appropriate for age behavior and/or intellectual deficits, presence of somnolence syndrome.)

ADDITIONAL NURSING DIAGNOSES

PAIN

Related to: Biologic injuring agents.

Defining Characteristics: (Specify: verbal descriptor of pain, headache in frontal or occipital area that is worse in the morning and becomes worse if head lowered or with straining, increased VS, restlessness, hostility, inability to relax.)

Goal: Child will experience decreased pain by (date and time to evaluate).

Outcome Criteria

✔ Child rates pain as less than (specify pain rating and scale used).

NOC: *Pain Level*

INTERVENTIONS	RATIONALES
Assess severity of headache, recurrence and progressive characteristics, precipitating factors and length of headache.	Provides information regarding presence of tumor as headache is a most common symptom in child.
Administer analgesic (specify) to treat or anticipate headache based on assessment.	(Action of drug.)
Provide toys, games for quiet play (specify).	Provides diversionary activity to detract from pain.
Apply cool compress to head for low to moderate pain.	Provides comfort and relief from headache, decreases facial swelling, if present.
After surgical intervention, opioids (morphine sulfate) may be initially used. Assess for side effects such as sedation and respiratory depression; use Naloxone to reverse.	Side effects occur rarely, opioids can be given safely with appropriate monitoring.
Determine the child's understanding of the word "pain" and ask family what word the child normally uses. Use a pain assessment tool appropriate for age and developmental level to identify intensity of pain.	Promotes better communication between child/family and nurse.
Plan a preventive approach to pain management around the clock; observe for signs of pain, both physiologic and behavioral.	Promotes early identification of pain which enhances pain relief measures.
Teach parents and child about analgesics, to administer in anticipation of headache and type to give (sustained release) (specify) and that it will help to control headache.	Controls pain before it becomes severe (action of drug).
Encourage child to restrain from coughing, sneezing, or straining during defecation.	Prevents straining that precipitates or intensifies headache.
Assist parents to develop activities that will not precipitate or increase headache pain.	Promotes stimulation for child's development needs.

NIC: *Pain Management*

Evaluation

(Date/time of evaluation of goal)

(Has goal been met? Not met? Partially met?)

(What is pain rating? Specify scale used.)

(Revisions to care plan? D/C care plan? Continue care plan?)

RISK FOR INJURY

Related to: Sensory, integrative, and effector dysfunction.

Defining Characteristics: (Specify: neuromuscular changes, neurosensory changes, behavioral changes, increased ICP, seizure activity, vital signs changes.)

Goal: Child will not experience injury by (date and time to evaluate).

Outcome Criteria

✔ Child does not exhibit increased ICP. Participates in teaching about treatment options (specify for child).

NOC: *Risk Detection*

INTERVENTIONS	RATIONALES
Assess head circumference in the infant/small child for increases as fluid obstruction caused by tumor will increase head size.	Provides data indicating an increase in ICP as tumor grows with a poorer prognosis because tumor size becomes large before diagnosis is made.
Assess vital signs including increased BP, decreased pulse pressure, pulse and respirations; take for 1 full minute when monitoring pulse and respirations.	Provides changes indicating presence of brain tumor depending on type and location of tumor.
Assess changes in gross and fine motor control, weakness, ataxia, spasticity, paralysis or change in balance, coordination.	Provides changes in neuromuscular status indicating presence of brain tumor.
Assess changes in vision (visual acuity, strabismus, diplopia, nystagmus), head tilt, papilledema.	Provides changes in neurosensory status indicating presence of brain tumor.
Assess for irritability, lethargy, loss of consciousness or coma, fatigue, napping.	Provides changes in behavior indicating presence of brain tumor.

INTERVENTIONS	RATIONALES
Assess for increased ICP including irritability, poor feeding, vomiting, head enlargement, lethargy, high-pitched cry (infant) or vomiting, diplopia, behavioral changes, change in VS, seizure activity.	Provides information about ICP change caused by brain distortion or shifting caused by tumor.
Alter environment by padding bed or crib, reduce light and stimulation.	Prevents injury if seizure activity possible.
Place in position of comfort with head elevated.	Promotes comfort and decreases increased ICP by gravity.
Teach parents and child about diagnostic procedures done to evaluate tumor presence; base information on child's age and past experiences (specify).	Promotes understanding of procedures to reduce.
Inform parents that surgery may be performed to remove the tumor as a reinforcement of physician information and that radiation and chemotherapy may be administered after surgery.	Prepared for surgery and possible postoperative therapy with information limited to sensitive, hopeful explanation; information about postoperative therapy should be postponed until this decision is made after surgery.

NIC: *Surveillance*

Evaluation

(Date/time of evaluation of goal)

(Has goal been met? Not met? Partially met?)

(Provide data about signs of increased ICP. Did child participate in teaching? Describe.)

(Revisions to care plan? D/C care plan? Continue care plan?)

ANXIETY

Related to: Change in health status and threat to self-concept.

Defining Characteristics: (Specify: increased apprehension as diagnosis is confirmed and condition worsens, expressed concern and worry about postoperative residual tumor and effects, hair removal before surgery, insomnia, social isolation.)

Goal: Clients will experience decreased anxiety by (date and time to evaluate).

Outcome Criteria

✔ Parents verbalize decreased anxiety.

✔ Child appears calm, without crying or irritability.

NOC: *Anxiety Control*

INTERVENTIONS	RATIONALES
Assess level of anxiety and need for information that will relieve it following surgery.	Provides information about degree of anxiety and need for interventions and support; allow for identification of fear and uncertainty about surgery and treatments and recovery, guilt about illness, possible loss of child, parental role and responsibility.
Encourage expression of concerns and inquire about condition of ill child and possible consequences and prognosis.	Provides opportunity to vent feelings, secure information needed to reduce anxiety.
Prepare family and/or child for diagnostic tests and surgery. Encourage child to draw a picture of the brain to clarify any misconceptions; encourage use of medical play (dolls, puppets, equipment) after procedures (specify for child).	Promotes understanding which decreases anxiety; may clarify misconceptions and increase feelings of control.
Encourage parents to stay with infant/child; encourage participation in care of infant/child.	Promotes care and support of child by parents.
If surgery planned, orient to special care unit, equipment and staff (specify how).	Reduces anxiety caused by fear of unknown.

INTERVENTIONS	RATIONALES
Teach parents and child about hair clipping and that hair will grow back in short period of time, to cover head with cap or scarf temporarily; that there is edema of the face and eyes after surgery; that a dressing will be applied that completely covers the head; use of a doll with head wrapped in a bandage may be useful in explaining the post-surgical dressing.	Promotes understanding of postoperative appearance to maintain self-image; support self-concept.
Teach parents and child that after surgery a headache and sleepy feeling may be present for a few days or even lethargy and coma may be present.	Provides an explanation of what to expect after surgery.
Clarify any information in lay terms and use aids that are age related if helpful to child (specify).	Prevents unnecessary anxiety resulting from misunderstanding or inconsistencies in information.

NIC: *Anxiety Reduction*

Evaluation

(Date/time of evaluation of goal)

(Has goal been met? Not met? Partially met?)

(Did parents verbalize decreased anxiety? Use quotes. Is child calm and not irritable? Describe behavior.)

(Revisions to care plan? D/C care plan? Continue care plan?)

BRAIN TUMOR

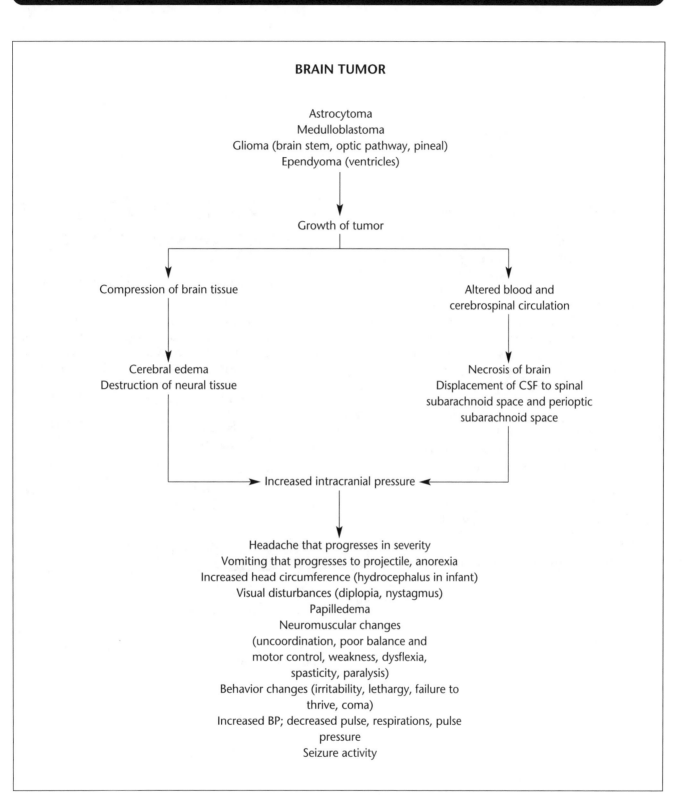

Astrocytoma
Medulloblastoma
Glioma (brain stem, optic pathway, pineal)
Ependyoma (ventricles)

Growth of tumor

Compression of brain tissue

Altered blood and
cerebrospinal circulation

Cerebral edema
Destruction of neural tissue

Necrosis of brain
Displacement of CSF to spinal
subarachnoid space and perioptic
subarachnoid space

Increased intracranial pressure

Headache that progresses in severity
Vomiting that progresses to projectile, anorexia
Increased head circumference (hydrocephalus in infant)
Visual disturbances (diplopia, nystagmus)
Papilledema
Neuromuscular changes
(uncoordination, poor balance and
motor control, weakness, dysflexia,
spasticity, paralysis)
Behavior changes (irritability, lethargy, failure to
thrive, coma)
Increased BP; decreased pulse, respirations, pulse
pressure
Seizure activity

CHAPTER 7.3

GUILLAIN-BARRÉ SYNDROME

Guillain-Barré syndrome (infectious polyneuritis) is an acute inflammation of the spinal and cranial nerves manifested by motor dysfunction that predominates over sensory dysfunction. The actual cause is unknown, but it is associated with a previously existing viral infection or vaccine administration. Neurologic symptoms include muscle cramps and paresthesia with weakness progressing to paralysis. The severity of the disease ranges from mild to severe with the course of the disease dependent on the degree of paralysis present at the peak of the condition. Recovery is usually complete and may take weeks or months. The disease most commonly occurs in children between 4 and 10 years of age. Treatment is symptom-dependent with hospitalization required in the acute phase of the disease to observe and intervene for respiratory or swallowing complications.

MEDICAL CARE

Anti-inflammatory (Corticosteroids): to reduce inflammation process and immune responses; Ibuprofen may or may not be helpful in early stages of disease.

Analgesics/Antipyretics: acetaminophen to relieve pain in muscles or elevated temperature if present.

Stool Softeners: given for easier elimination to prevent constipation and Valsalva's maneuver.

Oxygen Therapy: given with ventilatory support depending on ABGs revealing decreased PO_2 level.

Arterial Blood Gases: reveals O_2 and CO_2 and pH levels as indication of acidosis or respiratory failure or need for oxygen therapy.

Cerebrospinal Fluid Analysis: reveals protein concentration of more than 60 mg/dl and white blood cells of fewer than 10/cu mm.

Plasmapheresis: may be used to shorten length of illness and/or to lessen long-term disability.

COMMON NURSING DIAGNOSES

See DECREASED CARDIAC OUTPUT

Related to: Effects of autonomic dysfunction on cardiac activity.

Defining Characteristics: (Specify: variations in hemodynamic readings [tachycardia, bradycardia, hypotension, hypertension] decreased peripheral pulses, oliguria, cyanosis, pallor of skin and mucous membranes, ECG changes [arrhythmias], diaphoresis, dizziness, orthostatic hypotension.)

See INEFFECTIVE BREATHING PATTERN

Related to: Neuromuscular impairment.

Defining Characteristics: (Specify: altered chest expansion, respiratory depth changes, cyanosis, abnormal ABGs.)

See INEFFECTIVE AIRWAY CLEARANCE

Related to: Tracheobronchial obstruction.

Defining Characteristics: (Specify: abnormal breath sounds [crackles, wheezes], changes in rate or depth of respiration, paralysis in chest muscles, tachypnea, cough, dyspnea, inability to clear secretions from airway, inability to swallow secretions, weakness in speech, gag reflex, aspiration.)

See IMBALANCED NUTRITION: LESS THAN BODY REQUIREMENTS

Related to: Inability to ingest food, absorb nutrients.

Defining Characteristics: (Specify: anorexia, diarrhea, weakness of chewing and swallowing muscles, dysesthesia of hands with inability to feed self, weight loss, loss of muscle tone, paralysis [ascending].)

See DIARRHEA

Related to: Neuromuscular impairment.

Defining Characteristics: (Specify: increased frequency, loose, liquid stools, increased bowel sounds.)

 See IMPAIRED PHYSICAL MOBILITY

Related to: Neuromuscular impairment.

Defining Characteristics: (Specify: paralysis, inability to purposefully move within physical environment including bed mobility, transfer and ambulation, limited ROM, decreased muscle strength and control, trauma from falls.)

See HYPERTHERMIA

Related to: Illness causing autonomic instability.

Defining Characteristics: (Specify: increase in body temperature above normal range or decrease below normal range, warm or cool to touch.)

ADDITIONAL NURSING DIAGNOSES

 IMPAIRED URINARY ELIMINATION

Related to: Neuromuscular impairment.

Defining Characteristics: (Specify: paralysis, retention.)

Goal: Child will have improved urinary elimination by (date and time to evaluate).

Outcome Criteria

✔ Bladder is not palpable.

✔ Intake equals output.

NOC: *Urinary Elimination*

INTERVENTIONS	RATIONALES
Assess continuing extent of paralysis and effect on urinary elimination.	Provides information about effect of motor weakness that travels upward from extremities.
Assess for I&O q 4 to 8h and palpate bladder q 2h; assess for cloudy, foul-smelling urine.	Provides monitoring for I&O ratio and presence of urinary retention, UTI as paralysis progresses.

INTERVENTIONS	RATIONALES
Provide urinary elimination rehabilitation program; perform Credé's maneuver in gentle fashion if indicated.	Promotes urine elimination and return to normal pattern as soon as possible.
Catheterize as last resort; maintain indwelling catheter if needed to maintain elimination.	Relieves distention and retention.
Instruct parents in program to rehabilitate urinary function (specify).	Promotes urinary elimination and return to baseline pattern without retention and possible urinary bladder infection.
Teach parents to maintain fluid intake and monitor output in relation to intake.	Maintains I&O balance and enough intake to encourage urinary output.
Inform to report any reduction or absence of urinary elimination.	Prevents complication of neuromuscular impairment of disease and effect on urinary bladder function.

NIC: *Urinary Elimination Management*

Evaluation

(Date/time of evaluation of goal)

(Has goal been met? Not met? Partially met?)

(Is bladder palpable above symphysis after voiding? What is intake and output? Provide cc's and amount of time.)

(Revisions to care plan? D/C care plan? Continue care plan?)

 PAIN

Related to: Biologic injuring agent (inflammation of nerves).

Defining Characteristics: (Specify: communication of pain descriptors of discomfort in hands and feet, guarding behavior, alteration in muscle tone, autonomic responses of diaphoresis, VS changes.)

Goal: Child will experience decreased pain by (date and time to evaluate).

Outcome Criteria

✔ Child rates pain as less than (specify pain rating and scale used).

NOC: *Pain Level*

INTERVENTIONS	RATIONALES
Assess pain and ability to participate in activities.	Provides information about degree of pain or presence of progressive paralysis.
Reposition q 2h, support extremities and maintain clean, comfortable bed with eggcrate mattress and padding to bony prominences as needed; use good postural alignment, provide passive ROM.	Promotes comfort and reduces risks for skin impairment.
Administer analgesics (specify) based on pain assessment and respiratory status; evaluate effect.	Eliminates or controls pain and promotes comfort (action of drug).
Apply moist heat to painful areas as ordered.	Promotes circulation to area and relieves pain.
Reassure parents and child that pain decreases as motor changes become resolved or improve.	Provides information about length of time pain might be expected to continue.
Determine the child's understanding of the word "pain" and ask family members what word the child uses at home; use pain assessment tool appropriate for the child's age and developmental level to identify the intensity of pain.	Promotes better communication between the child/family and nurse.
Plan a preventive approach to pain around the clock; observe for signs of pain, physiologic and behavioral.	Promotes early identification of pain which enhances effective pain relief.

NIC: *Pain Management*

Evaluation

(Date/time of evaluation of goal)

(Has goal been met? Not met? Partially met?)

(What is pain rating? Specify scale used)

(Revisions to care plan? D/C care plan? Continue care plan?)

ANXIETY

Related to: Change in health status and threat to self-concept.

Defining Characteristics: (Specify: increased apprehension as condition worsens and paralysis spreads, expressed concern and worry about permanent effects of disease, treatments during hospitalization, expressed feeling of increased helplessness and uncertainty.)

Goal: Clients will experience decreased anxiety by (date and time to evaluate).

Outcome Criteria

✔ Parents and child verbalize decreased feelings of anxiety.

NOC: *Anxiety Control*

INTERVENTIONS	RATIONALES
Assess source and level of anxiety, how anxiety is manifested and need for information that will relieve it.	Provides information about degree of anxiety and need for interventions, sources may include fear and uncertainty about treatment and recovery, guilt about presence of illness, possible loss of parental role and responsibility while hospitalized.
Encourage expression of concerns and opportunity to ask questions about condition and recovery of ill child.	Provides opportunity to vent feelings, secure information needed to reduce anxiety.
Communicate therapeutically with parents and child and answer questions calmly and honestly.	Promotes supportive environment.
Assist parents and child to note improvements resulting from treatments.	Promotes positive attitude and optimistic outlook for recovery.
Encourage parents to stay with child and assist in care of child.	Allows for care and support of child instead of increasing anxiety that is caused by absence and lack of knowledge about child's condition.
Encourage child to participate in own care depending on ability and/or paralysis; allow to make choices about ADL as soon as possible.	Promotes independence and control and preserves developmental status.
Teach parents and child about disease process and behaviors, physical effects.	Provides information to relieve anxiety by knowledge of what to expect.
Discuss each procedure or type of therapy, effects of any diagnostic tests to parents and child as appropriate to age.	Reduces fear of unknown which may increase anxiety.

INTERVENTIONS	RATIONALES	INTERVENTIONS	RATIONALES
Teach parents and child that degree of severity varies but motor weakness and paralysis start with extremities and move upward with the peak reached in 3 weeks and improvement seen by 4 to 8 weeks.	Provides information about usual course of disease and length of illness.	Assess for presence of permanent disability or possibility of long-term recovery and effect on parents.	Identifies factors associated with long recovery period.
Clarify any information and answer questions in lay terms and use aids for visual reinforcement if helpful.	Prevents unnecessary anxiety resulting from inaccurate knowledge or beliefs or inconsistencies in information.	Encourage parents to express feelings and unmet needs and ability to meet and develop self-expectations.	Identifies potential for social deprivation of parents and development of strategies to achieve realistic expectations.
		Encourage touching and play activities between parents and child.	Enhances comfort and positive parental behaviors.
		Encourage and praise positive parental behaviors; support any participation in care or decision-making on behalf of the child.	Reduces anxiety for and enhances learning about child's needs and care.
		Teach parenting skills needed for long-term recovery period (specify).	Promotes parental knowledge and awareness of skills to be learned and implemented.
		Teach about physical therapy program including ROM, exercises, gait training, bracing (refer as indicated).	Facilitates muscle recovery and prevents contractures and permanent disability, promotes sense of confidence and control.
		Continue to inform and support parents during recovery period (provide telephone numbers).	Provides reassurance that recovery is slow and conserves parental emotional reserves.
		Refer to Guillain-Barré Syndrome Support Group for assistance or community agencies for support.	Provides information and support from those with experience with the disease.

NIC: *Anxiety Reduction*

Evaluation

(Date/time of evaluation of goal)

(Has goal been met? Not met? Partially met?)

(Did parents and child verbalize decreased feelings of anxiety? Use quotes.)

(Revisions to care plan? D/C care plan? Continue care plan?)

 # RISK FOR IMPAIRED PARENTING

Related to: Illness.

Defining Characteristics: (Specify: verbalization of decreased interactions with hospitalized child and inability to provide care, lack of control over situation, request for information about parenting skills for long recovery period or permanent residual disability.)

Goal: Child will receive appropriate parenting by (date and time to evaluate).

Outcome Criteria

✔ Parents participate in child's care.

✔ Parents identify agencies that offer assistance and support.

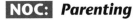 **NOC:** *Parenting*

NIC: *Support System Enhancement*

Evaluation

(Date/time of evaluation of goal)

(Has goal been met? Not met? Partially met?)

(Did parents participate in child's care? Describe. Which agencies did parents identify?)

(Revisions to care plan? D/C care plan? Continue care plan?)

GUILLAIN-BARRÉ SYNDROME

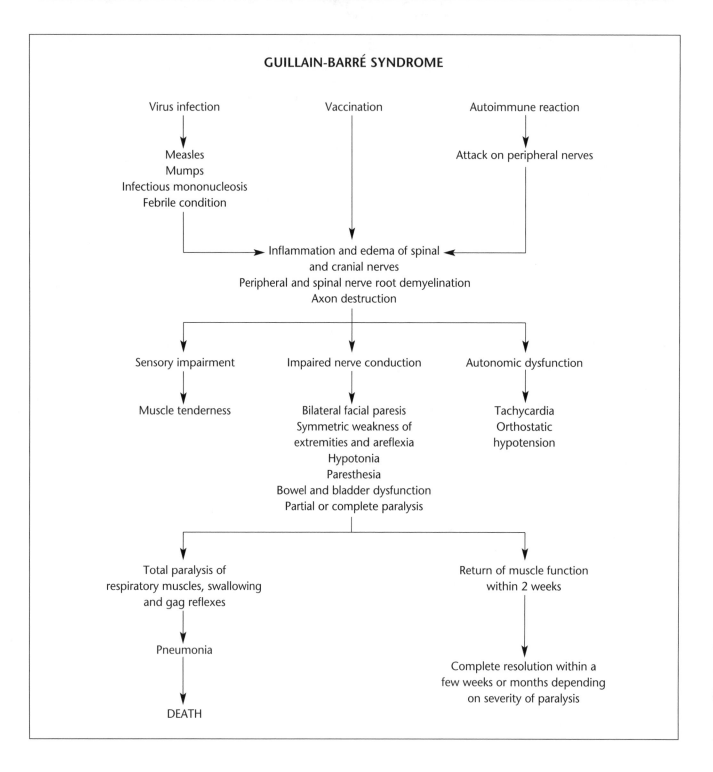

Virus infection

Vaccination

Autoimmune reaction

Measles
Mumps
Infectious mononucleosis
Febrile condition

Attack on peripheral nerves

Inflammation and edema of spinal
and cranial nerves
Peripheral and spinal nerve root demyelination
Axon destruction

Sensory impairment

Impaired nerve conduction

Autonomic dysfunction

Muscle tenderness

Bilateral facial paresis
Symmetric weakness of
extremities and areflexia
Hypotonia
Paresthesia
Bowel and bladder dysfunction
Partial or complete paralysis

Tachycardia
Orthostatic
hypotension

Total paralysis of
respiratory muscles, swallowing
and gag reflexes

Return of muscle function
within 2 weeks

Pneumonia

Complete resolution within a
few weeks or months depending
on severity of paralysis

DEATH

CHAPTER 7.4

MENINGITIS

Meningitis is the inflammation of the meninges and is the most common infection of the central nervous system (CNS). It may be bacterial or viral in origin. Bacterial infections may be caused by *Haemophilus influenzae* (type B), *Streptococcus pneumoniae*, *Neisseria meningitidis*, or *Staphlococcus aureus*. Those at greatest risk for this disease are infants between 6 and 12 months of age with most cases occurring between 1 month and 5 years of age. The most common route of infection is vascular dissemination from an infection in the nasopharynx or sinuses, or one implanted as a result of wounds, skull fracture, lumbar puncture, or surgical procedure. Viral (aseptic) meningitis is caused by a variety of viral agents and usually associated with measles, mumps, herpes, or enteritis. This form of meningitis is self-limiting and treated symptomatically for 3 to 10 days. Treatment includes hospitalization to differentiate between the two types of meningitis, isolation and management of symptoms, and prevention of complications.

MEDICAL CARE

Antipyretics: given to reduce fever.

Antibiotics: given to treat the infection, or specific to identified microorganisms as a result of culture and sensitivity tests.

Anticonvulsants: to prevent seizure activity.

Computerized Tomography Scan: reveals subdural effusion.

Cultures of Blood, Urine, Cerebrospinal Fluid, Nasopharynx: reveal causative organism.

Lumbar Puncture: reveals cloudy or purulent appearance, increased WBC predominant polymorphonuclear leukocytes, increased protein, decreased glucose in bacterial type; clear, normal or slight elevation of WBC with predominant lymphocytes, slight increased

glucose, slight protein, normal lactate dehydrogenase in viral type.

Electrolyte Panel: reveals decreased K^+ and increased Na^+, changes indicating dehydration.

Serum Osmolality: reveals increase if antidiuretic hormone secretion increased.

Complete Blood Count: reveals increased WBC.

Urinalysis: increased osmolarity if antidiuretic hormone secretion increased, increased sp. gr.

COMMON NURSING DIAGNOSES

See HYPERTHERMIA

Related to: Illness.

Defining Characteristics: (Specify: increase in body temperature above normal range, warm to touch, increased respiratory and pulse rate.)

See RISK FOR DEFICIENT FLUID VOLUME

Related to: Excessive losses.

Defining Characteristics: (Specify: vomiting, diarrhea.)

Related to: Deviations affecting intake of fluids.

Defining Characteristics: (Specify: decreased intake, fluid restrictions, change in level of consciousness.)

Related to: Failure of regulatory mechanisms.

Defining Characteristics: (Specify: secretion of antidiuretic hormone, increased sp. gr. and osmolality, reduced output, dehydration.)

See DISTURBED THOUGHT PROCESSES

Related to: Physiologic changes.

Defining Characteristics: (Specify: disorientation to time, place, persons, events, changes in consciousness,

behavior changes also important to monitor fluids and ventilation.)

ADDITIONAL NURSING DIAGNOSES

ANXIETY

Related to: (Specify: threat to or change in health status of child; threat to or change in environment [hospitalization of child].)

Defining Characteristics: (Specify: increased apprehension that condition of child might worsen, expressed concern and worry about actual hospitalization of child and seriousness of illness.)

Goal: Parents will experience decreased anxiety by (date and time to evaluate)

Outcome Criteria

✔ Parents verbalize decreased anxiety.

NOC: *Anxiety Reduction*

INTERVENTIONS	RATIONALES
Assess sources and level of anxiety, how anxiety is manifested, and need for information and support.	Provides information about the need for interventions to relieve anxiety and concern; sources may include fear and uncertainty about treatment and recovery, guilt for presence of illness, possible loss of parental role, and loss of responsibility when hospitalization necessary.
Encourage to express concerns and ask questions regarding condition of ill child.	Provides opportunity to vent feelings, secure information needed to reduce anxiety.
Encourage to be involved in care and decision-making regarding child's needs.	Promotes constant monitoring of child's condition for improvements or worsening of symptoms.
Encourage parent to stay with child or visit when able and call when concerned if hospitalized; assist in care (hold, feed, bathe, clothe and diaper), and provide information about child's daily routines.	Allows parent to care for and support child instead of increasing anxiety if not with child.

INTERVENTIONS	RATIONALES
Assess parental feelings of guilt from not suspecting the seriousness of the illness sooner; encourage them to openly discuss feelings.	Prevents or minimizes feelings of blame or guilt.
Teach about disease process and behaviors, physical effects and symptoms of disease (specify).	Relieves anxiety of parents.
Explain reason for procedures or type of therapy, effects of any diagnostic tests (specify).	Reduces fear of unknown which increases anxiety.
Teach parents about isolation precautions for at least 24 hours or until diagnosis is made and antibiotic therapy begins to take effect.	Provides opportunity to validate type of meningitis and to take measures to prevent transmission to others in contact with child.
Clarify any misinformation and answer questions in lay terms when parents able to listen, give same explanation as other staff and/or physician gave regarding disease process and transmission.	Prevents unnecessary anxiety resulting from inaccurate knowledge or beliefs or inconsistencies in information.

NIC: *Anxiety Reduction*

Evaluation

(Date/time of evaluation of goal)

(Has goal been met? Not met? Partially met?)

(Did parents verbalize decreased anxiety? Use quotes.)

(Revisions to care plan? D/C care plan? Continue care plan?)

RISK FOR INJURY

Related to: Internal factor of altered neurologic regulatory function.

Defining Characteristics: (Specify: increased intracranial pressure; early signs of lethargy, restlessness, increased head circumference, headache, vomiting, personality changes or late signs of decreased level of consciousness, change in posturing, widening of pulse pressure, projectile vomiting, decreased pulse and respirations, seizure, abnormal PERL, shrill cry, bulging fontanel, changes in vision.)

Goal: Child will not experience injury by (date and time to evaluate).

Outcome Criteria

✔ (Specify for child, e.g., no decrease in LOC; no vomiting or seizures.)

NOC: *Risk Detection*

INTERVENTIONS	RATIONALES
Assess neurologic status to include VS pattern, changes in consciousness, behavior patterns and pupillary/ocular responses appropriate for age (measure head circumference in infant) (specify when).	Provides information that offers clues to possible change in intracranial pressure caused by inflammation of the brain and associated edema.
Attach cardiac and respiratory monitor to assess for bradycardia and hypoxia.	Increased intracranial pressure will decrease pulse and respirations, widen the pulse pressure with pulse becoming irregular and respirations rapid and shallow as ICP progresses and the body attempts to decrease blood flow to brain.
Reposition q 2h, positioning child to optimize comfort with HOB slightly elevated, no pillow in bed, side-lying position if nuchal rigidity present; avoid sudden movements such as lifting the head; have oxygen and suctioning equipment on hand to be administered when needed.	Maintains airway patency and prevents obstruction by secretion which increases CO_2 retention and ICP.
Provide quiet environment free from bright lighting, minimize gentle handling and care of infant/child, allow for rest periods between care or procedures, restrict visiting if irritable.	Promotes comfort and rest and reduces irritability.
Administer antibiotics as prescribed (specify) as soon as ordered based on analysis of CSF, throat cultures.	Manages existing infection and prevents further spread of infection (action of drug).
Note any seizure activity including onset, frequency, duration and type of movements before, during, or after seizure; pad bed and remove objects/toys from bed and administer any ordered anticonvulsants.	Prevents injury during seizure which is a complication of meningitis.
Administer stool softeners, avoid use of restraints and prevent or reduce crying episodes.	Prevents Valsalva's maneuver that will increase ICP.

INTERVENTIONS	RATIONALES
Position with head elevated up to 30 degrees and maintain head alignment with sandbag.	Decreases intracranial pressure by allowing blood flow from brain by gravity or any obstruction of jugular drainage.
Stay with infant/child and sit near and speak in a low voice.	Provides limited stimulation to infant/child during acute stage of disease.
Inform parents of changes in condition, reasons for physical and mental changes and effects of the disease.	Promotes knowledge about possible manifestations of the disease and causes.
Explain causes of increased ICP and importance of preventing any further increases in ICP.	Allows for understanding of increased ICP and life-threatening nature of such a complication.
Inform of reason for seizure activity and other signs and symptoms of the disease and treatment necessitated by them.	Provides knowledge of seizure complications and actions and responsibility in prevention and/ or treatment of this activity.
Inform parents of risk for complications and need for monitoring for increased ICP; review signs and symptoms of increased ICP.	Allows for ongoing care and responsibility in preventing change in neurologic status.

NIC: *Surveillance*

Evaluation

(Date/time of evaluation of goal)

(Has goal been met? Not met? Partially met?)

(Provide data about outcome criteria chosen. What is LOC? Did child vomit? Are there signs of increased ICP? Describe.)

(Revisions to care plan? D/C care plan? Continue care plan?)

DEFICIENT KNOWLEDGE

Related to: Lack of exposure to information.

Defining Characteristics: (Specify: request for information about medications, signs and symptoms and behaviors to report, general care during convalescence of infant/child.)

Goal: Parents will obtain information about meningitis by (date and time to evaluate).

Outcome Criteria

✔ Parents verbalize understanding of cause and treatment plan.

NOC: *Knowledge: Treatment Regimen*

INTERVENTIONS	RATIONALES
Assess knowledge of disease and method to control and resolve disease; willingness and interest of parents to implement care.	Promotes plan of instruction that is realistic to ensure compliance of medical regimen; prevents repetition of information.
Provide information and explanations in clear language that is understandable; use pictures, pamphlets, video tapes, model in teaching about disease.	Ensures understanding based on readiness and ability to learn; visual aids reinforce learning.
Teach about administration of medications including (specify: action of drugs, dosages times frequency, side effects, expected results, methods to give medications); provide written instructions and schedule to follow and inform to administer full course of antibiotic to child.	Provides information for compliance in medication therapy to prevent or treat infection and seizure activity resulting from the disease; bacterial meningitis is treated with antibiotics, and viral meningitis may be treated with antibiotics until diagnosis is established.
Assist to plan feedings and/or develop menus to include nourishing fluids, caloric and basic four groups for age group.	Promotes optimal nutrition in a progressive manner as tolerable.
Reinforce to parents follow up to assess for potential hearing impairment.	Promotes identification of hearing loss (injury to 8th cranial nerve caused by meningitis).

INTERVENTIONS	RATIONALES
Inform parents as to the benefits of routine immunizations with *H. influenzae* (type B) vaccine, beginning at 2 months of age for a total of 3 doses.	May prevent the disease; data suggests the incidence of this form of meningitis has decreased since the vaccine was introduced; may decrease the spread of infection to unvaccinated infants.
Teach to promote adequate rest and activities that provide age appropriate play and stimulation (specify).	Rest important for convalescence and stimulating activities needed for continued development or to promote stimulation if developmental lag is present.
Teach to isolate other children in family for 24 hours if respiratory infection present or until culture is negative.	Prevents transmission of bacteria to others in family.
Teach to report elevated temperature, poor feeding or anorexia, irritability or other changes in behavior or level of consciousness, decrease in hearing acuity.	Reveals signs and symptoms of presence of or spread of infection.

NIC: *Teaching: Disease Process*

Evaluation

(Date/time of evaluation of goal)

(Has goal been met? Not met? Partially met?)

(What did clients verbalize about the cause of meningitis and the treatment plan? Use quotes.)

(Revisions to care plan? D/C care plan? Continue care plan?)

MENINGITIS

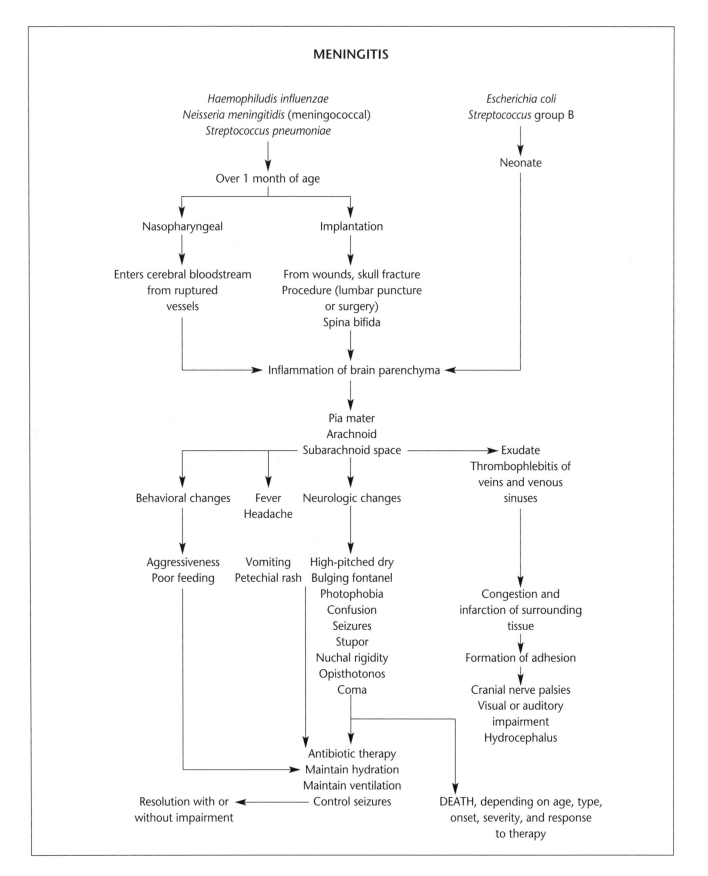

Haemophiludis influenzae
Neisseria meningitidis (meningococcal)
Streptococcus pneumoniae

Escherichia coli
Streptococcus group B

Neonate

Over 1 month of age

Nasopharyngeal

Implantation

Enters cerebral bloodstream
from ruptured
vessels

From wounds, skull fracture
Procedure (lumbar puncture
or surgery)
Spina bifida

Inflammation of brain parenchyma

Pia mater
Arachnoid
Subarachnoid space

Exudate
Thrombophlebitis of
veins and venous
sinuses

Behavioral changes

Fever
Headache

Neurologic changes

Aggressiveness
Poor feeding

Vomiting
Petechial rash

High-pitched dry
Bulging fontanel
Photophobia
Confusion
Seizures
Stupor
Nuchal rigidity
Opisthotonos
Coma

Congestion and
infarction of surrounding
tissue

Formation of adhesion

Cranial nerve palsies
Visual or auditory
impairment
Hydrocephalus

Antibiotic therapy
Maintain hydration
Maintain ventilation
Control seizures

Resolution with or
without impairment

DEATH, depending on age, type,
onset, severity, and response
to therapy

CHAPTER 7.5

SENSORY DEFICITS

Sensory deficits can lead to auditory or visual deprivation and affect the child's ability to interact with the environment. Cognitive, perceptive, communicative, and social skills may all be affected.

Vision disorders are common in children with the most prevalent problems of a refractive type (myopia or hyperopia) and others that include amblyopia, strabismus, cataracts, and glaucoma. Eye injury may occur as a result of trauma from blunt or sharp objects, or from infection resulting in conjunctivitis, keratitis, or even blindness or loss of the eye.

Auditory disorders are classified as conductive, sensorineural or mixed conductive-sensorineural hearing loss. Causes include damage to the inner ear structures or the auditory nerve from congenital defects, infection, ototoxic drugs, long-term excessive exposure to noises (sensorineural) or middle ear infection such as otitis media (conductive).

Hearing and vision screenings vary with the age of the infant/child and are performed as part of physical assessment of all children. Treatment focuses on the correction and rehabilitation of any actual or potential impairment.

MEDICAL CARE

Anti-inflammatories: to eye to reduce inflammation if present.

Antibiotics: to treat infection.

Vision Tests: Lighthouse Vision test or Blackbird Preschool Vision Test for children 3 to 4 years of age; Snellen E vision chart for children 5 to 6 years of age; Snellen vision chart for children 7 years and older who are familiar with the alphabet; Corneal Light Reflex test and Cover/Uncover test to reveal malalignment; visual tracking to identify muscle movement abnormalities; test for peripheral vision and amblyopia reveal objection to cover over eye or inability to see at a 90-degree angle from straight line of vision.

Hearing Tests: audiometry reveals degree of hearing loss and possible locale of defect in child 2 to 5 years of age based on behavior modification and over 5 years if child is able to cooperate; reaction to noise in infant; conductive tests (Rinne and Weber) in children of school-age reveals auditory acuity; tympanometry reveals middle ear air pressure and abnormalities but not reliable in young children; brain stem-evoked audiometry reveals hearing acuity in the infant or child by computer analysis of electrical or brain wave potentials that are initiated by the hearing process.

COMMON NURSING DIAGNOSES

See DELAYED GROWTH AND DEVELOPMENT

Related to: Effects of physical disability.

Defining Characteristics: (Specify: delay or difficulty in performing skills [motor, social, expressive] typical of age group, behavior and/or intellectual deficits, poor academic performance, reduced independence in performance of ADL.)

ADDITIONAL NURSING DIAGNOSES

DISTURBED SENSORY PERCEPTION: AUDITORY

Related to: (Specify: altered sensory reception, transmission and/or integration of neurologic disease or deficit, altered state of sense organ, inability to hear [partial or complete deafness].)

Defining Characteristics: (Specify: change in behavior pattern, anxiety, change in usual response to stimuli, altered communication pattern, auditory distortions, reduced auditory acuity, inappropriate responses.)

Goal: Client will experience improved hearing by (date and time to evaluate).

Outcome Criteria

✔ (Specify outcome criteria appropriate for individual child.)

NOC: *Risk Control: Hearing Impairment*

INTERVENTIONS	RATIONALES
Assess history of chronic otitis media, brain infection, use of ototoxic drugs, rubella or other intrauterine infections (viral), congenital defects of ear or nose, presence of deafness in family members, hypoxemia and increased bilirubin levels in low-birth weight infants.	Provides information about possible risks for conductive or sensorineural hearing loss.
Assess for auditory acuity: Infant: failure to waken to sounds; no response to loud noise; no response to sound made out of visual field; lack of startle and blink reflexes; failure to turn head to localize sound by 6 months; absence of babble by 7 months; lack of response to spoken words/failure to follow simple commands (older infant). Child: failure to respond to name or to locate sound; failure to respond to being read to or to sound of music; failure to respond to verbal speech; requesting repeat of message; gesturing instead of speech; shy, timid, inattentive; poor performance in school; failure to develop understandable language by 24 months; vocal play, head banging for increased vibratory sensation; stubborn attitude related to decreased comprehension; appear to be "in their own world."	Provides information of infant/child ability to hear using techniques that are age dependent.
Perform audiometry or other tests depending on age and preparation of technician.	Evaluates degree of hearing acuity and/or loss and type of hearing loss.
Face infant/child when speaking, speak distinctly and slowly without shouting to gain child's attention.	Provides opportunity to develop lip reading.

INTERVENTIONS	RATIONALES
Assist with use of hearing aid.	Promotes maximum benefit from aid hearing.
Encourage use of sign language, lip reading, cued speech, speech therapy and as much verbal communication as possible.	Promotes communication with others.
Provide for play and social interactions, self-care in all activities for age group, continued attendance at school.	Promotes independence for age group and security in interacting with peers.
Anticipate grief reaction after the diagnosis; facilitate expression of feelings and concerns.	Grief reaction is normal part of early adjustment phase; promotes adjustment to diagnosis.
Help child focus on sounds in the environment.	Maximizes child's hearing potential.
Recommend closed-captioned TV.	Provides enjoyment for the child; facilitates feelings of normalcy.
Encourage child to read books and practice responding to cues with language development or use of aids or methods.	Promotes effective communication and corrects or prevents impairments.
Encourage child to take responsibility for the care and use of the aid as soon as possible.	Promotes independence and self esteem.
Teach parents and child about type of tests to be performed and procedure to be followed by child.	Prevents anxiety caused by test and possible results if not done as part of normal child assessment and screening.
Alert parents to behavioral cues indicating hearing impairment.	Promotes identification of hearing loss for correction before development is affected.
Teach parents about hearing aid resources, types available and instruct in cleaning and care of aid and the proper adjustment for optimal benefit.	Assists with hearing aid selection if loss is conductive type.
Instruct child in methods to conceal hearing aid (specify).	Prevents negative effect of self-concept and image.
Refer parents and child of resources to learn lip reading or signing or speaking (specify).	Promotes a method of communication with others and especially those with hearing impairment.
Encourage parents and family to provide stimulation through language.	Promotes developmental process and language use.
Refer to appropriate community resources and support groups, as needed (specify).	Provides support to parents.

(continues)

(continued)

INTERVENTIONS	RATIONALES
Encourage parents to promote socialization with peers.	Promotes feelings of normalcy and self-esteem.
Assist parents to arrange for vision testing.	Poor sight may decrease the ability to learn lip reading or sign language.
Discuss with the family to maintain normalcy, including discipline and limit setting.	Promotes normal growth and development.
Assist parents and child to adjust environment and select toys that promote social interactions and increase hearing potential.	Encourages social interactions, development of friendships, and sense of belonging.
Encourage parents to notify school nurse and teacher of degree of hearing loss and methods of communications used by child.	Provides information that encourages a positive school experience and opportunity for learning in a regular classroom and socialization with classmates.

NIC: *Teaching: Disease Process*

Evaluation

(Date/time of evaluation of goal)

(Has goal been met? Not met? Partially met?)

(Provide data about the outcome criteria selected.)

(Revisions to care plan? D/C care plan? Continue care plan?)

DISTURBED SENSORY PERCEPTION: VISUAL

Related to: (Specify: altered sensory reception, transmission and/or integration of neurologic disease or deficit, altered state of sense organ, inability to see [partial or complete loss of sight].)

Defining Characteristics: (Specify: change in behavior pattern, anxiety, change in usual responses to stimuli, visual distortions, reduced visual acuity, myopia, hyperopia, lazy eye, cross-eye, cataracts, glaucoma, trauma to eye, frequent injury by walking into objects.)

Goal: Client will experience improved vision by (date and time to evaluate).

Outcome Criteria

✔ (Specify outcome criteria appropriate for individual child.)

NOC: *Risk Control: Visual Impairment*

INTERVENTIONS	RATIONALES
Assess history of rubella or syphilis of mother before birth of child, presence of genetic disorders in the family, excessive oxygen given to infant, congenital conditions that cause blindness, impairment caused by strabismus, cataract or glaucoma.	Provides information about risks for or presence of sight impairment or blindness.
Assess for risk of trauma to an eye from toys, missiles or projectiles into eye during games or play, excessive sunlight to eyes.	Eye trauma caused by accidents is most common cause of blindness in children and information provides safety education plan to prevent eye injury.
Assess for visual acuity: Infant: failure to follow light or object with eye movement and cessation of body movement; failure to fixate on mother's face; delay in posture and in developmental tasks; absence of binocularity; failure to move eyes together. Child: failure to respond to visual stimuli; squinting, blinking, rubbing of eyes; eye crossing after 6 months of age; headache after using eyes; failure to initiate eye contact, nystagmus, head tilt, holding reading material close to face, bumps into objects when walking or crawling; poor performance in school.	Provides information of infant/child ability to see using techniques that are age dependent.
Perform visual tests for acuity peripheral vision and muscle balance depending on age and intellectual development level; include tests for strabismus, amblyopia.	Evaluates degree of acuity and/or loss and possible causes with consideration for improving visual acuity with age.
Face infant/child when speaking, explain sounds and what is happening in the environment.	Promotes comfort and security with environment.
State name when approaching and explain any procedure before starting, use touch if acceptable.	Reduces anxiety and sudden contact that is unexpected.
Assist with use and care of glasses or patching one eye and encourage wearing of these as prescribed.	Promotes independence in use of aids for refractive disorders and strabismus.

INTERVENTIONS	RATIONALES
Provide for age related toys and social interactions within secure environment.	Promotes stimulation and development.
Provide well lit environment and familiar placement of objects to orient child to environment.	Promotes safety and security in the environment and prevents possible trauma from bumping into furniture or falling.
Emphasize the abilities and praise attempts and/or accomplishments.	Promotes self-esteem of child.
Talk softly to infant before contact; learn to read total body cues, not just eyes and visual cues; use gentleness of touch when when interacting with infant.	Promotes association of human voice with anticipated changes; prepares infant for changes.
Tell the child exactly what you will be doing before you do anything; reinforce this as you perform the procedure; warn of discomfort.	Promotes understanding and feelings of security and trust.
Allow the child to touch instruments and equipment whenever possible.	Promotes increased understanding through speech.
Use the child's name specifically when you want a response from him/her.	Promotes communication since visually impaired children lack the input of visual cues.
Teach parents and child about tests to be performed, what is being tested and procedure to be followed by child.	Prevents anxiety and promotes cooperation.
Discuss with parents the child's abilities and impairment and what might be expected of child; behaviors that might indicate a decrease in visual acuity.	Provides a realistic appraisal of visual ability of the child.
Assist parents to explore the possibility of rehabilitation to accomplish ADL skills, use of Braille, mobility aids, trained dogs.	Provides assistance to gain independence for the child.

INTERVENTIONS	RATIONALES
Encourage parents to treat child as others in family, setting limits, encouraging play and relationships with family members.	Promotes integration into the family and creates a sense of belonging.
Instruct in eye care, administration of eye medications (specify).	Promotes health of eye and compliance with medical regimen.
Encourage parents to notify school of sight deficit and to place in a front row, use large printed materials, proper lighting.	Encourages learning with optimal consideration for impairment.
Teach parents to plan for regular vision screening.	Monitors visual acuity for improvements or need for change in treatment; screening is often done in schools.
Initiate referral to an ophthalmologist for evaluation if acuity is not normal for age or if indication of a disorder is present.	Permits thorough examination of eyes to identify and treat any disorder.
Refer to national and community agencies and associations that supply educational materials, services for blind or partially sighted children.	Provides information and support for families of child with impaired vision.

NIC: *Teaching: Disease Process*

Evaluation

(Date/time of evaluation of goal)

(Has goal been met? Not met? Partially met?)

(Provide data about the outcome criteria selected.)

(Revisions to care plan? D/C care plan? Continue care plan?)

SENSORY DEFICITS

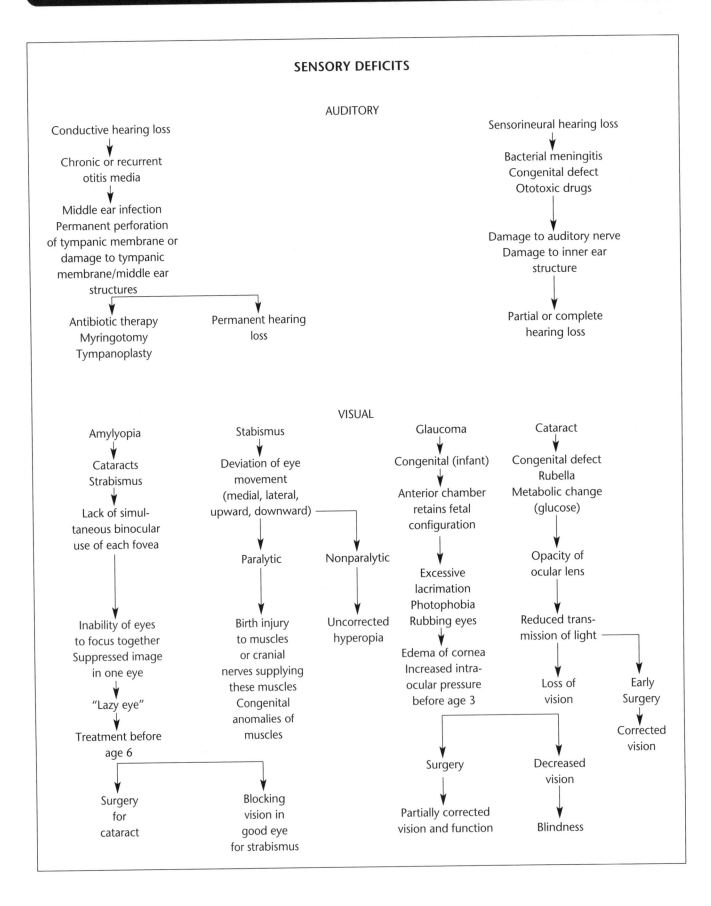

CHAPTER 7.6

REYE'S SYNDROME

Reye's syndrome is an acute encephalopathy, often including fatty infiltration of organs such as the liver, heart, lungs, pancreas, and skeletal muscle. It has been associated with a viral condition such as influenza or varicella and the use of aspirin as an analgesic/antipyretic, but the exact cause is not known. Serious complications of the disorder can include increased intracranial pressure from cerebral edema, high levels of ammonia from organ involvement, and mental dysfunction from progressive coma. Recovery is complete in most depending on severity of the condition but some neurologic and mental residual disability may occur. The most common group affected by this condition are those between 6 to 11 years of age although all ages are susceptible. Hospitalization with close observation is required with therapy to monitor and treat all vital functions affected by the condition and state of consciousness.

MEDICAL CARE

Sedatives/Anticonvulsants: promote CNS depression for sedation or to prevent or treat seizures.

Muscle Relaxants: induce sedation and relax muscles if mechanical assistive ventilation used.

Diuretics (Osmotic): mannitol (Osmitrol) to induce diuresis by increasing osmotic pressure of glomerular filtrate to prevent reabsorption of water.

Antibiotics: treat infection if present or specific antibiotic dependent on culture and sensitivities.

Anti-inflammatories: (corticosteroids) reduce inflammatory process, capillary dilation, and permeability.

Antacids: via nasogastric tube to maintain pH of over 4.0 to prevent gastrointestinal bleeding.

Liver Biopsy: reveals histologic results of impaired liver or pathology.

Enzymes: reveal increased glutamic oxaloacetic transaminase (SGOT), glutamic pyruvic transaminase (SGPT), lactic dehydrogenase (LDH), creatine phosphokinase (CPK), amylase, and lipase.

Ammonia: reveals increases of twice the normal level (hyperammonimia).

Glucose: reveals decreases with this disease (hypoglycemia) that may lead to brain damage.

Prothrombin/Partial Thromboplastin Times (PT, APPT): reveals prolonged times.

Cholesterol: reveals decreased level.

Uric acid: reveals increased level.

Arterial Blood Gases (ABGs): reveal levels that may indicate possible increases in cerebral edema or respiratory distress.

COMMON NURSING DIAGNOSES

See DECREASED CARDIAC OUTPUT

Related to: Mechanical or electrical effect on the heart.

Defining Characteristics: (Specify: variations in hemodynamic readings, ECG changes, arrhythmias, decreased peripheral pulses, oliguria, diuretic therapy, changes in perfusion of vital organs.)

See IMPAIRED GAS EXCHANGE

Related to: Assistive ventilatory use and oxygen supply.

Defining Characteristics: (Specify: hypercapnia, hypoxia, confusion, restlessness, irritability, inability to move secretions, cyanosis, retractions, changes in ABGs.)

See DISTURBED THOUGHT PROCESSES

Related to: Physiologic changes, encephalopathy.

Defining Characteristics: (Specify: cognitive dissonance, disorientation, changes in consciousness, hallucination, altered sleep patterns, coma, altered attention span and memory, lethargy, drowsiness.)

See HYPERTHERMIA

Related to: Illness.

Defining Characteristics: (Specify: increase in body temperature above normal range, increased respiratory and pulse rate, warm to touch.)

See RISK FOR DEFICIENT FLUID VOLUME

Related to: Medications.

Defining Characteristics: (Specify: diuretic therapy, altered intake, NPO status, increased urinary output, loss via nasogastric tube suctioning.)

See RISK FOR IMPAIRED SKIN INTEGRITY

Related to: Physical immobilization, hypothermia blanket, invasive procedures.

Defining Characteristics: (Specify: disruption of skin surfaces, redness, edema, discharge, warmth at insertion sites for IV, monitoring devices, redness or excoration at pressure points.)

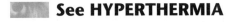
ADDITIONAL NURSING DIAGNOSES

ANXIETY

Related to: Threat of death; change in health status; change in environment (hospitalization).

Defining Characteristics: (Specify: apprehension and uncertainty about child's condition, feelings of inadequacy and increased helplessness about child cared for in intensive care unit, fear associated with severe acuity of condition, possible sequelae as a result of the disorder.)

Goal: Parents will experience decreased anxiety by (date and time to evaluate).

Outcome Criteria

✔ Parents verbalize decreased anxiety.

NOC: *Anxiety Control*

INTERVENTIONS	RATIONALES
Assess level of anxiety, need for information and support about severity and life threatening nature of the illness.	Provides information about severity of stress and anxiety, guilt about responsibility of delay in diagnosis and loss of parental role, fears and feelings about possible complications.
Allow expression of concerns and opportunity to ask questions about condition and recovery of child.	Provides opportunity to vent feelings, secure information needed to reduce anxiety.
Encourage parents to remain with child and participate in care if appropriate; if parents unable to stay, allow open visitation and frequent telephoning.	Promotes parent involvement and interaction with the child.
Encourage parents to bring a favorite toy, book or other items.	Promotes contact with familiar objects outside the hospital environment.
Provide for space to rest, bathe and relax if staying with child; provide quiet room if desired.	Promotes emotional support to parents to reduce anxiety.
Refer to clergy or social services as appropriate.	Provides support and assistance in dealing with severely ill child.
Explain reason for and what to expect for each procedure or type of therapy (lumbar puncture, IV lines, urinary catheter, NG tube, respirator).	Reduces fear and promotes understanding.
Provide honest information in understandable language and reinforce physician.	Prevents unnecessary anxiety resulting from inaccurate information or beliefs.
Teach parents about state of consciousness of child, stage of disease and signs and symptoms to expect.	Reduces fear and anxiety.

NIC: *Anxiety Reduction*

Evaluation

(Date/time of evaluation of goal)

(Has goal been met? Not met? Partially met?)

(Did parents verbalize decreased anxiety? Use quotes.) (Revisions to care plan? D/C care plan? Continue care plan?)

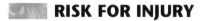 **RISK FOR INJURY**

Related to: Illness.

Defining Characteristics: (Specify: altered clotting factors, changes in orientation and consciousness, increased ICP, altered sleep pattern, cognitive dissonance, inability to close or blink eyes, hypoglycemic seizure activity, coma.)

Goal: Child will not experience injury by (date and time to evaluate).

Outcome Criteria

✔ (Specify appropriate outcome criteria based on individual child's condition.)

NOC: *Risk Detection*

INTERVENTIONS	RATIONALES
Assess for stage by noting signs and symptoms associated with the condition which range from vomiting, lethargy, and liver dysfunction to disorientation, deepening coma, loss of reflexes, and seizures.	Indicate stage as a basis for expected behaviors and need for specific care and preventive measures.
Assess vomiting, papilledema, ataxia, irritability, lethargy, apathy, confusion, change in level of consciousness, increased pulse, and decreased BP q 1h; if ICP monitor in place, note elevation above 20 mm Hg or any gradual increases for physician.	Indicates increasing ICP caused by cerebral edema and advancing stage of disease.
Elevate head of bed 30 degrees and maintain head and neck alignment.	Promotes cerebral circulation and reduces venous pressure; prevents neck flexion.
Administer osmotic diuretic, diretic, sedative, anticonvulsants, neuromuscular blocking agent IV separately or in combination as ordered (specify).	Administered to promote fluid output to reduce edema, prevent seizure activity, and induce sedation to reduce agitation and activity that increase ICP.
Provide clustering of care and procedures.	Promotes rest.

INTERVENTIONS	RATIONALES
Carry out seizure precautions of padding bed, removing objects from bed, maintain suction and oxygen at bedside.	Prevents injury during seizure and treats apnea if it occurs.
Monitor laboratory tests of increased prothrombin or partial thrombin time, fibrin split products, decreased platelets and serum glucose, decreased electrolyte levels (K⁺).	Provides information about coagulation defects from liver dysfunction, hypoglycemia metabolic dysfunction, and loss of electrolytes from diuretic therapy.
Monitor for occult blood in stool, gastric aspirate, skin for petechiae, hematoma, oozing or frank bleeding from any orifice or mucous membranes.	Provides information about possible bleeding from impaired liver function.
Administer antacid, vitamin K and/or blood as ordered.	Replaces blood loss and increases blood clotting capabilities; antacids are given to discourage gastrointestinal irritation and bleeding.
Instill eye drops (as ordered) or tape eyelids closed if paralyzed (specify).	Provides moisture to eyes if unable to blink or close eyes to prevent corneal damage.
Teach parents of every aspect of care and equipment used including comatosed status, effects of medications, IV therapy, NG tube care, use of catheter, use of monitoring devices (ICP, cardiac, CVP), intubation and ventilation.	Assist parents to deal with their child that is acutely ill.
Reassure parents that mild stimulation is allowed and that speaking and touching child is permitted.	Provides stimulation as child may be able to perceive tactile and auditory stimuli when unresponsive.
Teach parents that child will be reoriented to person, time and place when awakened from the coma.	Child may not be aware of the environment and realize that he or she has been hospitalized.
Assist parents to read labels for aspirin (salicylate) content and to avoid using these drugs (e.g., Pepto-Bismol) when child is ill.	Promotes prevention of syndrome as aspirin considered to be a causative factor.
Teach parents that deficits usually improve and resolve in 6 to 12 months during recovery and evaluation and rehabilitation may be needed.	Provides guidance as to what to expect as child progresses to wellness.

NIC: *Surveillance*

Evaluation

(Date/time of evaluation of goal)

(Has goal been met? Not met? Partially met?)

(Provide data about outcome criteria chosen.)

(Revisions to care plan? D/C care plan? Continue care plan?)

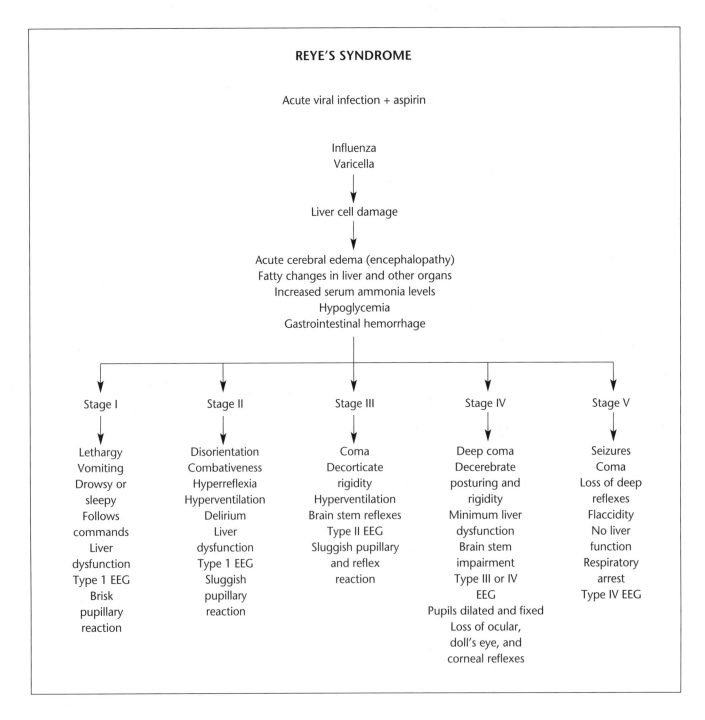

REYE'S SYNDROME

Acute viral infection + aspirin

Influenza
Varicella
↓
Liver cell damage
↓
Acute cerebral edema (encephalopathy)
Fatty changes in liver and other organs
Increased serum ammonia levels
Hypoglycemia
Gastrointestinal hemorrhage

Stage I	Stage II	Stage III	Stage IV	Stage V
Lethargy	Disorientation	Coma	Deep coma	Seizures
Vomiting	Combativeness	Decorticate	Decerebrate	Coma
Drowsy or	Hyperreflexia	rigidity	posturing and	Loss of deep
sleepy	Hyperventilation	Hyperventilation	rigidity	reflexes
Follows	Delirium	Brain stem reflexes	Minimum liver	Flaccidity
commands	Liver	Type II EEG	dysfunction	No liver
Liver	dysfunction	Sluggish pupillary	Brain stem	function
dysfunction	Type 1 EEG	and reflex	impairment	Respiratory
Type 1 EEG	Sluggish	reaction	Type III or IV	arrest
Brisk	pupillary		EEG	Type IV EEG
pupillary	reaction		Pupils dilated and fixed	
reaction			Loss of ocular,	
			doll's eye, and	
			corneal reflexes	

CHAPTER 7.7

SEIZURES

A seizure is a central nervous system (CNS) event characterized by an excessive level of neuronal electrical discharges in the brain. Seizures may be idiopathic or chronic and recurrent (epilepsy or acute acquired and nonrecurrent). Seizures can be partial or generalized with signs and symptoms dependent on the areas involved and range from varying degrees of motor, sensory and sensorimotor changes, and altered consciousness. Partial seizures may be classified as partial or complex partial and generalized seizures as tonic-clonic, absence, atonic or akinetic, myoclonic, and infantile spasms. Seizures occur at any age in children with epilepsy, but mostly in children over 3 years of age. Infantile spasms occur in infants between 3 to 9 months of age. Treatment focuses on prevention of subsequent seizure activity with medication regimen or surgical removal of a focal lesion, tumor, or hemorrhage. Febrile seizures occur in children between 3 and 5 months. The younger the age of the first episode, the more likely there will be recurrence. Status epilepticus is characterized by a seizure lasting more than 30 minutes or repeated seizures without regaining consciousness and is viewed as a medical emergency with a prognosis dependent on the length of the seizure activity and the effect on the brain.

MEDICAL CARE

Anticonvulsants: decrease or limit impulses and spread of electrical discharges in the brain.

Amphetamines: stimulate CNS and counteract drowsiness caused by anticonvulsant therapy.

Electroencephalogram (EEG): reveals abnormal electrical impulses to the brain in initial stage of seizure and characteristic patterns identifying type of seizure.

Skull X-rays: reveal head trauma if present.

Computerized Tomography Scan (CT): reveals abnormalities such as brain tumor, trauma, or infection as causes of seizure.

Ultrasound: reveals intraventricular hemorrhage if present as cause of seizure.

Brain Scan: reveals abnormality as source of seizure if present.

Lumbar Puncture: reveals abnormality in cerebrospinal fluid caused by bleeding trauma or infection responsible for seizure activity.

Complete Blood Count: reveals increased WBC if infection present.

Electrolyte Panel: reveals abnormal levels of calcium or phosphorus as cause of seizure if levels decreased.

Blood Glucose: reveals metabolic cause for seizure if decreased.

Lead Level: reveals increased level as cause of seizure.

COMMON NURSING DIAGNOSES

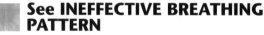

See INEFFECTIVE BREATHING PATTERN

Related to: (Specify: neuromuscular impairment, perception or cognitive impairment.)

Defining Characteristics: (Specify: dyspnea, tachypnea, changes in respiratory depth, cyanosis, cessation of breathing in status epilepticus, obstruction of airway by secretions during a seizure.)

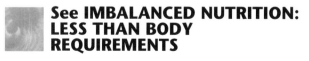

See IMBALANCED NUTRITION: LESS THAN BODY REQUIREMENTS

Related to: Rejection of diet.

Defining Characteristics: (Specify: weight under ideal for height and frame, poor eating patterns, anorexia, rejection of decrease in protein and carbohydrate and increase of fat in dietary intake.)

311

ADDITIONAL NURSING DIAGNOSES

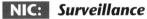 RISK FOR INJURY

Related to: (Specify: internal factors of biochemical regulatory function [seizure, tissue hypoxia], physical trauma [broken skin, altered mobility], psychological changes [orientation].)

Defining Characteristics: (Specify: seizure activity with change in consciousness, falls, muscle flaccidity or rigidity, aspiration of secretions, cyanosis, change in sensation in a body part, muscle weakness, presence of aura before seizure.)

Goal: Client will not experience injury by (date and time to evaluate).

Outcome Criteria

✔ Client sustains no physical injury from seizure.

NOC: *Risk Detection*

INTERVENTIONS	RATIONALES
Assess seizure activity including type of activity before, during, and after seizure, movements and parts of body involved (tonic and clonic), site of onset and progression of seizure, duration of seizure, pupillary changes, bowel or bladder incontinence, paralysis, sleep, alertness, or confusion after seizure, presence of aura.	Provides information that prepares environment for prevention of trauma or complications as a result of seizure.
Assess skin for color (pallor, flushed or cyanosis), respiratory rate, depth, and ease for signs of distress; have oxygen, suctioning equipment on hand.	Provides information about possible obstruction or aspiration of secretions if seizures are prolonged and affect ventilation.
Maintain sidelying position with side rails up, bed or crib padded, and articles removed from area near child.	Allows for secretions to drain and maintains airway patency; padding protects child from injury during seizure.
Avoid attempts to restrain any movements or putting anything in child's mouth; provide gentle support to head and arms if harm might result.	Restraint may result in fracture and inserting object in mouth increases stimuli.
Loosen clothing, assist child to floor if not in bed and place pad under head.	Prevents injury from fall.

INTERVENTIONS	RATIONALES
Stay with child during seizure, reorient when awake, and allow to rest or sleep after seizure.	Provides support and prevents any injury to child.
Administer and evaluate anticonvulsants obtaining blood levels as ordered (specify).	(Action of drugs.)
Assist parents to remain calm during seizure activity of child.	Allows parents to function appropriately to protect the child from injury.
Teach about information to record about seizure activity should it occur (specify).	Provides physician with important information needed to prescribe medical regimen.
Teach parents about care of child during seizure and precautions to take.	Ensures safe and effective actions to prevent injury.

NIC: *Surveillance*

Evaluation

(Date/time of evaluation of goal)

(Has goal been met? Not met? Partially met?)

(Did client have a seizure? Was any injury sustained?)

(Revisions to care plan? D/C care plan? Continue care plan?)

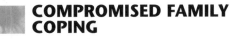 COMPROMISED FAMILY COPING

Related to: Situational crisis.

Defining Characteristics: (Specify: preoccupation of significant persons with anxiety, guilt, fear regarding child's disorder, display of protective behaviors by significant persons that are disproportionate to child's needs [too much or too little], recurrence of seizure activity, lack of support by family members to child.)

Related to: (Specify: inadequate or incorrect information or understanding by a primary person and/or significant persons.)

Defining Characteristics: (Specify: verbalizations by significant persons of inadequate knowledge base that interferes with care and support of infant/child.)

Goal: Family will cope effectively by (date and time to evaluate).

Outcome Criteria

✔ Family members identify stressors of child's illness.

✔ Family identifies 3 effective ways to cope with child's illness.

NOC: *Family Coping*

INTERVENTIONS	RATIONALES
Assess anxiety, fear, erratic behavior, perception of crisis situation by family members.	Provides information affecting family ability to cope with infant/child's recurring disorder.
Assess coping methods used and effectiveness; family ability to cope with ill member of family, stress on family relationships, developmental level of family, response of siblings, knowledge and attitudes about disorder and health practices.	Identifies coping methods that work and need to develop new coping skills; family attitudes and coping abilities directly affect child's health and feeling of wellness, members of family may develop emotional problems when stressed, and ill member may strengthen or strain family relationships.
Encourage expression of feelings and questions in accepting, nonjudgmental environment and assist family members to express problems and explore solutions responsibly.	Reduces anxiety and enhances family's understanding of infant/child's condition and provides opportunity to express feelings, problems, and problem-solving strategies by whole family.
Encourage family involvement in care during hospitalization and after discharge.	Provides for reduction of anxiety and fear.
Allow for open visitation, encourage telephone calls to hospital by family members.	Encourages bonding and assists in coping with infant/child's hospitalization.
Provide place for family members to rest, freshen up.	Promotes comfort of family.
Suggest social worker referral if needed.	Provides support and resources for financial or infant/child's care relief.
Give positive feedback and praise family efforts in developing coping and problem-solving techniques and caring for infant/child.	Encourages parents and family to participate in care and gain some control over the situation.
Assist to establish short- and long-term goals in maintaining child care and family integration of child into home routine.	Promotes inclusion of ill child in family routines and activities.

INTERVENTIONS	RATIONALES
Reinforce appropriate coping behavior.	Promotes behavior change and adaptation to care of infant/child prone to seizures.
Teach that overprotective behaviors may hinder growth and development.	Knowledge will enhance family understanding of condition and adverse effects of behavior.
Encourage to maintain health of family members and discuss needs of all family members; inform of methods to provide care and attention to all members.	Chronic anxiety, fatigue will affect health and care capabilities of family.
Suggest methods to maintain child's independence and role in the family.	Ensures acceptance of child into family routines.
Reassure parents that they do not pass this disorder directly onto their offspring, that intellectual functioning is not affected, that the child is not considered violent or insane, that the disorder is not contagious.	Explodes the many myths associated with the disorder.
Reinforce to parents that child should attend school and participate in activities with friends and peers.	Normalizes life of child as much as possible.
Teach parents that child needs to wear or carry identification and treatment information.	Provides information that may be needed in an emergency.
Refer to Epilepsy Foundation.	Provides information and support to family for chronic, long-term care.

NIC: *Support System Enhancement*

Evaluation

(Date/time of evaluation of goal)

(Has goal been met? Not met? Partially met?)

(What stressors did family identify? Which 3 coping mechanisms did family identify?)

(Revisions to care plan? D/C care plan? Continue care plan?)

DEFICIENT KNOWLEDGE

Related to: Lack of exposure to information about ongoing care.

Defining Characteristics: (Specify: expressed request for information about medication regimen, causes of seizures and when to report to physician.)

Goal: Parents will obtain information about care of child by (date and time to evaluate).

Outcome Criteria

✔ Parents verbalize understanding of cause of seizures.

✔ Parents verbalize correct medication plan for child.

NOC: *Knowledge: Treatment Regimen*

INTERVENTIONS	RATIONALES
Assess parents' and child's perceptions and knowledge about disorder, fears and misconceptions about disorder, nature and frequency of seizures, and factors that initiate seizures.	Provides information regarding long-term care of child with a seizure disorder and how to deal with seizures and the stigma attached to this disorder.
Teach about administration of anticonvulsants (specify name of drug(s), action of drug(s) and when given in combination, times, frequency, side effects, expected results, methods to give drugs) and provide written instructions to follow related to age group and a schedule to follow; give at most convenient times with meals or at bedtime with as few disruptions in routines and activities as possible; give in tablets, liquid extracts, emulsions, or crushed in syrup or jelly; avoid milk if giving phenytoin or phenobarbital and supplement vitamin D; replace prescription before running out of drug(s) and avoid skipping doses (specify).	Promotes compliance to drug regimen which is the most important treatment to prevent seizure.
Teach parents and child to report lethargy, ataxia, nausea, vomiting, hyperactivity, blood dyscrasia, stomatitis, tremor, nystagmus.	Indicates side effects of sedatives and anticonvulsants.
Teach parents about blood testing for therapeutic levels, blood count, liver function tests when instructed.	Prevents toxicity and other severe side effects of drug therapy by adjusting dosage or changing medications.

INTERVENTIONS	RATIONALES
Inform that seizures may be provoked by omission of medication administration, an illness or infection, too much activity, lack of sleep, excessive alcohol or drug intake, emotional stress, or other causes specific to child.	Promotes knowledge and understanding of causes of increased frequency of seizures.
Teach parents to supervise child in bathroom, avoid dangerous play and toys, avoid exposure to incidents that trigger seizure, pad areas in bed, or wear protective clothing if needed.	Provides precautions to prevent injury as a result of a seizure.
Encourage parents to notify school nurse and teacher of disorder and actions to take including telephone number to call.	Promotes knowledge and understanding to prevent injury and embarrassment to child.
Discuss any activity restrictions such as sports, rough play, need for someone in attendance.	Promotes knowledge of activity based on individual child and seizure activity and response to therapy.
Alert parents of possible changes in behavior, activity, or personality or changes in school performance or interactions with family and peers.	Indicates effects of anticonvulsants on behavior and learning.
Refer to resources offering assistance such as Epilepsy Foundation of America, community support groups.	Provides educational materials, employment, legal services, support, and counseling to families and children.

NIC: *Teaching: Prescribed Medication*

Evaluation

(Date/time of evaluation of goal)

(Has goal been met? Not met? Partially met?)

(What did parents say about the cause of the seizures? What did parents verbalize about medications for child?)

(Revisions to care plan? D/C care plan? Continue care plan?)

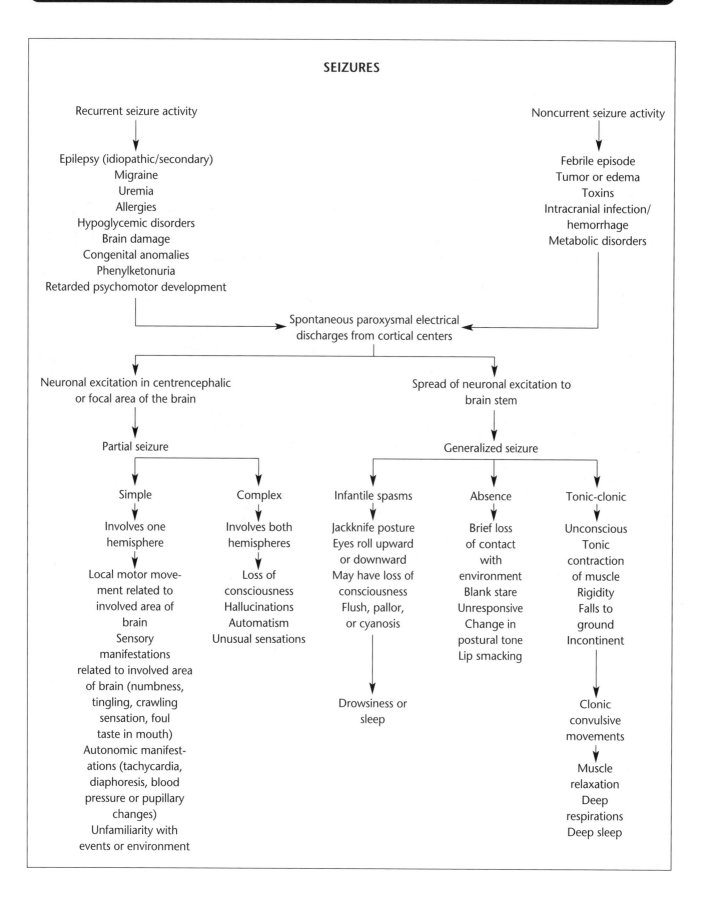

SEIZURES

Recurrent seizure activity

Noncurrent seizure activity

Epilepsy (idiopathic/secondary)
Migraine
Uremia
Allergies
Hypoglycemic disorders
Brain damage
Congenital anomalies
Phenylketonuria
Retarded psychomotor development

Febrile episode
Tumor or edema
Toxins
Intracranial infection/
hemorrhage
Metabolic disorders

Spontaneous paroxysmal electrical
discharges from cortical centers

Neuronal excitation in centrencephalic
or focal area of the brain

Spread of neuronal excitation to
brain stem

Partial seizure

Generalized seizure

Simple

Complex

Infantile spasms

Absence

Tonic-clonic

Involves one
hemisphere

Involves both
hemispheres

Jackknife posture
Eyes roll upward
or downward
May have loss of
consciousness
Flush, pallor,
or cyanosis

Brief loss
of contact
with
environment
Blank stare
Unresponsive
Change in
postural tone
Lip smacking

Unconscious
Tonic
contraction
of muscle
Rigidity
Falls to
ground
Incontinent

Local motor move-
ment related to
involved area of
brain
Sensory
manifestations
related to involved area
of brain (numbness,
tingling, crawling
sensation, foul
taste in mouth)
Autonomic manifest-
ations (tachycardia,
diaphoresis, blood
pressure or pupillary
changes)
Unfamiliarity with
events or environment

Loss of
consciousness
Hallucinations
Automatism
Unusual sensations

Drowsiness or
sleep

Clonic
convulsive
movements

Muscle
relaxation
Deep
respirations
Deep sleep

CHAPTER 7.8

SPINA BIFIDA

Spina bifida is a defect of the central nervous system that involves the failure of neural tube closure during embryonic development. There are two types of spina bifida: spina bifida occulta and spina bifida cystica. Spina bifida occulta is a defect in the closure without the herniation and exposure of the spinal cord or meninges at the surface of the skin in the lumbosacral area. Spina bifida cystica (meningocele or myelomeningocele) is a defect in the closure with a sac and herniated protrusion of meninges, spinal fluid and possibly some part of the spinal cord and nerves at the surface of the skin in the lumbosacral or sacral area.

Hydrocephalus is often associated with spina bifida cystica. The neurologic effects are related to the anatomic level and nerves involved in the defect and range from varying degrees of sensory deficits, to partial or total motor impairment resulting in flaccidity, partial paralysis of lower extremities, and loss of bladder and bowel control. Children with spina bifida cystica, especially myelomeningocele, are commonly afflicted with orthopedic abnormalities that may include hip dislocation, spinal curvatures, or clubfeet and may require assistive devices such as braces, special crutches, or wheelchairs for mobility.

Treatment includes surgical repair of defect as well as other anomalies depending on severity of the neurologic deficit and may be done during infancy or later. Other treatment focuses on prevention of complications, bowel and urinary management, and promotion of optimal growth and development.

MEDICAL CARE

Stool Softeners: prevent constipation and promote bowel rehabilitation.

Antispasmodics: increase capacity or urinary bladder in treatment of bladder spasticity.

Cholinergics: increase urinary bladder tone and prevent retention.

COMMON NURSING DIAGNOSES

See RISK FOR IMPAIRED SKIN INTEGRITY

Related to: Excretions and secretions.

Defining Characteristics: (Specify: urinary and/or fecal incontinence, redness and irritation of perineal and anal areas, disruption of skin in perineal and anal areas, leakage of CSF from sac, rupture of sac, use of diapers.)

Related to: Physical immobilization and pressure.

Defining Characteristics: (Specify: redness, excoriation at bony prominences or other pressure areas, skin breakdown at pressure points, inability to change position, paralysis.)

Related to: Altered sensation, circulation and skeletal prominence.

Defining Characteristics: (Specify: loss of tactile perception in extremities, pressure on bony prominences, lack of padded protection and massage of bony prominences, improper application of hot or cold.)

See IMPAIRED PHYSICAL MOBILITY

Related to: Neuromuscular impairment.

Defining Characteristics: (Specify: inability to purposefully move within physical environment, including bed mobility, transfer, and ambulation, imbalance, impaired coordination, partial or complete paralysis of lower extremities, flaccidity, spasticity, skeletal abnormalities [hip, feet, spine].)

See IMBALANCED NUTRITION: LESS THAN BODY REQUIREMENTS

Related to: Inability to ingest food.

Defining Characteristics: (Specify: NPO status following surgery, inadequate swallowing or sucking in presence of ICP, reduced muscle tone, abnormal eating pattern development.)

See CONSTIPATION

Related to: Neuromuscular impairment.

Defining Characteristics: (Specify: frequency less than usual, hard, formed stool, palpable mass, inability to maintain normal bowel elimination pattern, poor anal sphincter tone and ability to feel urge to defecate.)

See RISK FOR TRAUMA

Related to: (Specify: weakness, balancing difficulties, lack of safety precautions, cognitive or emotional difficulties, reduced muscle coordination, skeletal abnormalities.)

Defining Characteristics: (Specify: injury from falls, improper use of assistive aids, fractures, mental impairment, loss of tactile sensation, paralysis of extremities.)

See DELAYED GROWTH AND DEVELOPMENT

Related to: Effects of disorder or disability before of after surgery.

Defining Characteristics: (Specify: frequent hospitalizations, delay or difficulty in performing skills typical of age group [motor, social or expressive], inability to perform self-care or self-control activities appropriate for age, behavior and/or intellectual deficits.)

ADDITIONAL NURSING DIAGNOSES

RISK FOR INFECTION

Related to: Inadequate primary defenses [broken skin, inadequate bladder emptying].

Defining Characteristics: (Specify: breaks or leaks in meningeal sac, abrasion or irritation of sac, contamination of sac or surgical repair by urinary or stool incontinence.)

Goal: Client will not experience infection by (date and time to evaluate).

Outcome Criteria

✔ (Specify, e.g., sac is intact and moist. Incision clean, dry, and intact without redness, edema,

odor, or drainage; temperature <99° F, WBC < [specify for age].)

NOC: *Risk Detection*

INTERVENTIONS	RATIONALES
Assess sac for breaks or leakage of CSF, irritation of sac redness, swelling, purulent drainage at or around sac area, fever, irritability, nuchal rigidity, cloudy, foul-smelling urine.	Provides information about potential for infection of the sac site, meningitis if sac is ruptured, or is present.
Maintain the infant in prone position or side-lying, as permitted, with head lower than buttocks or hips slightly flexed with a pad between the knees; anchor position with sandbags.	Reduces pressure on the sac to prevent possible rupture and prevents rolling on side or back.
Apply a moist sterile dressing over the sac, use sterile saline or antibiotic solution; ointment if ordered may be applied.	Prevents drying of sac membrane that could predispose to break, or rupture of sac and contamination.
Reinforce moist dressing with dry sterile dressing and change when needed being careful to avoid damage to sac by removing moist dressing after it has dried.	Prevents contamination by capillary action through moisture.
Apply a shield over the sac dressing and tape a plastic sheet below the defect; following surgical closure on the defect, apply a transparent occlusive dressing over the area below the sac site.	Protects the sac from contamination by urine or feces.
Alter routine nursing care activities such as feedings, changing linens and comforting as needed.	Prevents trauma to sac.
Perform handwashing before any care or procedure involving the site before or after surgery and carry out sterile technique for all sac and wound care.	Prevents transmission of microorganisms to site.
Maintain cleanliness of anal area and apply a sterile shield between anus and sac or wound site.	Prevents contamination by feces caused by poor anal sphincter control which allows for dribbling and incontinence of stool.
Administer antibiotics as ordered (specify drug, dose, route, and time).	(Action of drug.)

(continues)

(continued)

INTERVENTIONS	RATIONALES
Following surgical repair of defect, note any changes in wound including redness, swelling, warmth, drainage, fever.	Indicates wound infection.
Following surgery, cleanse wound with antiseptic as ordered (specify) and change dressings when needed using sterile technique for at least 24 hours.	Promotes cleanliness of wound and prevents infection (action of drug).
Avoid ureteral contamination with stool, perform thorough perianal hygiene as needed.	Prevents urinary tract infection.
Teach parents about positioning infant, application of protection around sac (shield, foam rubber doughnut).	Prevents damage to the sac and possible infection.
Teach parents to cleanse the sac gently with moist cotton balls if soiled, avoid diapering the infant until after surgery and healing has taken place.	Protects sac from contaminants and maintains cleanliness.
Handle infant gently, hold and support back above the defect, or place on pillow in prone position to move from place to place.	Prevents pressure on the sac area.
Inform parents of signs and symptoms of infection of sac or surgical site, whichever is applicable, that should be reported.	Promotes early detection of infectious process for early treatment.
Teach handwashing technique, dressing change, use of clean or sterile linens, gloves, supplies when caring for sac area.	Prevents transmission of infectious organisms; sterile technique may not be needed in giving care after surgery is performed.

NIC: *Surveillance*

Evaluation

(Date/time of evaluation of goal)

(Has goal been met? Not met? Partially met?)

(Provide data about outcome criteria, e.g., describe sac or incision; what is temperature? WBCs?)

(Revisions to care plan? D/C care plan? Continue care plan?)

HYPOTHERMIA

Related to: Illness.

Defining Characteristics: (Specify: fluid and heat loss from large area of exposed sac, cool skin, body temperature lower than normal range.)

Goal: Infant will maintain temperature by (date and time to evaluate).

Outcome Criteria

✔ Temperature remains above (specify, e.g., 97.8° F).

NOC: *Thermoregulation*

INTERVENTIONS	RATIONALES
Assess temperature q 2 to 4h and note lack of stability; assess temperature of extremity.	Provides information as to source of temperature changes which may be low if infection is present.
Place infant in an isolette or provide radiant warmer based on hypothermia evaluation keeping sac moist postoperatively.	Provides warmth and reduces the heat loss causing hypothermia.
Teach parents to take temperature and report any decreases or increases.	Monitors for temperature instability detection for early intervention.
Teach parents in proper amount of clothing and room temperature for infant/child (specify).	Provides optimal environmental temperature.

NIC: *Surveillance*

Evaluation

(Date/time of evaluation of goal)

(Has goal been met? Not met? Partially met?)

(What is temperature?)

(Revisions to care plan? D/C care plan? Continue care plan?)

BOWEL INCONTINENCE

Related to: Neuromuscular involvement.

Defining Characteristics: (Specify: constant dribbling or involuntary passage of stool, reduced anal sphincter tone and control, skin integrity breakdown caused by continuous contact with liquid stool.)

Goal: Child will have decreased episodes of bowel incontinence by (date and time to evaluate).

Outcome Criteria

✔ Child participates in bowel control regimen.

✔ Child is able to control bowel elimination.

NOC: *Bowel Continence*

INTERVENTIONS	RATIONALES
Assess presence of neurogenic bowel, degree of incontinence, potential for rehabilitation.	Provides information about condition for use in plan of establishing bowel elimination routine.
Change diapers as quickly as feasible; cleanse perianal area carefully.	Dry, clean skin resists breakdown.
Apply barrier creams (specify) as ordered to perianal area during diapering.	Prevents skin breakdown (action).
Place child on a toilet or potty chair at the same time each day; use stimulation and suppository if helpful.	Establishes a routine for elimination to empty bowel.
Maintain fluid intake of up to 2,000 ml/day depending on age; include fiber and roughage in diet at regular times of the day.	Promotes bulk for easier and more manageable passage.
Apply padding in waterproof undergarments but avoid use of diapers.	Prevents embarrassment for the child if bowel elimination not controlled.
Teach parents and child about program for control of bowel incontinence (fluids, diet, routine toileting, use of stimulation).	Promotes success in bowel training.
Teach about behavior modification as a method to be used for bowel rehabilitation.	Promotes compliance with routine to control bowel incontinence.
Suggest clothing and undergarments to protect from staining accidents.	Promotes self-image and prevents embarrassing incidents.
Instruct parents on proper cleansing and diapering techniques of infant/toddler.	Promotes understanding to maintain good skin integrity.

NIC: *Bowel Incontinence Care*

Evaluation

(Date/time of evaluation of goal)

(Has goal been met? Not met? Partially met?)

(Does child participate in bowel control regimen? Has child achieved control? Provide data.)

(Revisions to care plan? D/C care plan? Continue care plan?)

IMPAIRED URINARY ELIMINATION

Related to: Neuromuscular defect.

Defining Characteristics: (Specify: incontinence, retention, neurogenic bladder with increased or decreased tone [flaccid or spastic], absence of awareness of bladder fullness, passing of urine or ability to stop flow of urine [reflex incontinence].)

Goal: Child will have improved urinary elimination by (date and time to evaluate).

Outcome Criteria

✔ (Specify outcome criteria appropriate for individual child: e.g., learns to perform self-catheterization or maintains a daily urinary elimination pattern.)

NOC: *Urinary Elimination*

INTERVENTIONS	RATIONALES
Assess presence of neurogenic bladder, degree of incontinence, potential for rehabilitation, age of child.	Provides information about condition for use in plan of establishing urinary elimination routine.
Assess urine for cloudiness, foul odor, fever, lethargy, dysuria, retention.	Indicates urinary bladder infection caused by urinary retention or residual resulting in urinary stasis and medium for bacterial growth.
Offer and encourage intake of 30 ml/lb/day including acid-containing beverages and dietary inclusion of foods high in acid content.	Promotes renal blood flow and acidifies urine to prevent infection.
Maintain clean genital and anal area after each elimination episode or as needed if incontinent.	Controls introduction of microorganisms into urethra and urinary bladder.
Catheterize after urination if indicated and ordered.	Moves residual urine if unable to empty bladder completely.
Perform scheduled rehabilitation program of placing child on toilet or potty chair at same times each day.	Establishes a routine for urinary elimination if this is a possibility.

(continues)

(continued)

INTERVENTIONS	RATIONALES
Perform intermittent catheterization q 3 to 4h if indicated to resolve incontinence.	Ensures emptying of bladder to prevent incontinence and infection.
Perform Credé's maneuver if indicated.	Promotes emptying of bladder.
Administer antispasmodic, smooth muscle relaxant, anticholinergic as ordered (specify drug, dose, route, and time).	Improves bladder storage and continence by increasing bladder (action).
Teach parents and child (age dependent) in use of external urinary device or procedure for intermittent self-catheterization; demonstrate and allow for return demonstration.	Provides method for emptying bladder routinely or managing incontinence by use of collecting device connected to a closed system.
Teach about rehabilitative program of toileting and using Credé's method.	Provides an alternate method of controlling incontinence although may be temporary.
Encourage parents to avoid use of diapers for child over 3 years of age; suggest pad and water-proof undergarment as an alternative.	Causes embarrassment for child.
Inform parents of other methods available including implantation of an artificial sphincter, creation of an artificial reservoir, or creation of a urinary diversion to control incontinence.	Provides information about procedures that can be done if intermittent catheterization is not successful.
Teach parents and child about changes in urine characteristics indicating bladder infection and measures to take to prevent this complication.	Allows for early interventions to control infection and eventual renal complications.
Encourage to monitor fluid intake/day, weights and changes to report, foods and fluids that are acidic including citrus fruits, meat, eggs, cheese, prunes, breads.	Maintains a monitoring system to ensure control of possible complications.

NIC: *Urinary Elimination Management*

Evaluation

(Date/time of evaluation of goal)

(Has goal been met? Not met? Partially met?)

(Provide data about specific outcome criteria for child; e.g., did child learn self-catheterization or maintain a bladder elimination pattern?)

(Revisions to care plan? D/C care plan? Continue care plan?)

DISTURBED BODY IMAGE

Related to: Biophysical, psychosocial factor of child.

Defining Characteristics: (Specify: urinary/bowel incontinence, partial or complete paralysis, recurring hospitalizations, change in social, verbal expression of negative feelings about body and functional disabilities, feelings of helplessness and hopelessness, inability in performing ADL.)

Goal: Child will experience improved body image by (date and time to evaluate).

Outcome Criteria

✔ Child expresses feelings about disability.

✔ Child identifies at least 1 positive thing about own body.

NOC: *Body Image*

INTERVENTIONS	RATIONALES
Assess child for feelings about abilities and disabilities in ADL, social interaction, effect on self-concept.	Provides information about potential for independence in thinking and functioning.
Encourage independence and maximize functioning with use of aids for bathing, grooming, dressing, eating, mobility, toileting, and praise any attempts at self-care activities.	Promotes ADL capability by use of assistive aids as needed depending on disability.
Encourage expression of feelings and concerns and support communication of child with parents and peers.	Provides opportunity to vent feelings to reduce anxiety and negative feelings.
Provide touch and hugging, age-appropriate activities with other children.	Conveys caring and concern for child and enhances socialization.
Stress and mention positive accomplishment; avoid negative comment.	Enhances body image and confidence.
Instruct in use of assistive aids for ADL.	Promotes independence and enhances body image.

INTERVENTIONS	RATIONALES
Encourage parents to maintain support and care for child.	Encourages acceptance of child.
Advise parents to maintain same behavior rules for child as other children in family and to integrate care and activities into family routines.	Provides sense of belonging to family.

NIC: *Self-Esteem Enhancement*

Evaluation

(Date/time of evaluation of goal)

(Has goal been met? Not met? Partially met?)

(What feelings about disability did child verbalize? What positive thing about body did child identify? Use quotes.)

(Revisions to care plan? D/C care plan? Continue care plan?)

 ## INTERRUPTED FAMILY PROCESSES

Related to: Situational crisis of long-term condition of child.

Defining Characteristics: (Specify: family system unable to meet physical, emotional needs of its members, inability to express or accept wide range of feelings, family unable to deal with or adapt to chronic condition and disabilities of child in a constructive manner, excessive involvement with child by family members, guilt expressed by family members, lack of support from family and friends, irritability and impatience as a response by family members to child.)

Goal: Family will adapt to child's disability and begin to move forward by (date and time to evaluate).

Outcome Criteria

✔ Family discusses disability and effect on individuals and the family system.

✔ Family identifies ways to cope with chronic illness.

✔ Family members exhibit positive feelings for each other.

NOC: *Family Normalization*

INTERVENTIONS	RATIONALES
Assess family ability to cope with child, stress on family relationships, developmental level of family, response of siblings, knowledge of health practices, family role behavior and attitude about long-term care, economic pressures, resources to care for long-term condition and grieving process, signs of depression, feelings of powerlessness and hopelessness.	Provides information about family attitudes and coping abilities that directly affect the child's health and feeling of well-being; chronic condition affecting a child in a family may strengthen or strain relationships and members may develop emotional problems when family is stressed.
Assess anxiety level of family and child, perception of crisis situation, coping and problem-solving methods used and effectiveness.	Identifies need to develop new coping skills and realistic behaviors in goal setting and interventions necessary for family and child to adapt to crisis.
Encourage expression of feelings and provide factual, honest information about care with or without surgical repair, abilities and disabilities.	Allows reduction in anxiety and enhances family understanding of condition and child's needs.
Assist to identify helpful techniques to use to problem solve and cope with problem and gain control over the situation.	Provides support for problem solving and management of situation.
Provide anticipatory guidance for crisis resolution.	Assists family to adapt to situation and develop new coping mechanisms.
If hospitalizations frequent, assign same personnel to care for child if appropriate.	Promotes trust and communication with family members.
Support and encourage parental and family caretaking efforts.	Provides positive reinforcement of roles and reduces stress in family members.
Encourage family members to express feelings and reaction to appearance and condition of infant/child.	Relieves anxiety and concern and allows a show of acceptance for their responses.
Communicate empathy for patient and family.	Promotes coping and positive adjustment to illness.
Be aware of cultural differences in coping behaviors; needs differ according to cultural and ethnic backgrounds.	Promotes cultural and developmental normalcy.

(continues)

(continued)

INTERVENTIONS	RATIONALES
Assist family with identifying realities of disabilities and suggest contact with community agencies, clergy, social services, physical and occupational therapy including Spina Bifida Association of America.	Provides support, information and assistance.
Assist to discuss family dynamics and need to tolerate conflict and individual behaviors.	Assists to understand the family behaviors leading to resolution.
Reinforce positive coping behaviors.	Promotes behavior change and adaptation to care of child.
Teach that overprotective behavior may hinder growth and development and that child should have limits and rules to live by.	Enhances family understanding of condition and need for integration of child into family activities.
Encourage to maintain health of family members and social contacts.	Prevents adverse effect of chronic anxiety, fatigue, and isolation on health and care capabilities of family.
Explain causes, treatment and prognosis of condition; inform parents that they are not at fault for development of the congenital defect.	Reduces guilt and provides information about condition.
Inform parents that surgery may be performed within 48 hours after birth or be delayed to age of 3 months or until further neurologic function is assessed, to allow for better epithelialization to occur, and to reduce the possibility of the development of hydrocephalus; use this information as reinforcement of physician information.	Provides information to assist family in decision about surgical procedure.
Inform need for follow-up appointments with physician and therapists.	Ensures compliance with medical regimen.

NIC: *Family Involvement*

Evaluation

(Date/time of evaluation of goal)

(Has goal been met? Not met? Partially met?)

(Did family discuss disability and the effect on the family? Provide quotes. What ways did the family identify to cope with illness? Describe family behaviors towards each other.)

(Revisions to care plan? D/C care plan? Continue care plan?)

RISK FOR INJURY

Related to: Repeated exposure to latex products and development of latex allergy.

Defining Characteristics: (Specify: child exhibits symptoms such as: sneezing, coughing, rashes, hives, wheezing when handling products made of rubber (balloons, tennis balls, Band-Aids) or when exposed to hospital products that contain latex such as gloves, catheters, and so forth.)

Goal: Child will not experience injury by (date and time to evaluate).

Outcome Criteria

✔ Child will not be exposed to latex in any form.

NOC: *Risk Detection*

INTERVENTIONS	RATIONALES
Identify children with latex allergy; children with this allergy should wear a form of identification such as a medical bracelet.	Promote expediency in treatment if a reaction occurs; may prevent an allergic reaction.
Maintain an environment that is latex-free, especially with high-risk populations (children with spina bifida, for example). Do not allow latex balloons in hospital environment.	Prevent development of latex allergy; prevent allergic reaction in those who are already sensitized.
Keep emergency equipment nearby, including equipment needed to treat an anaphylactic reaction.	Promote prompt emergency treatment.
Ask all patients admitted about reactions to latex allergy during all initial interviews.	Promotes screening of all patients which may prevent severe allergic reactions in otherwise low-risk patients.

NIC: *Surveillance*

Evaluation

(Date/time of evaluation of goal)

(Has goal been met? Not met? Partially met?)

(Was child exposed to latex?)

(Revisions to care plan? D/C care plan? Continue care plan?)

SPINA BIFIDA

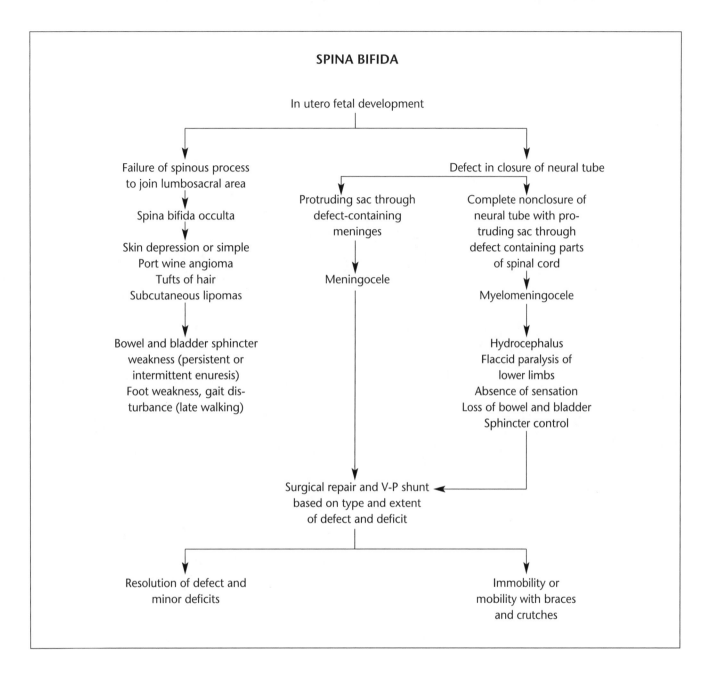

In utero fetal development

Failure of spinous process
to join lumbosacral area

Spina bifida occulta

Skin depression or simple
Port wine angioma
Tufts of hair
Subcutaneous lipomas

Bowel and bladder sphincter
weakness (persistent or
intermittent enuresis)
Foot weakness, gait dis-
turbance (late walking)

Defect in closure of neural tube

Protruding sac through
defect-containing
meninges

Meningocele

Complete nonclosure of
neural tube with pro-
truding sac through
defect containing parts
of spinal cord

Myelomeningocele

Hydrocephalus
Flaccid paralysis of
lower limbs
Absence of sensation
Loss of bowel and bladder
Sphincter control

Surgical repair and V-P shunt
based on type and extent
of defect and deficit

Resolution of defect and
minor deficits

Immobility or
mobility with braces
and crutches

UNIT 8

HEMATOLOGIC SYSTEM

CHAPTER 8.0

HEMATOLOGIC GROWTH AND DEVELOPMENT

The hematologic system includes the blood (plasma and cells) and the blood-forming tissues/organs (red bone marrow, lymph, lymph nodes, spleen, thymus, and tonsils). The cellular portion of the blood contains the erythrocytes (RBC), leukocytes (WBC), and thrombocytes (platelets). The plasma portion contains water and solutes, which include albumin, electrolytes, and proteins (clotting factors, fibrinogen, globulins, and antibodies). The system provides the body with specialized cells to transport oxygen, nutrients, and other substances to all the tissues; assist in clotting to prevent blood loss; and provide protection to the body from infectious agents (immunologic function). Children are vulnerable to disorders common to the system such as anemia, immunologic disorders, hemostatic problems, and malignancies involving the lymphatic system and blood cell production.

GROWTH AND DEVELOPMENT

- Blood volume of full-term newborn averages 300 ml.
- Fetal hemoglobin is present for 5 months; adult hemoglobin forms at 13 weeks of age.

- Hemoglobin is at its lowest between 4 and 6 months of age because maternal iron stores in the infant have been used up and this accounts for the lower hemoglobin at 6 months of age.
- Erythrocyte production increases rapidly after birth and results in an increase in reticulocytes (immature RBC).
- The life span of a RBC is 120 days, of a granulocyte 4 to 5 days, of an agranulocyte a half-life is 60 to 90 days, and of a platelet 8 to 10 days.
- Cell-mediated immune responses are deficient in the infant; immunoglobulin A (IgA) appears in the blood serum at 1 month of age and adult levels are reached at 10 years of age.
- Phagocytic action of neutrophils and monocytes is not at full strength in the newborn, so inflammatory response is less effective than in an older infant or child.
- By 5 months of age, immunoglobulin level is based on antibodies made by the infant's own system, but the child/adult level is not attained until 1 year of age.
- Lymphoid tissue (thymus, tonsils, adenoids, spleen, lymph nodes) grows rapidly during infancy and reaches peak growth at 12 years of age; it filters and traps pathogens before they enter the bloodstream.

CHAPTER 8.1

HIV/AIDS

Acquired immunodeficiency syndrome (AIDS) is caused by HIV (human immunodeficiency virus). HIV has been found in blood and bodily fluids (semen, saliva, vaginal secretions, urine, breast milk, and tears). Transmission of HIV can occur by 3 primary modes: exposure by sexual contact, IV exposure to blood, or perinatal exposure from an HIV-infected mother to her infant. In children and adolescent age groups 3 populations have been identified: 1) children exposed in utero from an infected mother; 2) children who have received blood products, especially children treated with hemophilia (before testing of blood products began in 1985); and 3) adolescents who are infected after engaging in high-risk behaviors (i.e., sharing of needles for injection of drug use; accidental needle sticks; unprotected sex and multiple sexual partners). Polymerase chain reaction (PCR) tests are very accurate in detecting HIV in infected infants (95% by 1 month).

Diagnosis of AIDS in children under 13 years of age, based on the Centers of Disease Control (CDC) criteria, include the presence of one of the following: 1) confirmed HIV in blood or tissues; 2) symptoms meeting the CDC criteria; or 3) HIV antibody and one or more of the following disorders: secondary infectious diseases, recurrent bacterial infections, or secondary cancers. Diagnosis of AIDS in children over 13 years of age and above is based on the CDC adult criteria. Children with HIV infection usually have detectable HIV antibody 6 to 12 months after exposure (except for infants of HIV-positive mothers). The diagnosis process for infants of HIV seropositive mothers, in the first 15 months of life, is difficult because of the presence of maternal antibody.

Infants with perinatal acquired AIDS are normal at birth but may develop symptoms within the first 18 months of life. Clinical manifestations in children include: fever; decreased CD4 count; anemia; decreased WBC count (less than 3,000 cells/mm^3); neutropenia (absolute neutrophil count of less than 1,500 cells/mm^3); thrombocytopenia; myelosuppression; vitamin K deficiency; hepatitis; pancreati-

tis; stomatitis and esophagitis; meningitis; retinitis (common with low CD4 counts); otitis media and sinusitis (chronic or recurrent); lymphadenopathy; hepatosplenomegaly; recurrent bacterial infections (especially, *Streptococcus pneumoniae* and *Haemophilus influenzae*); Mycobacterium infections (MAC) or tuberculosis; cytomegalovirus (CMV); failure to thrive (in infants); chronic diarrhea; neurologic involvement, (developmental delays and microcephaly in infants, or loss of motor skills in the older child); and pulmonary infections (*Pneumocystis carinii* [PCP], lymphocytic interstitial pneumonitis [LIP], and pulmonary lymphoid hyperplasia [PLH]). Kaposi sarcoma, a hallmark of adults with HIV, is rare in children with HIV. A major success in pediatric HIV is the recognition that a majority (from 25% to 8%) of perinatal transmissions can be prevented with prophylactic zidovudine therapy.

MEDICAL CARE

Diagnostic Tests for HIV in Children: enzyme-linked immunosorbent assay (ELISA) detects HIV antibodies; Western blot (detects serum antibody bound to specific HIV antigens); immunofluorescence assays. Because of the presence of maternal antibodies for newborns, the polymerase chain reaction (PCR assay) is required.

Medical Management: there is no cure for HIV. Medical care is directed at slowing the virus, preventing and treating the opportunistic infections, nutritional support, and symptomatic treatment. Combination drug therapy with antiviral therapy is recommended, with at least two antiviral drugs.

Antiretroviral Medications: drugs and treatment regimens are continually evolving. Currently recommended drugs include nucleoside analogue reverse transcriptase inhibitors (NRTIs, e.g., zidovudine), non-nucleoside analogue reverse transcriptase inhibitors (NNRTIs), and protease inhibitors (PIs).

IVIG (intravenous gamma globulin): may be helpful to decrease opportunistic infections.

Trimethoprim-Sulfamethoxasole: used for prevention/ treatment of *Pneumoncystis carinii*.

Immunizations: Immunizations should be given as recommended for all children, except no chicken-pox (varicella) vaccine, inactivated poliovirus (IPV) instead of oral poliovirus (OPV); and pneumococcal and influenza vaccine are recommended; Varicella zoster immune globulin should be given within 96 hours of chickenpox exposure.

Acyclovir: as prophylaxis for herpes infections.

Complete Blood Count (CBC): reveals increased WBC in infections, decreased T-helper lymphocytes.

Immunoglobulins (Ig): reveal increased levels.

COMMON NURSING DIAGNOSES

See INEFFECTIVE AIRWAY CLEARANCE

Related to: (Specify: infection, obstruction, secretions, decreased energy, and fatigue.)

Defining Characteristics: (Specify: abnormal breath sounds; changes in rate, ease, and depth of respirations; tachypnea; fever; weakness; ineffective cough with or without sputum.)

See INEFFECTIVE BREATHING PATTERN

Related to: Illness.

Defining Characteristics: (Specify: increase in body temperature above normal range, increased respiratory rate, tachycardia.)

See DIARRHEA

Related to: Inflammation, irritation of bowel.

Defining Characteristics: (Specify: chronic, increased frequency of loose, liquid stools; cramping; abdominal pain.)

See IMBALANCED NUTRITION: LESS THAN BODY REQUIREMENTS

Related to: (Specify: inability to ingest, digest, or absorb nutrients.)

Defining Characteristics: (Specify: anorexia, weight loss, lack of interest in feeding, failure to thrive, child's growth begins to slow or weight begins to decrease.)

See DELAYED GROWTH AND DEVELOPMENT

Related to: Neurologic involvement (75% to 90% of HIV infected children).

Defining Characteristics: Developmental delays or, after achieving normal development, loss of motor milestones; microcephaly (in HIV infected infants); and abnormal neurologic examination findings.

ADDITIONAL NURSING DIAGNOSES

ANXIETY

Related to: (Specify: change in health status, threat of death, threat to self-concept, fear of interpersonal transmission and contagion.)

Defining Characteristics: (Specify: increased apprehension and fear of diagnosis; expressed concern and worry about early death, effect of lifestyle changes on physical and emotional status, possible opportunistic infections.)

Goal: Clients will experience decreased anxiety by (date and time to evaluate).

Outcome Criteria

✔ Clients explore feelings about the child's illness.

✔ Clients report decreased anxiety.

NOC: *Anxiety Control*

INTERVENTIONS	RATIONALES
Assess level of anxiety of parents and child and how it is manifested; and need for information that will relieve anxiety.	Provides information about source and level of anxiety and need for interventions to relieve it; sources for the child may be procedures, fear of mutilation or death, unfamiliar environment of hospital, and may be manifested by restlessness and inability to play, sleep, or eat.
Refer for special counseling or social services as needed.	Reduces anxiety, supports family coping with illness, and promotes adjustment to lifestyle changes.

INTERVENTIONS	RATIONALES
Encourage open expression of concerns about illness, procedures, treatments, and prognosis.	Provides opportunity to vent feelings and fears to reduce anxiety.
Communicate with child at appropriate age level and answer questions calmly and honestly; use pictures, models, and drawings for explanations.	Promotes understanding and trust.
Allow child as much input in decisions about care and routines as possible.	Allows child more control and independence in situations.
Encourage parents to stay with child and have open visitation, provide a telephone number to call for information.	Promotes parental care and support.
Teach parents and child about the disease process, treatments, and therapy.	Promotes understanding that will relieve fear and anxiety.
Explain all procedures, treatments, and care in simple, direct, honest terms, and repeat as often as necessary; reinforce physician information if needed; provide specific information as needed.	Supplies information about all diagnostic procedures and tests.
Reassure parents and child that all information about the disease will be kept confidential.	Decreases anxiety associated social attitudes about the disease and those infected with it.
Refer to local and national AIDS groups and agencies to contact for assistance.	Provides information and support from those in similar circumstances.

NIC: *Anxiety Reduction*

Evaluation

(Date/time of evaluation of goal)

(Has goal been met? Not met? Partially met?)

(Did clients explore feelings about child's illness? Did clients report decreased anxiety? Use quotes.)

(Revisions to care plan? D/C care plan? Continue care plan?)

ANTICIPATORY GRIEVING

Related to: (Specify: perceived potential loss of infant/child by parents, perceived loss of physiopsychosocial well-being by child.)

Defining Characteristics: (Specify: expression of distress at potential loss, fatal prognosis of the disease, premature death of child.)

Goal: Clients will begin the grieving process by (date and time to evaluate).

Outcome Criteria

✔ Clients verbalize the stages of the grieving process.

✔ Clients identify support systems they may use for grief.

NOC: *Family Coping*

INTERVENTIONS	RATIONALES
Assess stage of grief process, problems encountered, feelings regarding long-term illness and potential loss.	Provides information about stage of grieving; time to work through the process varies with individuals as they move toward acceptance.
Provide emotional and spiritual comfort in an accepting environment and avoid conversations that will cause guilt or anger.	Provides for emotional needs of parents and child as appropriate, and helps them to cope with illness and its implications without adding stressors that are difficult to resolve.
Encourage parents' and child's responses and expressions of feelings such as concern, fear, anxiety, or guilt.	Promotes ventilation of feelings.
Assist in identifying and using effective coping mechanisms and in understanding situations over which they have no control.	Promotes constructive use of coping skills.
Allow for discussion of likelihood of child's death with parents and child, if appropriate, and encourage them to discuss this with family members, friends.	Presents realistic view of probable outcome of illness.
Refer to social, psychological, clergy services, or counseling as appropriate.	Provides support and information to child and family if need assistance.
Teach parents about stage of grieving process and of behaviors that are common in resolving grief.	Promotes understanding of feelings and behaviors that are manifested by grief.
Assist parents and child to identify coping skills, problem-solving skills, and approaches that may be used.	Promotes coping ability over period of prolonged illness and assists in resolving family stress.

(continues)

(continued)

INTERVENTIONS	RATIONALES
Refer to AIDS groups and agencies for social, economic, legal aid; family and friends for support.	Provides support for family and child as needed.

NIC: *Grief-Work Facilitation*

Evaluation

(Date/time of evaluation of goal)

(Has goal been met? Not met? Partially met?)

(Did clients verbalize the stages of grieving? Did clients identify support systems? Use quotes.)

(Revisions to care plan? D/C care plan? Continue care plan?)

RISK FOR INFECTION

Related to: Inadequate secondary defenses (immunosuppression).

Defining Characteristics: (Specify: presence of infective organism, opportunistic infectious process and malignancy, expressed need for information about transmission prevention.)

Goal: Client will not experience opportunistic infection by (date and time to evaluate).

Outcome Criteria

✔ Temperature remains (specify for child).

✔ WBC level remains > (specify for child).

✔ CD4 T-lymphocyte level remains > (specify).

NOC: *Risk Control*

INTERVENTIONS	RATIONALES
Assess CBC lab values; assess CD4 T-lymphocyte counts; assess blood culture for opportunistic infections; assess vital signs, as ordered, to identify changes in respirations or lung sounds.	To identify abnormal range of lab values related to infection or anemia; early recognition of organisms will expedite appropriate treatment of infections; early recognition of signs of pulmonary infections will expedite treatment for pulmonary changes.

INTERVENTIONS	RATIONALES
Assess for fever, malaise, fatigue, night sweats, weight loss, chronic diarrhea, oral infection or lesions, pain in joints and muscles, lymphadenopathy, upper and lower respiratory infections.	Provides information about signs and symptoms of infection during the (prodromal) stage of AIDS with responses that are age-dependent at onset of AIDS in infants/children: long-term opportunistic infections, including *Pneumocystis carinii* pneumonia, Kaposi's sarcoma, and lymphoma.
Provide protective isolation for immunosuppressed child; use gloves, mask, and gown for visitors; and during care, proper handwashing when needed.	Protects child from contact with infectious process in others.
Wear gloves for all care, when in contact with body fluids (changing diapers, handling any secretions or excretions); do not recap needles; clean all spills and disinfect article or area; use bleach solution in home; wash, disinfect, or dispose of all contaminated articles used; double bag all linens and specimens with proper precautionary labeling.	Prevents transmission of virus to personnel or caretaker; follows guidelines published by the Centers for Disease Control.
Use medical or surgical asepsis for all procedures and care as appropriate.	Prevents transmission of pathogens to child.
Administer medications as ordered to control disease progression or treat any infection as ordered (specify).	Prevents or treats infectious process, compensates for immunosuppression by improving functioning of immune system (action of drug).
Restrict contact with persons with infections or illnesses, have child to share room with another child who does not have an infection.	Prevents transmission of infection to child.
Teach parents and child of possible source for infection and risk of spread or transmission of infection.	Promotes understanding and cooperation in treatments and procedure, prevents spread of existing infection or risk of new infection.
Teach parents and child about isolation to prevent contact with sources of potential infections (i.e., infected persons or contaminated articles).	Promotes compliance with isolation techniques.

INTERVENTIONS	RATIONALES
Inform parents and child of diagnostic and reporting methods, signs and symptoms of specific diseases, risk factors in acquiring or transmitting disease and potential complications.	Provides information about the disease causes, treatment, and preventive measures.
Teach parents and child about high-calorie protein diet with food selections and sample menus.	Assists in maintaining nutritional status necessary to fight infection.
Teach parents and child to avoid family members, friends, peers, or others with infections or illnesses.	Prevents exposure to others with infection that may be transmitted to child with a compromised immune system.
Teach parents and child hand-washing technique.	Prevents transmission of pathogens via the hands.
Using written guidelines offered by Centers for Disease Control, instruct in care of bodily fluids, use of gloves, cleansing and care of articles used, disposal methods, care of linens, clothing, specimens, mode of transmission to others.	Prevents transmission of virus to others.
Encourage parents to contact school nurse and discuss child's needs and guidelines for school attendance.	Promotes safety of child and possible contacts; attendance is recommended by physician as long as child has control of body secretions, and does not bite or have open lesions.
Teach parents and child about immunization needed to prevent infectious disease.	Protects child from infectious diseases (pneumonia and influenza).
(If appropriate, inform child of precautions to take if sexually active [condom use] or if using drugs [not sharing needles].)	Prevents transmission of virus to others by taking appropriate precautions.

NIC: *Surveillance*

Evaluation

(Date/time of evaluation of goal)

(Has goal been met? Not met? Partially met?)

(What is temperature? What is WBC level? CD4 T-lymphocyte level?)

(Revisions to care plan? D/C care plan? Continue care plan?)

SOCIAL ISOLATION

Related to: (Specify: altered state of wellness, unaccepted social behavior, low blood count precautions, repeated hospitalizations, social stigma of HIV, physical limitations.)

Defining Characteristics: (Specify: protective isolation; absence of support by family, friends, others; seeks to be alone; expresses feelings of rejection, indifference of others; aloneness; withdrawal; displays behavior unaccepted by dominant culture; evidence of altered state of wellness.)

Goal: Clients will experience increased social support by (date and time to evaluate).

Outcome Criteria

✔ (Specify for clients, e.g., child returns to school, family reports support from friends, etc.)

NOC: *Social Involvement*

INTERVENTIONS	RATIONALES
Assist child to identify personal strengths to facilitate enhanced coping.	To increase child's self-competence and increase child's self-esteem.
Assess child and family for feelings about stigma associated with the disease, rejection by others.	Provides information about extent of isolation felt by the family and child.
Provide accepting, warm environment for child and parents to express their feelings.	Promotes trust and comfort to enhance adaptation to presence of positive testing or actual symptoms of the disease.
Encourage child to interact with peers, attend school and activities.	Promotes feeling of belonging, and provides growth and development.
Reinforce peers, school nurse and personnel about AIDS and safe activities for child and other children.	Provides information and education about AIDS.
Discuss with child and parents misconceptions that the public has and ways to correct the situation by providing information about causes and mode of transmission and by answering questions and concerns.	Promotes correct information dissemination and dispels myths about the disease, thereby reducing fear and rejection by others.

(continues)

(continued)

INTERVENTIONS	RATIONALES
Reassure parents and child that confidentiality will be maintained at school and elsewhere if needed.	Protects child from stigma associated with the disease.

NIC: *Support System Enhancement*

Evaluation

(Date/time of evaluation of goal)

(Has goal been met? Not met? Partially met?)

(Provide data based on the outcome criteria selected, e.g., did child return to school? Did family report support of friends? Use quotes.)

(Revisions to care plan? D/C care plan? Continue care plan?)

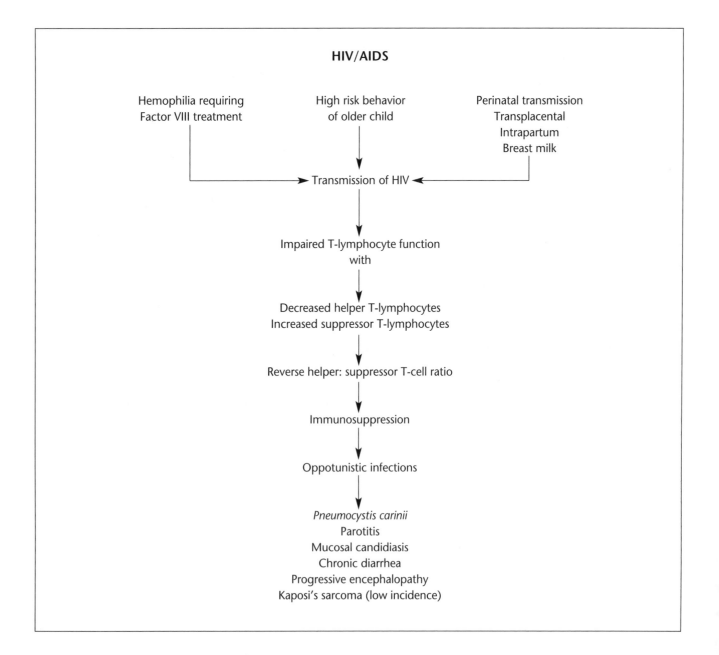

HIV/AIDS

Hemophilia requiring
Factor VIII treatment

High risk behavior
of older child

Perinatal transmission
Transplacental
Intrapartum
Breast milk

→ Transmission of HIV ←

Impaired T-lymphocyte function
with

Decreased helper T-lymphocytes
Increased suppressor T-lymphocytes

Reverse helper: suppressor T-cell ratio

Immunosuppression

Oppotunistic infections

Pneumocystis carinii
Parotitis
Mucosal candidiasis
Chronic diarrhea
Progressive encephalopathy
Kaposi's sarcoma (low incidence)

CHAPTER 8.2

ANEMIA

Anemia is the most common group of hematologic disorders of infancy and childhood. The term anemia refers to a reduction in either the total number of circulating red blood cells (RBC) or a decrease in the concentration of hemoglobin (Hgb). The etiology of anemia is divided into 3 categories: 1) excessive blood loss (acute or chronic hemorrhage), 2) increased destruction of RBCs (or hemolysis), or 3) impaired or decreased rate of production (or bone marrow failure). The following three types of anemia are included here: iron deficiency, sickle cell anemia, and aplastic anemia.

Iron deficiency anemia is primarily caused by an inadequate intake of dietary iron. The iron stores of the full-term infant normally meet the infant's nutritional needs until 6 months of age. In comparison, the iron stores for the premature infant normally is depleted by 2 to 3 months of age (milk is iron-poor). Treatment consists of iron supplementation and optimum nutrition.

Sickle cell anemia (Hgb SS) is referred to as a genetic disease of autosomal dominant inheritance (and a sickling hemoglobinopathy syndrome). Hgb SS is caused by the substitution of a single amino acid (valine replaces glutamic acid) at the sixth position of the B-chain. It occurs primarily in the black race and symptoms appear usually after 4 to 6 months of age because of the presence of fetal hemoglobin earlier. Treatment consists of prevention/treatment of sickle cell pain crisis; and supportive/symptomatic measures.

Aplastic anemia is defined as bone marrow failure characterized by the reduction or absence of the solid elements of the blood (red cells, white cells, and platelets). There are two types: primary (congenital or Fanconi anemia, an inherited autosomal recessive trait) or secondary (acquired, caused by exposure to toxins in the environment or a complication of an infection). Symptoms occur in the acquired type after exposure to a toxin or infection and in the congenital type usually after 17 months of age. Treatment is directed at restoration of bone marrow function, by two approaches: immunosuppressive therapy and replacement of the bone marrow through bone marrow transplantation.

MEDICAL CARE

DIAGNOSTIC EVALUATION FOR IRON DEFICIENCY ANEMIA

Red Cell Smear: examines the red cell shape and content (i.e., MVC and MCH).

Free Erythrocyte Protoporphyrin (FEP): elevated FEP is associated with an inadequate iron supply.

Serum-Iron Concentration (SIC): measures circulating iron (normal: 70% ug/dl in infants).

Total Iron-Binding Capacity (TIBC): measures transferrin (iron-binding globulin) for iron transport. Transferrin saturation: divide the SIC by the TIBC and multiplying by 100; (10%—suggests anemia).

TREATMENT FOR IRON DEFICIENCY ANEMIA

Iron Supplements: ferrous sulfate for prevention/ treatment of iron deficiency.

Vitamin C Supplements: may enhance iron absorption.

DIAGNOSTIC EVALUATION FOR SICKLE CELL ANEMIA

Stained Blood Smear: will reveal a few sickled RBCs; it is not 100% accurate.

Sickle-Turbidity Test (Sickledex): a reliable screening method for the sickle cell trait or disease.

Hemoglobin Electrophoresis: is an accurate, rapid, and specific test for detecting the homozygous and heterozygous forms of sickle cell anemia.

TREATMENT FOR SICKLE CELL ANEMIA

Hydration: given for hemodilution to treat/prevent sickle cell crisis.

Analgesics: to prevent/treat pain crisis.

Immunizations: should receive all recommended childhood immunizations; should also receive: pneumococcal (at 2 years of age and a booster at 5 years of age); *Haemophilus influenzae*, type B (is given to all infants at 2 months of age); and meningococcal vaccine (at 2 years of age).

Folate Replacement: is given for the treatment of aplastic type of sickle cell crisis.

Blood Transfusions: packed RBC transfusions are used to replace prematurely destroyed red cells and to diminish the percentage of hemoglobin S (sickled hemoglobin). It is primarily used with severe complications (i.e., stroke, progressive hypoxia, pulmonary disease, or in severe hemolysis).

DIAGNOSTIC EVALUATION FOR APLASTIC ANEMIA

Red Cell Indices: examine an elevated MCV (mean corpuscular volume of the RBC).

Hgb Electrophoresis: will reveal an abnormally high fetal hemoglobin.

Chromosomal Studies: will reveal multiple chromosomal abnormalities.

CBC: evaluation of lab values characteristic of anemia, leukopenia, and decreased platelet count.

Bone Marrow Aspiration: examination confirms hypocellularity and fatty replacement of bone marrow (conversion of red bone marrow to yellow, fatty bone marrow).

TREATMENT FOR APLASTIC ANEMIA

Anti-Lymphocyte Globulin (ALG) or antithymocyte globulin (ATG): suppresses T-cell-dependent autoimmune responses, (based on theory that aplastic anemia is caused by an autoimmune response).

Androgens: may be used with ATG, may stimulate erythropoiesis.

Immunoglobulin: (IV) has been successful in the acquired type of aplastic anemia (of infectious origin).

Bone Marrow Transplantation: is the treatment of choice for severe aplastic anemia. It is the only mode of treatment which may result in a cure of this disease. Prognosis is highly correlated with the number of pretransplant transfusions (better to consider early in the course of the disease).

COMMON NURSING DIAGNOSES

See INEFFECTIVE TISSUE PERFUSION

Related to: Impaired oxygen-carrying capacity of the blood.

Defining Characteristics: (Specify: *in iron deficiency anemia:* irritability, anxiety, blood loss in the stool, hypochronic RBCs, normal or near normal RBC count, decreased serum ferritin and iron; *in sickle cell anemia:* pallor, weakness, anorexia, easy fatigability, jaundice and developmental delays; *in aplastic anemia:* pallor, fatigue, weakness, loss of appetite, normochromic, normocytic RBCs in reduced numbers, leukopenia, thrombocytopenia [risk of spontaneous bleeding or bleeding after mild to severe trauma].)

See RISK FOR DEFICIENT FLUID VOLUME

Related to: Impaired kidney function to concentrate urine (in the sickle cell patient).

Defining Characteristics: (Specify: dilute urine or low specific gravity; diuresis; enuresis; dehydration [dry mucous membranes; dry diapers and sunken fontanel in the infant]; prone to dehydration from environmental factors [i.e., overheating].)

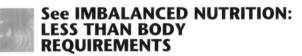

See IMBALANCED NUTRITION: LESS THAN BODY REQUIREMENTS

Related to: Inadequate ingestion of iron.

Defining Characteristics: (Specify: in iron deficiency: underweight or may be overweight [because of excessive cow's milk ingestion]; fecal loss of blood; pallor; poor muscle development; prone to infections; inadequate intake of iron-rich foods; weakness.)

See RISK FOR IMPAIRED SKIN INTEGRITY

Related to: Allergic response.

Defining Characteristics: (Specify: itching, rash, urticaria, face and lymph node swelling; sclerosing from extravasation at venous access when receiving ATG.)

ADDITIONAL NURSING DIAGNOSES

PAIN

Related to: Tissue anoxia.

Defining Characteristics: (Specify: communication of pain descriptors, guarding and protective behavior of area, soft tissue swelling, warmth over painful area, crying, clinging behavior.)

Goal: Client will experience decreased pain by (date and time to evaluate).

Outcome Criteria

✔ Pain rating is decreased to (specify level and pain scale used).

NOC: *Pain Level*

INTERVENTIONS	RATIONALES
Assess for location, severity, and duration of pain (specify frequency).	Provides information about pain caused by vaso-occlusion resulting from RBC sickling, ischemia, and necrosis in soft tissue, joints, abdomen, back, or wherever occlusion occurs.
Administer analgesics as ordered (specify); administer intermittently over 24-hour period before pain becomes severe rather than wait for request or complaint from child.	Controls pain and promotes comfort.
Provide rest periods, refrain from disturbing child unless necessary.	Decreases stimuli that increase pain and promotes rest, decreases oxygen expenditure.
Apply dry heat to area and note response of pain decrease.	Promotes vasodilation and circulation to area to reduce pain.
Maintain position of comfort, handle painful areas gently, and support with pillows.	Promotes comfort and prevents pain from movement.
Inform parents and child of cause of pain, methods to control it.	Provides information and rationale for treatment.

INTERVENTIONS	RATIONALES
Teach parents to avoid situations that cause stress for the child, and clothing or positions that restrict and impede blood flow.	Provides measures to control sickling, which results in pain.

NIC: *Pain Management*

Evaluation

(Date/time of evaluation of goal)

(Has goal been met? Not met? Partially met?)

(What is pain rating? Specify scale used.)

(Revisions to care plan? D/C care plan? Continue care plan?)

ACTIVITY INTOLERANCE

Related to: Generalized weakness, imbalance between oxygen supply and demand.

Defining Characteristics: (Specify: reduced oxygen delivery to tissues from reduced RBC or RBC sickling; fatigue; verbalization of weakness; changes in respiratory rate, depth, and ease; irritability; low tolerance to activity; increased pulse.)

Goal: Child will increase activity to (specify level and date and time to evaluate).

Outcome Criteria

✔ (Specify for child, e.g., is able to play a game; feed self, etc.)

NOC: *Activity Tolerance*

INTERVENTIONS	RATIONALES
Assess temperature, respirations, and pulse; changes in behavior (irritability, lightheadedness, short attention span); if easily fatigued, unable to sleep, or weak; ability to tolerate any activity or ADL.	Provides information about VS changes caused by hypoxia and about behavior changes caused by reduced oxygenation of the brain.
Assist with activities that require exertion and are beyond tolerance and ability.	Minimizes physical exertion, which increases oxygen to tissues.
Provide rest periods, plan care and activities around rest/sleep.	Decreases oxygen expenditure to enhance tissue oxygenation.

(continues)

(continued)

INTERVENTIONS	RATIONALES
Provide appropriate quiet play and activities, and allow interaction with child of same age, if possible (specify).	Promotes diversionary activity and prevents withdrawal.
Administer oxygen therapy as ordered (specify).	Provides supplemental oxygen, if needed, to treat hypoxia.
Administer transfusion of blood, packed RBC, platelets as ordered (specify).	Replaces blood or blood components depending on type of anemia and need.
Teach parents and child how to conserve energy and increase endurance of child, including placing articles within reach, anticipating needs and assisting before child attempts activity, allowing for rest; remain with child as needed.	Provides information to prevent fatigue by minimizing physical activity or exertion, which utilizes more oxygen.
Encourage parents to avoid stressful situations.	Promotes quiet environment for child.

NIC: *Energy Management*

Evaluation

(Date/time of evaluation of goal)

(Has goal been met? Not met? Partially met?)

(What is child able to do? Provide data related to outcome criteria.)

(Revisions to care plan? D/C care plan? Continue care plan?)

RISK FOR INFECTION

Related to: (Specify: decreased Hgb and decreased immune system functions; in aplastic anemia: immunosuppressive therapy, ATG, and steroids; in sickle cell anemia: splenic dysfunction.)

Defining Characteristics: (Specify: temperature elevation [greater than or equal to a temperature of 101° F or 38.5° C]; elevated WBC counts; positive cultures for bacterial organisms; positive throat, urine or blood culture; changes in respirations and sputum characteristics; cloudy, foul-smelling urine.)

Goal: Child will not experience infection by (date and time to evaluate).

Outcome Criteria

✔ Temperature remains <99° F.

✔ Child denies pain or swelling in any area.

NOC: *Risk Control*

INTERVENTIONS	RATIONALES
Assess temperature, signs, symptoms, and laboratory tests indicating infectious process, irritability and malaise, swelling in soft tissue or lymph nodes.	Provides information about infection in a child made susceptible by steroid and globulin therapy, particularly in aplastic anemia, or pneumococcal and salmonella infections in child with sickle cell anemia.
Provide protective isolation if neutrophil count is less than 500/cu mm; use mask and gown and good handwashing when caring for child.	Prevents transmission of pathogens to a susceptible child.
Obtain culture of body fluid for examination.	Identifies pathogens and sensitivity to antibiotic therapy if an infection is present.
Teach parents and child to limit contact with persons who are ill or have respiratory infections.	Prevents exposure to those with infections or illness that may be transmitted to child with anemia.
Instruct in handwashing technique and when to use it, including before meals, after using bathroom.	Prevents exposure to infectious agents transmitted by hands or hard surfaces.
Inform parents of recommended childhood immunizations; and of acquiring the following vaccines when the child is 2 years of age or older: meningococcal and pneumococcal.	Prevents infectious disease in the susceptible child.
Teach parents to report any temperature elevation, changes in respirations and pulse, pain or swelling in any area.	Indicates possible infection that may be controlled with early intervention.

NIC: *Surveillance*

Evaluation

(Date/time of evaluation of goal)

(Has goal been met? Not met? Partially met?)

(What is temperature? Does child deny pain or swelling?)

(Revisions to care plan? D/C care plan? Continue care plan?)

RISK FOR INJURY

Related to: (Specify: abnormal blood profile [thrombocytopenia] reaction to transfusion or ATG administration.)

Defining Characteristics: (Specify: fever; restlessness; chills; shortness of breath; chest pain; tachycardia; hypotension; headache; thrombocytopenia at 20,000/cu mm level; bruising; petechiae; bleeding from mucous membranes; blood in urine, sputum, stool; nosebleed; blood in vomitus; stomatitis.)

Goal: Client will not experience injury by (date and time to evaluate).

Outcome Criteria

✔ No evidence of bleeding.

NOC: *Risk Detection*

INTERVENTIONS	RATIONALES
Assess for signs of bleeding from any site as manifested in skin changes; also, blood from nose, oral cavity, urinary or gastrointestinal tract, and factors that precipitate or increase bleeding.	Provides information indicating blood loss as tendency increases with therapy for aplastic anemia.
Assess blood in urine with dipsticks and hematests (specify when).	Identifies occult blood in urine or stool.
Protect child from trauma by padding bed and toys, using soft toothbrush and towels or swabs for cleaning mouth, avoiding rectal temperature and injections.	Prevents bleeding in skin layers, deeper tissues, or mucous membranes.
Discontinue transfusion if allergic reaction occurs, notify physician.	Prevents irreversible reaction to blood or blood products.
If ordered, perform skin test for ATG before dose, administer steroid daily 30 minutes before ATG, which is given in normal saline IV.	Alerts to possible sensitivity to horse serum and protects from allergic reaction to ATG.
Teach parents and child about activities to avoid while on therapy, such as contact sports or activities that cause falls.	Prevents trauma, which causes bleeding when tendency is present.

INTERVENTIONS	RATIONALES
Advise parents to avoid aspirin and aspirin products.	Encourages bleeding by its effect on platelet aggregation.
Instruct parents to report any bleeding from any site, nosebleed that will not stop, blood in urine or stool.	Provides for early interventions to control bleeding.

NIC: *Surveillance*

Evaluation

(Date/time of evaluation of goal)

(Has goal been met? Not met? Partially met?)

(Is there any evidence of bleeding? What was looked for?)

(Revisions to care plan? D/C care plan? Continue care plan?)

DEFICIENT KNOWLEDGE

Related to: Lack of information about anemia.

Defining Characteristics: (Specify: request for information about pathophysiology of anemia, changes that occur, preventive measures and treatments.)

Goal: Clients will obtain information about anemia by (date and time to evaluate).

Outcome Criteria

✔ Parents verbalize understanding of (specify type of anemia) and treatment plan.

NOC: *Knowledge: Disease Process*

INTERVENTIONS	RATIONALES
Assess for knowledge level of type of anemia, cause, treatment, prevention.	Provides information needed for appropriate teaching content for parents and child.
Teach about RBC physiology and the changes that occur in the anemia the child has.	Promotes understanding of RBC function to provide a rationale for signs, symptoms, and treatments.
Teach parents about genetic counseling for sickle cell anemia.	Provides information about risk of offspring having the disease.
Teach parents and child about bone marrow transplant treatment if appropriate.	Provides information of this therapy if child has aplastic anemia.

(continues)

(continued)

INTERVENTIONS	RATIONALES
Instruct child to carry or wear identification information, including condition, treatments, and physician's name and telephone number.	Provides information in the event of an emergency.
Teach parents and child about dietary intake of iron, including foods such as iron-rich formula for infant, meats, whole grains, green leafy vegetables, dried fruits.	Provides iron intake or replacement in iron-deficiency anemia.
Administer oral iron replacement (specify dose) as ordered, and instruct to take with orange juice to promote absorption; give iron preparation between meals, avoid administering with milk, use straw or dropper, and have child rinse mouth after ingestion.	Provides iron replacement therapy.
Refer parents and child to National Association for Sickle Cell Disease and other community agencies and groups for family, parents or child.	Provides information and support for child and family with sickle cell or aplastic anemia.

INTERVENTIONS	RATIONALES
Reinforce to parents importance of child attending school and participating in family activities.	Treats child as member of family and integrates him or her into social, mental, and physical activities, that will enhance growth and development needs.
Teach risks to avoid, including signs and symptoms of infection, bleeding, hypoxia, malnutrition, immunizations, high altitudes, side effects of steroid therapy, emotional and physical stress.	Prevents complications of disease.

NIC: *Teaching: Disease Process*

Evaluation

(Date/time of evaluation of goal)

(Has goal been met? Not met? Partially met?)

(What did parents say about the cause of the child's anemia? What did parents verbalize about treatment for child?)

(Revisions to care plan? D/C care plan? Continue care plan?)

ANEMIA

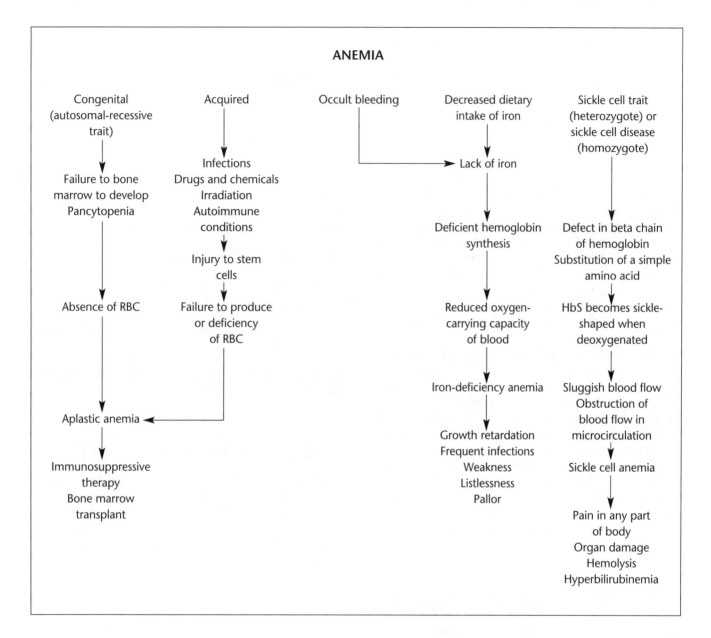

CHAPTER 8.3

HEMOPHILIA

Hemophilia, an X-linked disorder, is a congenital hereditary bleeding disorder caused by an abnormal gene that produces a defective clotting factor protein with little or no clotting ability. The two most common forms of this disorder are: 1) factor VIII deficiency (hemophilia A, or classic hemophilia) and 2) factor IX deficiency (hemophilia B, or Christmas disease). Because both of these disorders are X-linked, the female is the carrier and the disorder is manifested only in males.

Hemophilia is classified into the following three groups, based on the severity of factor deficiency, mild (5–50%), moderate (1–5%) and severe (1%). Hemophiliacs are at risk for prolonged bleeding or hemorrhage as a result of minor trauma. Individuals with severe hemophilia, or less than 1% clotting factor, are also at risk to suffer from spontaneous bleeding without trauma or more severe prolonged bleeding after trauma. Bleeding can occur at any part of the body. Hemarthrosis, or bleeding into the joint spaces, is the most common complication of severe hemophilia. The knee joint is the most frequent joint involved.

MEDICAL CARE

DIAGNOSTIC EVALUATION

In the hemophilia patient, the following tests will be within the normal range: prothrombin time, fibrinogen level, thrombin level, and platelet count; the following tests will be abnormal: prolonged PTT and low levels of clotting factor (for factor VIII or IX).

Partial Thromboplastin Time Test (PTT): measures activity of thromboplastin.

Thromboplastin Generation Test (TGT): measures blood's ability to generate thromboplastin. Specific for determination of specific factor deficiencies, especially factor VIII and IX.

Prothrombin Test (PT): measures activity of prothrombin and detects deficiencies only for factor V, VII, X, fibrinogen, and prothrombin.

Platelet Test: total number of circulating platelets.

Bleeding Time: measures time interval for bleeding from small superficial wound to cease.

Factor VIII: antihemophilic factor A or antihemophilic globulin (AHG).

Factor IX: antihemophilic factor B or plasma thromboplastin component (PTC).

THERAPEUTIC MANAGEMENT

Replacement of the Deficient Clotting Factor: Factor VIII and Factor IX (IV): (monoclonal), (reconstituted with sterile water immediately before use); DDAVP: (1-deamino-8-D-arginine vasopressin), a synthetic form of vasopressin that is the treatment of choice for hemophilia.

Corticosteroids: are used to treat inflammation in the joints; Ibuprofen is used for pain management.

Oral Use of EACA or Amicar (Epsilon aminocaproic acid): promotes clotting, it is used in children (>1 year of age) for mucous membrane bleeding; also for pre-procedural and postprocedural oral surgery (a dose of factor replacement must be given first).

Porcine Preparations: prevents inhibitor antibodies (30% will develop inhibitor antibodies against factor replacements).

Regular Program of Exercise: active range-of-motion is recommended to strengthen muscles around joints and may decrease the number of spontaneous bleeding episodes.

TREATMENTS NOT CURRENTLY RECOMMENDED

Cryoprecipitate: has not been recommended (since 1988) because it cannot be treated to safely eliminate hepatitis or HIV viruses.

NSAIDS: (such as aspirin, Indocin, or Butazolidin) are not recommended because they inhibit platelet function.

COMMON NURSING DIAGNOSES

See IMPAIRED PHYSICAL MOBILITY

Related to: Pain and discomfort with the onset of bleeding episodes; and hemarthrosis.

Defining Characteristics: (Specify: pain in affected joint, and decreased ability to move the joint; immobilized joints [first 24 to 48 hours after a bleeding episode], potential contractures in affected joints.)

See RISK FOR IMPAIRED SKIN INTEGRITY

Related to: Spontaneous bleeding episodes or bleeding episodes related to trauma.

Defining Characteristics: (Specify: bleeding into soft tissue, muscles, and most frequently, joint capsules.)

ADDITIONAL NURSING DIAGNOSES

PAIN

Related to: Hemarthrosis.

Defining Characteristics: (Specify: a feeling of stiffness, tingling or aching in the affected joint, followed by a decrease in the ability to move a joint, verbal descriptors of pain, irritability, crying, restlessness.)

Goal: Client will experience decreased pain by (date and time to evaluate).

Outcome Criteria

✔ Pain rating is decreased to (specify level and pain scale used).

NOC: *Pain Level*

INTERVENTIONS	RATIONALES
Assess for joint pain, swelling and limited ROM.	Bleeding episodes should be treated at the onset of discomfort, which requires replacement of the deficient factor.
Immobilize joints and apply elastic bandages to the affected joint if prescribed; elevate affected extremity/joint; avoid heat application.	Immobilization is mandatory for comfort and to avoid further bleeding; elastic bandage most often prevents muscle bleeding; elevation of affected extremity/joint will minimize swelling; heat application will promote vasodilatation and that may prolong bleeding time; ice packs promote vasoconstriction to active bleeding sites, but must be used cautiously to prevent skin damage in young children.
Administer analgesics for pain (specify as ordered).	Administer ibuprofen for pain management; avoid NSAIDS (aspirin), as they may inhibit platelet function.
Provide bed cradle over painful joints and/or other sites of bleeding.	Prevents pressure of linens on affected sites, especially joints (i.e., hemarthrosis).
Maintain immobilization of the affected extremity during the acute phase (24 to 48 hours); apply a splint or sling to the affected extremity if prescribed.	Prevents increase of pain and potential increased bleeding time caused by movement.
Inform child of cause of pain and interventions to relieve it; how medications must be administered via mouth, while injections are avoided; to avoid taking aspirin or aspirin product for pain.	Promotes understanding of pain responses and methods to reduce it.
Instruct child to support and protect painful areas and in the importance of immobilization.	Promotes comfort and prevents further bleeding into joints.

NIC: *Pain Management*

Evaluation

(Date/time of evaluation of goal)

(Has goal been met? Not met? Partially met?)

(What is pain rating? Specify scale used.)

(Revisions to care plan? D/C care plan? Continue care plan?)

RISK FOR INJURY

Related to: Decreased clotting factor (VIII or IX).

Defining Characteristics: (Specify: prolonged bleeding anywhere from or in the body; spontaneous bleeding episodes; mild to severe bleeding episodes after trauma; hemarthrosis [bleeding to the joint and swelling of the joint]; affected bleeding site will display warmth, redness, swelling, and pain with limited movement.)

Goal: Client will not experience injury by (date and time to evaluate).

Outcome Criteria

✔ No evidence of bleeding.

✔ Joints are not swollen, warm, or red.

NOC: *Risk Control*

INTERVENTIONS	RATIONALES
Assess signs and symptoms of bleeding; hemarthrosis (stiffness, tingling, or pain); subcutaneous and intramuscular hemorrhage; oral bleeding; epistaxis (is not a frequent sign); petechiae (are uncommon).	Early detection of bleeding episodes will delay initiation of factor replacement therapy and will minimize complications; oral bleeding is often caused by trauma to the gums; petechiae is caused by low platelet function versus a deficient clotting factor.
Provide appropriate oral hygiene (use of a water irrigating device; use of a soft toothbrush or softening the toothbrush with warm water before brushing; use of sponge-tipped toothbrush).	Implementation of appropriate oral hygiene will minimize trauma to the gums.
Advise adolescents to use an electric shaver versus manual razor devices (with blades).	High risk of bleeding is related to use of razor blades; minimal risk of bleeding is associated with use of electric shaver.
Substitute the subcutaneous route for intramuscular injections; utilize venipuncture blood drawing technique for all required blood testing samples versus use of a finger or heel puncture.	Both of these measures are associated with less bleeding after implementing a subcutaneous injection or venipuncture blood sample.
Utilize appropriate toys (soft, not pointed or small sharp objects); for infants, may need to use padded bed rail sides on crib; avoid rectal temperatures.	All of these recommendations will minimize and/or prevent bleeding episodes due to trauma.

INTERVENTIONS	RATIONALES
Implement the following measures to control and stop all bleeding episodes: 1) apply pressure (10 to 15 mins); 2) immobilize and elevate affected extremity above the heart; 3) application of cold pack (if prescribed); 4) institute factor replacement therapy (based on medical protocol); 5) institute DDAVP (it can be given IV or intranasally).	To allow clot formation. To decrease blood flow to control bleeding. To promote vasoconstriction, but use caution with small children to avoid tissue damage. To control and stop bleeding episode and to prevent crippling effects from joint bleeding.
Other recommended adjunct measures: 1) complete bed rest for intramuscular hemorrhage of lower spine area and non-weight bearing support; 2) assess laboratory values for blood clotting factors (VIII or IX) and vital signs; 3) stop passive range-of-motion exercises after an acute episode of bleeding.	To minimize hemorrhage in muscles of lower spine (i.e., attaching to trochanter or femur). These values determine current hemodynamic status and factor replacement therapy guidelines or protocols. To avoid injury to the affected extremity or joint and to avoid recurrence of bleeding to these.
Teach to wear appropriate medical identification and to notify medical personnel of diagnosis.	To prepare medical personnel, family members and others of accurate information in the event of an emergency.
Teach parents, family members and affected child: signs and symptoms of bleeding; and appropriate measures to control bleeding at home.	Empowers others with accurate information to recognize and control bleeding episodes; to prevent bleeding; and to prevent crippling effects of bleeding.
Limit use of helmets and padding of joints during participation in contact sports activities.	Daily use of these measures may cause the child to feel ostracized or may create emotional discomfort.
Recommend non-contact sports activities such as swimming, hiking, or bicycling.	These activities are considered a safe activity by the Hemophilia Foundation.
Avoid contact sports such as football, soccer, ice hockey, karate.	Contact sports will predispose the child to injury and bleeding episodes.
Maintain close supervision during play time to minimize injuries.	To prevent bleeding related to trauma in the child's environment (i.e., school or park).
Teach parents related to home health maintenance: 1) the affected child should receive all routine immunizations (use subcutaneous route, recommend pressure and elastic bandage after injections); 2) reinforce	To protect the child from childhood communicable diseases (but use subcutaneous route administration to prevent prolonged bleeding). To minimize oral trauma. To minimize emotional distress

INTERVENTIONS	RATIONALES
importance of appropriate dental hygiene program; 3) reinforce the provision of a safe but normal home environment, such as safety measures that are employed for all children of different ages are recommended; example: for the toddler, gates over stairs but avoid restraining the toddler's attempt to master motor skills; for the older child, participating in sports activities (use helmets and padding); 4) provide a home environment free of hazards, including clear pathways, and supervise child during ambulation and play without being overprotective.	during the child's progression through the different developmental stages. To minimize risk of trauma in the home by falls; infants and toddlers frequently fall or sustain injuries.
Instruct parents and child, if age appropriate, to administer factor VIII via IV if signs and symptoms appear, or before dental visits or other possible invasive procedures; instruct in mixing the precipitate, drawing into syringe, venipuncture, and application of pressure following IV, and allow for return demonstration.	Prevents or manages bleeding by factor replacement.
Teach parents to include iron-rich foods in diet; provide list of foods and sample menus.	Maintains iron level to prevent anemia.
Teach parents and child of possible reactions to IV concentrate administration and that blood is tested for AIDS.	Reduces anxiety caused by risk of infections such as hepatitis and AIDS from replacement products.

NIC: *Surveillance*

Evaluation

(Date/time of evaluation of goal)

(Has goal been met? Not met? Partially met?)

(Is there any evidence of bleeding? Are joints red, swollen, or warm?)

(Revisions to care plan? D/C care plan? Continue care plan?)

COMPROMISED FAMILY COPING

Related to: (Specify: inadequate or incorrect information or understanding, prolonged disease or disability

progression that exhausts the physical and emotional supportive capacity of caretakers.)

Defining Characteristics: (Specify: expression and/or confirmation of concern and inadequate knowledge about long-term care needs, problems and complications, anxiety and guilt, overprotection of child.)

Goal: Family will cope effectively with child's illness by (date and time to evaluate).

Outcome Criteria

✔ Family identifies 3 effective coping mechanisms related to chronic illness of child.

✔ Family members establish short term and long-term goals for family.

NOC: *Family Coping*

INTERVENTIONS	RATIONALES
Assess family's coping methods and their effectiveness; family interactions and expectations related to long-term care, developmental level of family; response of siblings; knowledge and use of support systems and resources; presence of guilt and anxiety; overprotection and/or overindulgent behaviors.	Identifies coping methods that work and the need to develop new coping skills and behaviors, family attitudes; child with special long-term needs may strengthen or strain family relationships and an undue degree of overprotection may be detrimental to child's growth and development (disallowing school attendance or peer activities, avoiding discipline of child, and disallowing child to assume responsibility for ADL.
Encourage family members to express problem areas and explore solutions responsibly.	Reduces anxiety and enhances understanding; provides family an opportunity to identify problems and develop problem solving strategies.
Help family establish short- and long-term goals for child and integrate child into family activities, include participation of all family members in care routines.	Promotes involvement and control over situations and maintains role of family members and parents.
Provide assistance of social worker, counselor, or other as needed.	Gives support to the family faced with long-term care of child with a serious illness.
Suggest community agencies and contact with the National Hemophilia Foundation or other families with a child with hemophilia.	Provides information and support to child and family.

(continues)

(continued)

INTERVENTIONS	RATIONALES
Encourage family members to express feelings, such as how they deal with the chronic needs of family member and coping patterns that help or hinder adjustment to the problems.	Allows for venting of feelings, which relieves guilt and anxiety and helps determine need for information and support.
Provide information regarding long-term care and treatments.	Enhances family understanding of medical regimen and responsibilities of family members.
Teach family that overprotective behavior may hinder growth and development and that child should be treated as normally as possible.	Promotes understanding of importance of making child one of the family and the adverse effects of overprotection of the child.

NIC: *Family Involvement*

Evaluation

(Date/time of evaluation of goal)

(Has goal been met? Not met? Partially met?)

(What 3 coping mechanisms did the family identify? What are the short- and long-term goals established by the family? Provide quotes.)

(Revisions to care plan? D/C care plan? Continue care plan?)

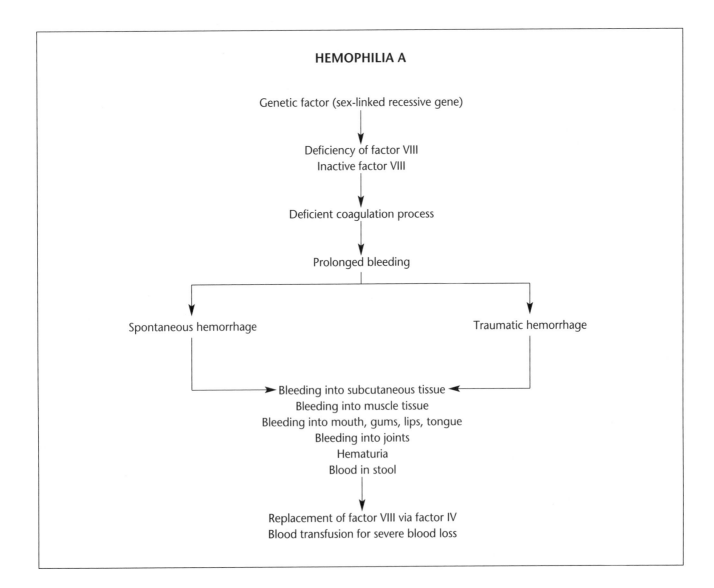

HEMOPHILIA A

Genetic factor (sex-linked recessive gene)

↓

Deficiency of factor VIII
Inactive factor VIII

↓

Deficient coagulation process

↓

Prolonged bleeding

Spontaneous hemorrhage   Traumatic hemorrhage

→ Bleeding into subcutaneous tissue ←
Bleeding into muscle tissue
Bleeding into mouth, gums, lips, tongue
Bleeding into joints
Hematuria
Blood in stool

↓

Replacement of factor VIII via factor IV
Blood transfusion for severe blood loss

CHAPTER 8.4

ITP

Idiopathic thrombocytopenic purpura (ITP) is an acquired hemorrhagic blood disorder. It is characterized by excessive destruction of platelets (thrombocytopenia) and purpura (a discoloration caused by petechiae beneath the skin). Etiology is unknown but it is believed to be an autoimmune response to disease-related antigens. ITP is classified into two forms: 1) acute form, which arises usually after an upper respiratory infection, measles, mumps, or chickenpox; and 2) chronic form, which is unresponsive to treatment (with persistent thrombocytopenia) beyond 6 months of diagnosis. Classic signs and symptoms of ITP may include: easy bruising with petechiae, and/or ecchymosis over bony prominences; bleeding from mucous membranes (i.e., epistaxis, bleeding gums); hematuria; hematemesis; hemarthrosis; hematomas over the lower extremities. ITP is seen most frequently between the ages of 2 and 10 years in children. It is rarely seen in infants less than 6 months of age. Treatment is primarily supportive as the course of this disease is self-limiting.

MEDICAL CARE

Diagnostic Evaluation of ITP: Platelet count (below 20,000 mm^3 to 30,000 mm^3); bone marrow aspiration (to rule out malignant infiltration of the marrow); abnormal platelet function (prolonged bleeding time, tourniquet test, and clot retraction); higher than normal levels of megakaryocytes; all other blood studies are typically normal. Also, lab studies are performed to rule out systemic lupus erythematosus, lymphoma, and leukemia.

Gamma Globulin (IVIG) (IV): can be expensive.

Corticosteroids: sometimes helpful in increasing the platelet count.

Anti-D Antibody Therapy: may increase platelet count after 48 hours.

Blood Transfusions: packed red blood cells are given to replace blood lost in symptomatic children with ITP. Platelet transfusions are seldom administered.

Splenectomy: reserved for symptomatic children with the chronic form of ITP or used as an emergency treatment when life-threatening hemorrhage occurs. Usually only performed in children older than 5 years.

Pain Control: acetaminophen products are substituted for salicylates.

COMMON NURSING DIAGNOSES

See RISK FOR INJURY

Related to: Autoimmune destruction of platelets.

Defining Characteristics: (Specify: petechiae, ecchymoses, hematomas, damage from trauma.)

See HYPERTHERMIA

Related to: Infection.

Defining Characteristics: (Specify: elevated temperature (above 38.5° C); elevated WBC counts indicating infection; and/or the presence of a positive culture for a bacterial organism.)

ADDITIONAL NURSING DIAGNOSES

ALTERED PROTECTION

Related to: Abnormal blood profile (thrombocytopenia).

Defining Characteristics: (Specify: platelet count below 20,000 cu mm/dL, petechiae, ecchymoses, bleeding from any mucous membrane area, hematomas on legs.)

Goal: Child will be protected from effects of thrombocytopenia by (date and time to evaluate).

Outcome Criteria

✔ No bleeding from any source.

NOC: *Abuse Protection*

INTERVENTIONS	RATIONALES
Assess for bleeding from gums, hematemesis, hematuria, hemathrosis, hematomas, epistaxis, or evidence of easy bruising, petechial rash.	Provides information and data indicating low platelet level and increased tendency for bleeding.
Avoid trauma to tissues by avoiding use of hard toothbrush or dental floss, taking rectal temperatures, performing unnecessary invasive procedures, and if administering an IM injection, applying pressure for 5 minutes to site.	Prevents bleeding caused by trauma to sensitive areas.
Administer medications (specify) as ordered.	Administered to children who are at highest risk for excessive bleeding.
Administer packed RBCs as ordered and monitor for responses, expected and adverse reactions.	Administered to replace blood loss or increase platelets.
Provide support in a warm, accepting environment for parents and child.	Promotes trust and comfort during periods of stress.
Teach parents and child about cause of disorder, reason for treatment and signs and symptoms indicating presence or relapse of disease.	Provides information about the disease needed to understand treatments and care.

INTERVENTIONS	RATIONALES
Inform parents and child to avoid rough contact play; blowing nose hard; straining at defecation; toys with sharp edges; using hard toothbrush; eating hard, rough foods.	Prevents trauma that causes bleeding.
Teach parents and child about medications and to avoid aspirin and aspirin over-the-counter products.	Promotes compliance in drug therapy to prevent relapses in bleeding; aspirin prevents platelet aggregation.
Teach child to avoid those with upper respiratory infections or any illness.	Prevents risk for infection in susceptible child.
Teach about and allow return demonstration of urine and stool testing for blood using dipstick and hematest; inform to report other signs of bleeding including fatigue, pallor, headache, and blood in sputum or vomitus.	Identifies presence of bleeding in gastrointestinal or urinary tract or any other area.

NIC: *Surveillance*

Evaluation

(Date/time of evaluation of goal)

(Has goal been met? Not met? Partially met?)

(Is there any evidence of bleeding? What types of bleeding were ruled out?)

(Revisions to care plan? D/C care plan? Continue care plan?)

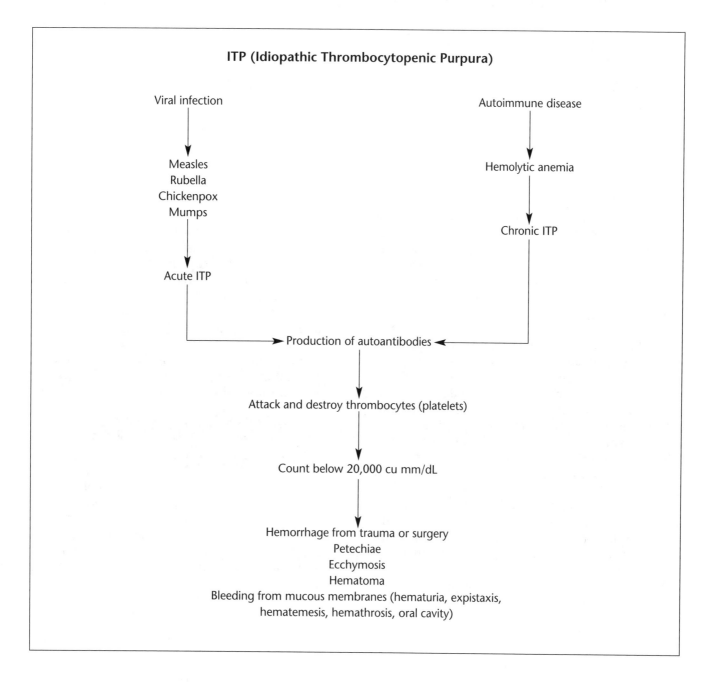

ITP (Idiopathic Thrombocytopenic Purpura)

Viral infection

Measles
Rubella
Chickenpox
Mumps

Acute ITP

Autoimmune disease

Hemolytic anemia

Chronic ITP

Production of autoantibodies

Attack and destroy thrombocytes (platelets)

Count below 20,000 cu mm/dL

Hemorrhage from trauma or surgery
Petechiae
Ecchymosis
Hematoma
Bleeding from mucous membranes (hematuria, expistaxis,
hematemesis, hemathrosis, oral cavity)

CHAPTER 8.5

LEUKEMIA AND LYMPHOMA

Leukemia is a malignant hemopoietic disease which is characterized by an unrestricted proliferation of poorly differentiated lymphocytes called blast cells that replace normal blood marrow elements. It occurs more frequently in male children after age 1 year. The peak age of onset is between 2 and 6 years. In children, the two most common forms of leukemia are: acute lymphoid leukemia (ALL) and acute myelogenous leukemia (AML).

Pathologic effects of leukemia include the replacement of normal bone marrow elements by leukemic cells which results in clinical manifestations of anemia, neutropenia, and thrombocytopenia. Symptoms related to anemia may result in fatigue, weakness, pallor, and lethargy. Neutropenia predisposes the child to febrile episodes and infection. Symptoms related to thrombocytopenia may result in cutaneous bruises or purpura, petechiae, epistaxis, melena, and gingival bleeding. Other common symptoms related to leukemic infiltration include: hepatosplenomegaly and lymphadenopathy; bone and joint pain; anorexia; abdominal pain; weight loss. Other symptoms, that are very rare, may include: hematuria, gastrointestinal bleeding, or central nervous system (CNS) bleeding. Prognosis is based on age and initial WBC at diagnosis, sex, histologic type of the disease, number of chromosomes, the DNA-index, morphology and cell-surface immunologic markers.

Lymphoma encompasses a group of neoplastic diseases that arise from the lymphoid and hemopoietic systems. There are two types: Hodgkin's disease and non-Hodgkin's lymphoma (NHL). NHL occurs more frequently and is the third most common childhood malignancy. In both types, it is observed in children under 15 years of age, and boys are affected more than girls. The peak incidence of NHL is between the ages of 7 and 11 years. Characteristics of Hodgkin's disease include: differentiated cells; pattern of infiltration is specific; subacute and a prolonged onset; and localized disease is present at the time of diagnosis. Characteristics of NHL include: undifferentiated cells; pattern of infiltration is diffuse; rapid onset; and widespread involvement at the time of diagnosis.

Clinical manifestations of Hodgkin's disease exhibit: 60% to 90% of cases presenting with cervical or supraclavicular adenopathy; the enlarged lymph node will be painless, firm, and movable; 50% of cases will also have mediastinal involvement with symptoms of airway obstruction; anorexia; weight loss; malaise; lethargy, and fever. Clinical manifestations of NHL depend on site of involvement: 1/3 of cases, intra-abdominal site, with mediastinal, peripheral nodal, right quadrant pain, with or without fever, 1/4 of cases, mediastinal site, with respiratory symptoms.

MEDICAL CARE

FOR LEUKEMIA

Treatment of leukemia involves multimodal therapy, including the use of chemotherapeutic agents with or without cranial irradiation in 3 phases. 1) Remission Induction Therapy includes corticosteroids (usually prednisone), vincristine (Oncovin), L-asparaginase, with or without doxorubicin; 2) CNS Prophylactic Therapy includes intrathecal methotrexate; 3) Maintenance Therapy (or Consolidation) includes weekly methotrexate and daily 6-mercaptopurine.

Supportive Therapies: for the treatment of side effects induced by the chemotherapy agents.

Prophylactic Antibiotic Therapy: to reduce the incidence of infections. Infection is a frequent threat resulting from immunosuppression effects of chemotherapy agents.

Granulocyte Colony-Stimulating Factors (GCSF): filgrastim (Neupogen) IV or subcutaneously 24 hours after chemotherapy is discontinued and is given for 10 to 14 days. GCSF directs granulocyte development, which decreases the duration of the neutropenia.

Replacement of Blood Elements: for the treatment of anemia, agranulocytopenia, and thrombocytopenia.

Prevention and Treatment of Oral Ulcers (Stomatitis): Peridex is the most commonly used mouth rinse to prevent or treat Candida and bacterial infections. Other mouth rinses that can be used include normal saline or baking soda solutions. Antifungal and antibacterial mouthwashes (nystatin) are used after mouth rinses 30 minutes after using Peridex. Use a soft sponge toothbrush (Toothette).

Severe Oral Infections: Acyclovir may be used to treat severe oral lesions.

Treatment of Oral Ulcer Pain: utilization of analgesics such as Chloraseptic lozenges, Orabase, or opiates.

Prevention and Management of Nausea and Vomiting: administration of antiemetic before the chemotherapy begins (30 minutes to 1 hour) and every 2, 4, or 6 hours for at least 24 hours after chemotherapy.

Diagnostic Evaluation of Leukemia (includes the following):
Complete Blood Count: decreased white blood cells, red blood cells, and platelets.

Physical Examination: liver, spleen, lymph nodes and the mediastinal area; weight loss; bone or joint pain; petechiae; abdominal pain.

Bone Marrow Aspiration: reveals hypercellularity with 60% to 100% blast cells.

Lumbar Puncture: evaluates the presence of central nervous system (CNS) leukemia.

Number of Chromosomes: number of chromosomes (ploidy or the DNA index) in the lymphoblasts. Better prognosis: DNA index of more than 1.16 and more than 46 chromosomes.

Cytogenic Abnormalities: presence of translocation of portions of one chromosome (e.g., the Philadelphia chromosome). Presence of the Philadelphia chromosome is least favorable.

Enzymes: lactic dehydrogenase (LDH), serum glutamic oxaloacetic transaminase (SGOT) and serum glutamic pyruvic transaminase (SGPT).

Monoclonal Antibodies: used to detect the presence of the common ALL antigen (CALLA) on leukemic cells. A positive CALLA is associated with a good prognosis.

Cell-Surface Immunologic Markers: B-cell (early pre B-cell, pre B-cell or B-cell) or T-cell.

Urine Tests: blood urea nitrogen (BUN), creatinine, and uric acid may be elevated.

Computerized Tomography Scans (CT): may reveal infiltrated sites with leukemic cells, such as the kidneys, testes, prostrate, ovaries, gastrointestinal tract, and lungs.

FOR LYMPHOMA

Medical Care for Hodgkin's Disease and NHL:
Diagnostic Evaluation for Hodgkin's Disease:
Laboratory Studies: CBC, erythrocyte sedimentation rate (ESR), serum copper and iron levels, serum ferritin and transferrin, renal and liver function tests, baseline thyroid function tests, T and B lymphocyte levels, PPD skin test.

Evaluation Includes: chest X-ray; CT scan of the mediastinal, pulmonary and upper abdominal area; ultrasound of neck and abdomen; isotope scanning; MRI; lymphangiogram (LAG); lymph node biopsy.

Diagnostic Evaluation for Non-Hodgkin's Disease:
Laboratory Studies: CBC with differential, liver and renal function studies, electrolyte, calcium, phosphorus, magnesium, lactate dehydrogenase (LDH), uric acid, EBV titers and urinalysis.

Evaluation Includes: bone marrow aspiration, lumbar puncture, lymph node biopsy, radiographic studies, CT scans of the lungs and gastrointestinal tract.

Supportive Therapies for Both Types: are similar to the care discussed in the leukemia child.

Treatment for Hodgkin's Disease: radiation and chemotherapy.

Chemotherapy Agents for Hodgkin's Disease: (2 regimens) **1) MOPP:** mechlorethamine, vincristine, prednisone, and procarbazine; **2) ABVD:** (for advanced disease) adriamycin, bleomycin, vinblastine, and dacarbazine.

Treatment for Non-Hodgkin's Disease: chemotherapy and radiation therapy.

Chemotherapy Agents for NHL: similar to leukemia.

COMMON NURSING DIAGNOSES

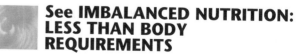

See IMBALANCED NUTRITION: LESS THAN BODY REQUIREMENTS

Related to: (Specify: loss of appetite; and/or pain in mouth; induced malabsorption or enteropathy [caused by abdominal radiation, chemotherapy, abdominal surgery, or frequent antibiotic use]; and anorexia-inducing substances [secreted by tumor cells]; xerostomia (irreversible dryness of mouth], destruction of microvilli of taste buds and/or lining of salivary glands [all can be caused by radiation therapy].)

Defining Characteristics: (Specify: anorexia, nausea, vomiting, stomatitis, mucositis, decreased salivation, cachexia, fatigue, diarrhea, alterations in taste, gustatory changes, weight loss, abdominal pain, psychologic and sociocultural factors.)

See RISK FOR DEFICIENT FLUID VOLUME

Related to: Excessive losses.

Defining Characteristics: (Specify: vomiting and diarrhea; blood losses (i.e., hemorrhagic cystitis, epistaxis, hemoptysis.)

See DIARRHEA

Related to: (Specify: surgery, radiation, chemotherapy, increased emotional stress, use of nutritional supplements, lactose intolerance, fecal impaction, tumor growth, infection or antibiotics.)

Defining Characteristics: (Specify: abnormal increase in quantity, frequency, and fluid content of stool.)

See RISK FOR IMPAIRED SKIN INTEGRITY

Related to: (Specify: delayed wound healing, immobility, external exposure to radiation, administration of chemotherapy and antibiotics.)

Defining Characteristics: (Specify: radiation effects: erythema, dryness, itching, increased pigmentation, dry desquamation, necrotic tissue; chemotherapy and antibiotic induced side effects: local phlebitis, stomatitis, mucositis, maculopapular rash, hyperpigmentation, nail changes, pruritus, dermatitis, alopecia, photosensitivity, acne, erythema, poor wound healing.)

See RISK FOR INFECTION

Related to: (Specify: disease process; immunosuppression caused by required chemotherapy; prolonged antibiotic and prednisone therapy; skin breakdown, serious bacterial, viral fungal, and protozoan infections; surgery and/or splenectomy; invasive proce-

dures; GI obstruction; malnutrition, inadequate serum protein level.)

Defining Characteristics: (Specify: increase in body temperature above normal range [>38.3° C or 101° F], neutropenia; inadequate number of neutrophils: severe risk of infection [<500/mm^3] or moderate risk of infection [<1000 mm^3]; presence of pathogens may or may not be identified from blood cultures.)

ADDITIONAL NURSING DIAGNOSES

FEAR

Related to: Diagnostic tests, procedures, treatments, diagnosis and prognosis.

Defining Characteristics: (Specify: child: crying, screaming, combative behaviors, anger, withdrawn behaviors, and verbalized fears; parents: fear, guilt, depression, anxiety.)

Goal: Child will experience decreased fear by (date and time to evaluate).

Outcome Criteria

✔ Child is calm.

✔ Child reports feeling less afraid.

NOC: *Fear Control*

INTERVENTIONS	RATIONALES
Assess child and parents' level of anxiety and fear.	Provides information about fears.
Explain to the child what will take place and what the child will feel, see, and hear during various procedures.	To increase the child's sense of control before and during procedures.
Encourage child and parents to be involved with procedure (specify).	To promote the child's and parents' sense of control.
Remain nonjudgmental regarding the child's behaviors and fears.	Encourages supportive relationship child's behavior.
Teach parents and child about the disease process and treatments, including radiation chemotherapy and its benefits and side effects (nausea, vomiting, diarrhea, stomatitis, alopecia are possibilities but are temporary).	Provides information that will relieve fear and anxiety; understanding of treatments and effect on body image.

INTERVENTIONS	RATIONALES
Explain all procedures, treatments, and care in simple, direct, honest terms and repeat as often as necessary; reinforce physician information if necessary and provide specific information as needed.	Supplies information about diagnostic procedures and tests, such as CBC, platelets with chemotherapy; and scans and X-rays for diagnosis.
Introduce child to another who has same disease.	Provides information and support from a peer with the same condition and who has empathy.

 Anxiety Reduction

Evaluation

(Date/time of evaluation of goal)

(Has goal been met? Not met? Partially met?)

(Describe child's behavior. Did child report feeling less fearful? Use quotes.)

(Revisions to care plan? D/C care plan? Continue care plan?)

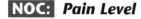 **PAIN**

Related to: (Specify: disease-related, treatment-related and procedure-related.)

Defining Characteristics: (Specify: multidimensional aspects of the cancer pain experience in children with cancer include components of assessment of cognitive of self-report, physiologic responses, behavioral manifestations, and the child's developmental level.)

Goal: Child will experience less pain by (date and time to evaluate).

Outcome Criteria

✔ Ranks pain as less than (specify level and pain scale being used).

NOC: *Pain Level*

INTERVENTIONS	RATIONALES
Assess the following three areas: 1) self-report responses of the child's pain (use words and pain assessment tools that help the child to describe pain (specify);	Provides information about pain that varies with age, developmental level of child and is unique to a particular child's learned emotional responses;

INTERVENTIONS	RATIONALES
2) behavioral manifestations (i.e., crying, facial expressions, muscle tension, screaming, pain verbalization, physical resistance, favors affected body parts, more common to observe during procedure-related pain or acute episodes); and 3) physiologic responses (evaluation of sweating palms, increased heart and respiratory rates, increased blood pressure, use along with self-report and behavioral assessments).	degree of pain and fatigue influence ability of child to perceive and identify discomfort.
Assess need for pain management.	Ensures consistency of pain management strategies.
Administer analgesics as prescribed (specify), on a preventive pain schedule, and monitor side effects of analgesics.	Ensures effective pain management; promotes comfort and rest; fosters a trusting and caring relationship between the child, family, and health care team.
Apply EMLA cream to sites to be used for intrusive painful procedures (i.e., venipuncture, bone marrow aspiration, lumbar puncture, implanted port access, subcutaneous and intramuscular injections); it must be applied 1 hour before the procedure to be effective.	Minimizes pain related to intrusive procedures; ensures child's safety during scheduled intrusive procedures.
Evaluate effectiveness of pain relief from all pain medication used.	Ensures effective pain control and management.
Promote rest and avoid disturbing child unnecessarily.	Decreases stimuli that increase pain, and promotes rest to conserve energy.
Maintain body alignment and support, and immobilize limbs with pillows and sand bags.	Promotes comfort and prevents contractures.
Apply heat (moist or dry) to painful areas.	Relieves pain by promoting circulation to the area.
Provide toys and activities for quiet play appropriate for age; use music, relaxation techniques; remain with child when pain is most acute.	Provides diversion and distraction from pain.
Inform child of cause of pain and interventions to relieve it, of how medications are administered and actions to expect; to report pain before it becomes severe.	Promotes understanding of pain response and methods to reduce it.

(continues)

(continued)

INTERVENTIONS	RATIONALES
Educate child and parents on various distraction techniques (i.e., counting, music, imagery, deep breathing, self-talk, positioning, reassurance, prayer, massage, therapeutic touch, relaxation).	Enhances trust between the nurse, child and the family; also, may minimize the child's pain perceptions and foster a sense of control during intrusive procedures.

NIC: *Pain Management*

Evaluation

(Date/time of evaluation of goal)

(Has goal been met? Not met? Partially met?)

(What is pain rating? Specify scale used.)

(Revisions to care plan? D/C care plan? Continue care plan?)

 IMPAIRED ORAL MUCOUS MEMBRANES

Related to: (Specify: administration of chemotherapy agents, side effect of radiotherapy, long-term administration of antibiotics.)

Defining Characteristics: (Specify: oral ulcers [stomatitis] are red, eroded, painful areas in the mouth and pharynx; and similar lesions [as stomatitis] that may extend along the esophagus and in the rectal area.)

Goal: Child will experience healing mucous membranes by (date and time to evaluate).

Outcome Criteria

✔ Mucous membranes are intact without lesions.

NOC: *Tissue Integrity: Skin and Mucous Membrane*

INTERVENTIONS	RATIONALES
Assess mouth daily for oral ulcers, pain, ability to ingest foods; provide meticulous oral hygiene, to prevent oral breakdown and to promote healing (start as soon as a drug is used that causes oral ulcers): use a softsponge toothbrush or toothette, administer	To effectively treat oral ulcers and to promote healing; to prevent bacterial and *Candida* infections; to prevent trauma to oral mucosa.

INTERVENTIONS	RATIONALES
frequent mouth rinses, at least every 4 hours and after meals; mouth rinses commonly used include Peridex, normal saline with or without sodium bicarbonate solution.	
Administer nystatin mouthwashes as ordered after mouth rinses; restrict oral intake for 30 minutes after taking this mouthwash.	To maintain oral integrity; to treat bacterial and fungal infections.
Administer Acyclovir (topically or IV) for oral herpes lesions as ordered.	To prevent or treat herpetic infections.
Apply local anesthetics to ulcerated areas before meals and as needed to relieve pain; topical agents include: Ora-base; can be applied directly to oral lesions as ordered or swished and spit.	To relieve pain associated with oral ulcers.
Apply lip balm (daily).	To prevent cracking and fissuring of lips; to maintain lip integrity.
Encourage a bland, soft diet and selection of foods by child.	To minimize oral discomfort and irritation; enhances sense of control, independence, decreases sense of helplessness; may increase child's level of nutrition.
Avoid using lemon glycerin swabs.	To prevent irritation of mouth ulcers decay of teeth.
Avoid juices containing ascorbic acid, hot, cold, or spicy foods.	To prevent discomfort to oral ulcers.
Avoid use of hydrogen peroxide as a mouth rinse.	It will delay healing of oral ulcers by breaking down protein.
Avoid use of milk of magnesia.	To prevent drying of oral mucosa.
Provide education to parents and child: 1) chemotherapy and radiation may cause oral ulcers; 2) effective oral hygiene strategies to prevent and treat oral ulcers; 3) child may require hospitalization (for hydration, parental nutrition, pain control of oral ulcers) if stomatitis interferes with food or fluid intake.	Promotes understanding of oral stomatitis, significance of daily oral hygiene, and pain control for oral ulcers.

NIC: *Surveillance*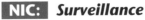

Evaluation

(Date/time of evaluation of goal)

(Has goal been met? Not met? Partially met?)

(Is there any evidence of mucous membrane impairment or new lesions?)

(Revisions to care plan? D/C care plan? Continue care plan?)

RISK FOR INJURY

Related to: (Specify: disease process; immunosuppression, thrombocytopenia and other side effects from chemotherapy and radiation treatments.)

Defining Characteristics: (Specify: fever [>38.3° C or 101° F], secondary infections; fatigue; anemia [hemoglobin level <11 g]; neutropenia [absolute neutrophil count <1000/mm³]; risk of hemorrhage or bleeding tendencies [platelet count of 20,000/mm³]; side effects of chemotherapy.)

Goal: Child will not experience injury by (date and time to evaluate).

Outcome Criteria

✔ Temperature remains <101° F.

✔ No evidence of bleeding.

NOC: *Risk Detection*

INTERVENTIONS	RATIONALES
Assess for bleeding from any site, WBC, platelet count, Hct, absolute neutrophil count, and febrile episodes.	Provides information about frank bleeding or blood profile abnormalities that predispose to bleeding caused by bone marrow suppression and immuno-suppression resulting from chemotherapy or radiation therapy.
Avoid trauma by not using hard toothbrush or dental floss, not taking rectal temperatures, not performing unnecessary invasive procedures.	Prevents bleeding during chemotherapy regimen, which alters platelet and clotting factors.
Carry out handwashing technique before giving care, use mask and gown when appropriate, provide a private room, monitor for any signs and symptoms of infection, especially pulmonary.	Prevents transmission of pathogens to a compromised immune system during chemotherapy if neutrophil count is less than 1000/cu mm.

INTERVENTIONS	RATIONALES
Teach parents and child to avoid rough play or sports, straining at defecation, blowing nose hard.	Prevents trauma that causes bleeding.
Teach parents and child to avoid those with upper respiratory infection or any illness.	Prevents risk for infection in the highly susceptible child.
Teach parents to report any fever, behavior changes, headache, dizziness, fatigue, pallor, slow oozing of blood from any area, exposure to a communicable disease.	Indicate complications associated with an abnormal blood profile.
Show and allow for return demonstration of urine and stool testing for blood using dipstick and hematest.	Identifies presence of bleeding in gastrointestinal or urinary tract.

NIC: *Surveillance*

Evaluation

(Date/time of evaluation of goal)

(Has goal been met? Not met? Partially met?)

(What is temperature? Is there any evidence of bleeding?)

(Revisions to care plan? D/C care plan? Continue care plan?)

DISTURBED BODY IMAGE

Related to: Side effects of chemotherapy and radiation therapy.

Defining Characteristics: (Specify: loss of hair; moon face; weight loss or gain; hyperpigmentation; skin rash or erythema; acne; skin thickening; or peeling of skin.)

Goal: Child will experience improved body image by (date and time to evaluate).

Outcome Criteria

✔ Child expresses feelings about how he or she looks.

✔ Child identifies at least 1 positive thing about own body.

NOC: *Body Image*

INTERVENTIONS	RATIONALES
Assess child for feelings about multiple restrictions in lifestyle, chronic illness, difficulty in school and social situations, inability to keep up with peers and participate in activities.	Provides information about status of self-concept and body image, that may require special attention.
Encourage expression of feelings and concerns and support communication with parents, teachers and peers.	Provides opportunity to vent feelings and reduce negative feelings about changes in appearance.
Avoid negative comment and stress positive activities and accomplishments.	Enhances body image and confidence.
Note withdrawal behavior and signs of depression.	Reveals responses to body image changes and possible poor adjustment to chances.
Show support and acceptance of changes in appearance of child; provide privacy as needed.	Promotes trust and demonstrates respect for child.
Encourage parents to maintain support for child.	Encourages acceptance of the child with special needs (must deal with long-term steroid therapy and its side effects, lifelong activity restrictions).
Teach parents and child about the risk for hair loss; correct misinformation and suggest ways to cope with body changes.	Provides correct information to assist in dealing with negative feelings about body.
Encourage parents to be flexible in care of child; to integrate care and routines into family activities, and allow child to participate in peer activities.	Promotes child's sense of well-being and of belonging and having control of life events by allowing participation in normal activities for age and enhancing developmental task achievement.
Assist parents and child to deal with peers and perceptions of appearance and how to tell others about change in appearance.	Prevents stigmatization of child by those who are not apprised of the child's disease; attitude of others will affect child's body image.
Suggest a cap, scarf, or other head covering.	Preserves body image by covering head if alopecia is present.
Suggest psychological counseling or child-life worker, and inform of functions performed by these professionals.	Assists in improving self-esteem and in learning, coping and problem solving skills.

NIC: *Self-Esteem Enhancement*

Evaluation

(Date/time of evaluation of goal)

(Has goal been met? Not met? Partially met?)

(What feelings about disability did child verbalize? What positive thing about their body did child identify? Use quotes.)

(Revisions to care plan? D/C care plan? Continue care plan?)

INEFFECTIVE COPING AND COMPROMISED FAMILY COPING

Related to: (Specify: for the child: separation from family, friends, home, and school activities; loss of control, altered self-image, altered body image, altered self-esteem, and altered sense of self-confidence. For the parents: uncertainty of child's future, sense of helplessness and powerlessness, multiple family stressors and demands [related to child's health care needs].)

Defining Characteristics: (Specify: for the child: depression, anxiety, withdrawn, excessive outbursts of temper, insecurity, sleep and/or eating disturbances, regressive behaviors, behavioral problems [acting out], denial, difficulties in interpersonal relationships, nonadherence with treatment. For parents: shock, disbelief, anger, guilt, numbness, denial, ambivalence, bargaining, overprotectiveness, grief for the loss of their healthy child, anticipatory grief for the potential loss of their child.)

Goal: Family and child will cope more effectively by (date and time to evaluate).

Outcome Criteria

✔ Family and child identify stressors.

✔ Family and child verbalize 3 effective coping mechanisms to use.

NOC: *Coping*

INTERVENTIONS	RATIONALES
Assess effectiveness of family coping methods; family interactions and expectations related to long-term, developmental level of family; response of	Provides information identifying successful coping methods or the need to develop new coping skills, behaviors and family attitudes; child with over-

INTERVENTIONS	RATIONALES
siblings; knowledge and use of support systems and resources; presence of guilt, anxiety, overprotective and/or overindulgent behaviors.	protection (e.g., not allowing child to attend school, participate in activities with peers, or assume responsibilities for ADL; avoiding disciplining of child) may be at risk in growth and development.
Encourage family members to express stressors and explore solutions responsibly.	Reduces anxiety and enhances understanding; allows family to identify problems and develop problem solving strategies.
Assist family in establishing short- and long-term goals for child and in integrating child into family activities; include participation of all family members in care routines.	Promotes involvement and control over situations, and maintains role of family members and parents.
Provide assistance of social worker, counselor, clergy, or other as needed.	Provides support to the family faced with long-term care of child with a serious, life-threatening illness.
Suggest community agencies and the American Cancer Society, that can provide contacts with families that have a child with leukemia or lymphoma.	Provides information and support to child and family.
Allow family members to express feelings on how they deal with the chronic needs of family member and on coping patterns that help or hinder adjustment to the problems.	Allows for venting of feelings to determine need for information and support, and relieves guilt and anxiety.

INTERVENTIONS	RATIONALES
Inform family of requested and needed information regarding long-term care and treatments.	Enhances family understanding of medical regimen and responsibilities of family members.
Inform family that overprotective behavior may hinder growth and development and that child should be treated as normally as possible.	Promotes understanding of importance of making child one of the family and the adverse effects of overprotection of the child.
Assist child and family to identify at least 3 coping mechanisms they can use to cope with the stressors of the child's illness.	Empowers the clients to take control of coping methods and find alternatives.

NIC: *Family Involvement*

Evaluation

(Date/time of evaluation of goal)

(Has goal been met? Not met? Partially met?)

(What stressors did the child and family identify? What 3 coping mechanisms did the child and family verbalize? Provide quotes.)

(Revisions to care plan? D/C care plan? Continue care plan?)

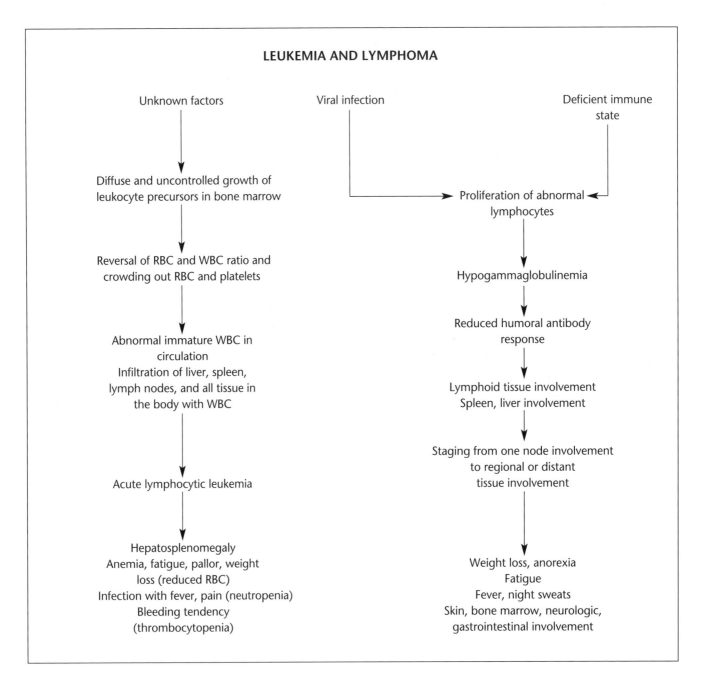

LEUKEMIA AND LYMPHOMA

Unknown factors

Viral infection

Deficient immune state

Diffuse and uncontrolled growth of leukocyte precursors in bone marrow

Proliferation of abnormal lymphocytes

Reversal of RBC and WBC ratio and crowding out RBC and platelets

Hypogammaglobulinemia

Reduced humoral antibody response

Abnormal immature WBC in circulation
Infiltration of liver, spleen, lymph nodes, and all tissue in the body with WBC

Lymphoid tissue involvement
Spleen, liver involvement

Staging from one node involvement to regional or distant tissue involvement

Acute lymphocytic leukemia

Hepatosplenomegaly
Anemia, fatigue, pallor, weight loss (reduced RBC)
Infection with fever, pain (neutropenia)
Bleeding tendency (thrombocytopenia)

Weight loss, anorexia
Fatigue
Fever, night sweats
Skin, bone marrow, neurologic, gastrointestinal involvement

UNIT 9

ENDOCRINE SYSTEM

CHAPTER 9.0

ENDOCRINE GROWTH AND DEVELOPMENT

The endocrine system includes the cells of certain glands that produce hormones; the organ or tissue sites that receive the hormone; and the transport system of the blood, lymph, and extracellular fluids that move the hormones from the point of origin to the point of utilization. Hormones may regulate general cell physiologic activities or may affect specific cells of the body. Glands included in this system are the pituitary, thyroid, parathyroid, adrenal, isles of Langerhans, ovaries, and testes. The system regulates and integrates functions with the neurologic system that assist the body to adjust behavior, growth, development, and sexual reproduction. In children, abnormal conditions involving these glands are caused by oversecretion or undersecretion of hormones or by a problem in the response to these hormones by the receiving organ or tissue. These abnormalities may result from congenital or acquired factors. They are usually treated by partial or complete surgical removal of the gland and/or drug therapy to replace hormone deficiencies.

GROWTH AND DEVELOPMENT

- Endocrine glands are well developed at birth, but their functions are immature.

- Secondary sex characteristics usually develop between 10 and 18 years of age in girls and between 12 and 20 years of age in boys; menarche usually occurs between 12 and 13 years of age.

CHAPTER 9.1

INSULIN-DEPENDENT DIABETES MELLITUS

Insulin-dependent diabetes mellitus (IDDM) is a metabolic disorder caused by a deficiency of insulin. The deficiency is thought to occur in those individuals who are genetically predisposed to the disease and who have experienced a precipitating event, commonly a viral infection or environmental change, that causes an autoimmune condition affecting the beta cells of the pancreas. It is treated by injection of insulin and regulation of diet and activity that maintain body functions. Complications that occur from improper coordination of these include hypoglycemia and hyperglycemia which, if untreated, lead to insulin shock or ketoacidosis. Long-term effects of the disease include neuropathy, nephropathy, retinopathy, atherosclerosis, and microangiopathy.

MEDICAL CARE

Insulin Replacement: given to control blood glucose concentrations; administered one, two, or more times/day individually prescribed for child.

Blood Glucose: reveals levels greater than 120 mg/dL in a fasting specimen and 200 mg/dL or greater in a random specimen; 300 mg/dL level in ketoacidosis.

Ketones: reveal increase in the blood and urine.

Urine Glucose: reveals glycosuria.

COMMON NURSING DIAGNOSES

See IMBALANCED NUTRITION: LESS THAN BODY REQUIREMENTS

Related to: Inability to metabolize glucose.

Defining Characteristics: (Specify: loss of weight with adequate food intake, lack of interest in food, inadequate intake, insufficient insulin, too much insulin.)

See RISK FOR IMPAIRED SKIN INTEGRITY

Related to: (Specify: injections and blood glucose monitoring, altered metabolic state, sensation, nutritional state.)

Defining Characteristics: (Specify: disruption of skin surfaces with daily injections [lipodystrophy], failure to rotate sites, weight loss, poor wound healing, dry skin.)

See RISK FOR DEFICIENT FLUID VOLUME

Related to: Osmotic diuresis.

Defining Characteristics: (Specify: output greater than intake, decreased urine output, dry skin and mucous membranes, poor skin turgor, dehydration with electrolyte depletion [K^+, Na^+, Cl^-, Mg^{2+}, PO^{3-}] with ketoacidosis, polyuria, polydipsia.)

ADDITIONAL NURSING DIAGNOSES

RISK FOR INJURY

Related to: (Specify: hyperglycemia or hypoglycemia.)

Defining Characteristics: (Specify: hyperglycemia—fatigue, irritability, headache, abdominal discomfort, weight loss, polyuria, polydipsia, polyphagia, dehydration, blurred vision; hypoglycemia—nervousness, sweating, hunger, palpitations, weakness, dizziness, pallor, behavior changes, uncoordinated gait.)

Goal: Client will not experience injury from hyperglycemia or hypoglycemia.

Outcome Criteria

✔ Blood glucose levels remain between 60 mg/dL and 120 mg/dL.

✔ Urine is free of ketones and glucose.

NOC: *Risk Detection*

INTERVENTIONS	RATIONALES
Assess for signs and symptoms of hyperglycemia, blood glucose level, urinary glucose and ketones, pH and electrolyte levels.	Provides information about complication caused by increased glucose levels resulting from improper diet, an illness, or omission of insulin administration; glucose is unable to enter the cells, and protein is broken down and converted to glucose by the liver, causing the hyperglycemia; fat and protein stores are depleted to provide energy for the body when carbohydrates are not able to be used for energy.
Administer insulin SC as ordered (specify), rotate sites, increase dosage as indicated by glucose levels; decrease food intake during an infection or illness and adjust insulin dosage during an illness.	Provides insulin replacement to maintain normal blood glucose levels without causing hypoglycemia; two or more injections may be given daily SC with a portable syringe pump or by intermittent bolus injections with a syringe and needle.
Provide diet with calories that balance expenditure for energy (specify) and correspond to type and action of insulin, and snacks between meals and at bedtime as appropriate.	Provides child's nutritional needs for proper growth and development using the exchange system developed and approved by the American Diabetic Association (ADA), or by carbohydrate counting—monitoring carbohydrate intake only, maintaining consistent level at meals and snacks, and adjusting insulin as needed (requires close collaboration with physician).
Promote exercise program consistent with dietary and insulin regimen; teach to increase carbohydrate intake before vigorous activities.	Aids in the utilization of dietary intake, regular activity may reduce amount of insulin required; a decrease in insulin and increased carbohydrate intake before vigorous exercise or activity may prevent hypoglycemia.
Assess for signs and symptoms of hypoglycemia, blood-glucose level.	Provides information about episodes of hypoglycemia resulting from increased activity without additional food intake or omission or incomplete ingestion of meals, incorrect insulin administration, illness.

INTERVENTIONS	RATIONALES
Provide rest and immediate source of a simple carbohydrate such as honey, milk, or fruit juice followed by a complex carbohydrate such as bread in amounts of 15 gm; repeat intake in 10 minutes for expected response of a reduced pulse rate; administer IV 50 percent glucose or glucagon IM if hypoglycemia is severe.	Alleviates the symptoms of hypoglycemia as soon as symptoms are noted; glucagon releases the glycogen stored in the liver to assist in restoring glucose levels; IV glucose is administered when condition is severe and child is unable to take glucose source PO. Glucagon, a hormone, releases stored glycogen from the liver and raises blood glucose in 5 to 15 minutes.
Teach parents and child signs and symptoms to note, reasons why they occur, and interventions to correct the complication.	Provides information about abnormal blood glucose levels causing complications of hyperglycemia, hypoglycemia, and the consequences.
Teach parents and child to regulate insulin, manage dietary intake, and exercise to accommodate needs of individual child.	Maintains child's growth and development needs while preventing complications.
Teach parents and child to adjust insulin administration based on blood-glucose testing and glycosuria, during an illness or after changes in food intake or activities.	Prevents and/or treats hyperglycemia; avoids serious complication of ketoacidosis.
Teach parents and child to administer a quick-acting carbohydrate followed by a longer-acting carbohydrate and to have Lifesavers, sugar cubes, Insta-glucose on hand at all times; instruct parents that, in the case of severe hypoglycemia, if the child is unconscious or unable to take oral fluids, to rub honey or syrup on the child's buccal surface until alert enough to take fluids/foods by mouth.	Prevents and/or treats hypoglycemia.
Inform parents and child to report erratic blood and urine test results, difficulty in controlling blood glucose levels, presence of an infection or illness.	Prevents more serious complications and long-term effects of the disease; poor control leads to serious and severe consequences in a few hours.

NIC: *Surveillance*

Evaluation

(Date/time of evaluation of goal)

(Has goal been met? Not met? Partially met?)

(What is blood-glucose level? Is there any evidence of ketonuria or glucosuria?)

(Revisions to care plan? D/C care plan? Continue care plan?)

DEFICIENT KNOWLEDGE

Related to: Lack of information about disease.

Defining Characteristics: (Specify: new diagnosis of IDDM; request for information about pathology, insulin therapy, dietary requirements, activity/exercise needs, blood and urine testing, personal hygiene and health promotion.)

Goal: Clients will obtain information about child's illness and treatment by (date and time to evaluate).

Outcome Criteria

✔ Clients verbalize understanding of IDDM.

✔ Clients demonstrate correct blood-glucose monitoring insulin administration, dietary management, and exercise planning.

✔ Clients identify signs and symptoms of hypo- and hyperglycemia and correct response.

NOC: *Knowledge: Disease Process*

INTERVENTIONS	RATIONALES
Assess parents and child for knowledge of disease and ability to perform procedures and care, for educational level and learning capacity, and for developmental level.	Provides information needed to plan teaching program; children 8 to 10 years of age may be able to take responsibility for some of the care.
Teach about cause of disease, disease process and pathology; use pamphlets and other aids appropriate for age of child and level of comprehension of parents.	Provides basic information that may be used as a rationale for treatments and care and allows for different teaching strategies.
Provide a quiet, comfortable environment; allow time for teaching small amounts at a time	Prevents distractions and facilitates learning.

INTERVENTIONS	RATIONALES
and for reinforcement, demonstrations and return demonstrations; start teaching 1 day following diagnosis and limit sessions to 30 to 60 minutes.	
Include as many family members in teaching sessions as possible.	Promotes understanding and support of family and feeling of security for child.
Instruct parents and child in insulin administration including storing insulin, drawing up insulin into syringe, rotating vial instead of shaking, drawing clear insulin first if mixing 2 types in same syringe, injecting SC, rotating sites, adjusting dosages, reusing syringe, and needle, and disposing of them.	Promotes accurate administration of insulin, which prevents complications.
(Instruct in use of syringe-loaded injector.)	Provides temporary method of insulin administration if child is afraid to puncture skin.
(Instruct parents and child in operation and use of a portable insulin pump to adjust insulin delivery.)	Provides continuous subcutaneous insulin infusion.
Teach parents and child about collection and testing of blood for glucose 4 times a day (before meals and before bed), with a lancet and blood-testing meter or a reagent strip compared to a color chart; collection and testing of urine with ketostix or Clinitest (specify).	Monitors glucose and ketone levels in blood and urine.
Teach parents and child about dietary planning with emphasis on proper meal times and adequate caloric intake according to age as ordered (offer food lists for free foods and exchanges according to the basic four groups and assist in preparing sample menus). Teach that food intake depends on activity, and describe methods to judge amounts of foods; provide list of acceptable food items from "fast food" restaurants, published by the ADA.	Provides information about an important aspect of total care of the child with diabetes according to the American Diabetic Association guidelines.

(continues)

(continued)

INTERVENTIONS	RATIONALES
Teach parents and child about role of exercise and alterations needed in food and insulin intake with increased or decreased activity.	Provides information about usual activity pattern and effect on dietary intake and insulin needs.
Teach parents and child about skin problems associated with diabetes, need for regular dental examinations, foot care, protection of and proper care of nails, prevention of infections and exposure to infections, eye examinations, immunizations.	Provides information about common problems resulting from long-term effects of the disease.
Instruct parents and child in record-keeping for insulin, test results, responses to diet and exercise, noncompliance in medical regimen and effects.	Provides a method to enhance self-care and demonstrates the need to notify physician for treatment evaluation and possible change.
Encourage child to wear or carry identification and information about the disease, treatment, and physician name.	Provides information in event of emergency.

NIC: *Teaching: Disease Process*

Evaluation

(Date/time of evaluation of goal)

(Has goal been met? Not met? Partially met?)

(Did clients verbalize understanding of IDDM? Did clients demonstrate correct glucose monitoring, insulin administration, diet management, and exercise planning? Did clients identify signs and symptoms of hypo- and hyperglycemia and correct response? Use quotes.)

(Revisions to care plan? D/C care plan? Continue care plan?)

COMPROMISED FAMILY COPING

Related to: (Specify: inadequate or incorrect information or understanding, prolonged disease or disability progression that exhausts the physical and emotional supportive capacity of caretakers.)

Defining Characteristics: (Specify: expression and/or confirmation of concern and inadequate knowledge about long-term care needs, problems and complications, anxiety and guilt, overprotection of child.)

Goal: Family will cope effectively by (date and time to evaluate).

Outcome Criteria

✔ Family explores feelings about long-term needs of child.

✔ Family identifies support systems and coping skills.

NOC: *Family Coping*

INTERVENTIONS	RATIONALES
Assess family coping methods and effectiveness, family interactions and expectations related to long-term care, developmental level of family, response of siblings, knowledge and use of support systems and resources, presence of guilt and anxiety, overprotection and/or overindulgence behaviors.	Identifies coping methods that work and the need to develop new coping skills and behaviors, family attitudes; child with special long-term needs may strengthen or strain family relationships, and that overprotection may be detrimental to child's growth and development (e.g., not allowing child to attend school or participate in peer activities; avoiding discipline of child; and not allowing child to assume responsibilities for care).
Encourage family members and child to express problem areas, anxiety and explore solutions responsibly.	Reduces anxiety and enhances understanding; provides family an opportunity to identify problems and develop problem-solving strategies.
Assist family to establish short- and long-term goals for child and to integrate child into family activities, include participation of all family members in care routines.	Promotes involvement in and control over situations and maintains role of family members and parents.
Provide assistance of social worker, counselor, clergy, or other as needed.	Provides support to the family faced with long-term care of child with a chronic illness.
Suggest community agencies and contact with the American Diabetic Association or other families with a diabetic child.	Provides information and support to child and family.
Allow family members to express feelings, to tell how they deal with the chronic needs of family member, and to describe coping patterns that help or hinder adjustment to the problems.	Allows for venting of feelings to determine need for information and support and to relieve guilt and anxiety.

INTERVENTIONS	RATIONALES
Teach family about long-term care and treatments.	Enhances family understanding of medical regimen and responsibilities of family.
Teach family that overprotective behavior may hinder growth and development so they should treat child as normally as possible.	Promotes understanding of importance of making child one of the family and demonstrates the adverse effects of overprotection of the child.
Discuss importance of follow-up appointments for physical examinations, laboratory tests.	Promotes positive outcome when family collaborates with the physician and health team to monitor disease.

NIC: *Family Involvement*

Evaluation

(Date/time of evaluation of goal)

(Has goal been met? Not met? Partially met?)

(Did family explore feelings about long-term needs of child? What support systems and coping mechanisms did the family identify? Provide quotes.)

(Revisions to care plan? D/C care plan? Continue care plan?)

INSULIN-DEPENDENT DIABETES MELLITUS (IDDM)

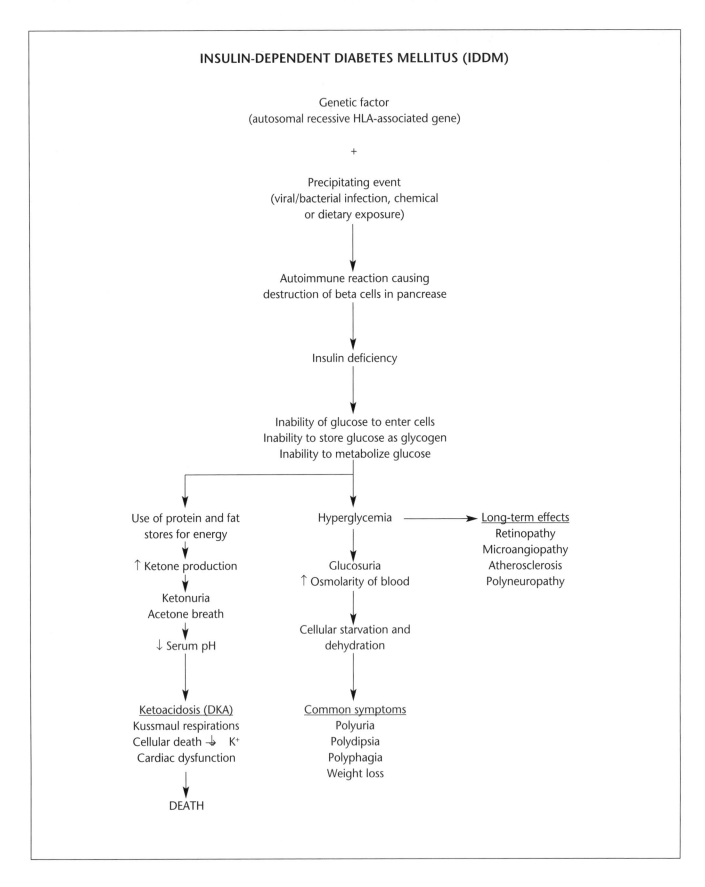

CHAPTER 9.2

HYPOTHYROIDISM

Hypothyroidism is the result of inadequate thyroid hormone production to maintain body processes. It may be the result of congenital thyroid abnormality and therefore present in infancy or it may become notable during the first two years of life. It appears later when production is inadequate to maintain body processes as rapid growth increases the need for hormones. Acquired causes of the condition may be thyrotoxicosis, thyroidectomy, irradiation, infections, and dietary deficiency of iodine. Secretions of the thyroid gland include thyroid hormone (thyroxine, T4 and triiodothyronine, T3) which are bound to proteins in the blood (thyroxine-binding globulin, TBG) and thyrocalcitonin (maintains calcium levels in blood). The hormones are controlled by the thyroid-stimulating hormone (TSH) that is secreted by the anterior pituitary gland. Treatment of hypothyroidism is by thyroid hormone replacement, which involves prompt intervention in the infant and gradually increasing amounts of hormone administration in the child. Treatment is maintained throughout life to ensure restoration of thyroid deficiency.

MEDICAL CARE

Hormones: levothyroxine sodium (Synthroid) as replacement therapy for diminished or absent thyroid function.

Vitamins: vitamin D to ensure calcium levels during periods of growth requiring increased demands.

Lab Tests: T3 (triodothyronine), T4 (thyroxine), TBG (thyroxine-binding globulin), TSH (thyroid-stimulating hormone) by RIA (radioimmunoassay testing) reveals decreases indicating hormone deficiency.

Protein-Bound Iodine: reveals increases after 2 months of age.

Bone X-ray: reveals bone age and effect of thyroid deficiency or treatment.

Scan: reveals presence of gland with location, size, and shape of the organ; radioactive iodine uptake by thyroid gland is scanned and displayed on a screen for examination.

COMMON NURSING DIAGNOSES

See RISK FOR IMPAIRED SKIN INTEGRITY

Related to: Internal factor of altered metabolic state (hypothyroidism).

Defining Characteristics: Skin pale, cool, dry, and scaly.

See IMBALANCED NUTRITION: LESS THAN BODY REQUIREMENTS

Related to: Inability to ingest or digest food; decreased body processes.

Defining Characteristics: Poor feeding, choking, thick tongue in infant; lethargy, reduced metabolic process, anorexia in child.

 ### See CONSTIPATION

Related to: Less than adequate physical activity, decreased body process.

Defining Characteristics: Lethargy, decreased peristalsis, fatigue, reduced activity level.

ADDITIONAL NURSING DIAGNOSES

DEFICIENT KNOWLEDGE

Related to: Lack of information about disorder.

Defining Characteristics: Request for information about cause and treatment of the disorder, thyroid replacement.

Goal: Clients will obtain information about child's illness and treatment by (date and time to evaluate).

Outcome Criteria

✔ Clients verbalize understanding of cause and treatment for hypothyroidism.

NOC: *Knowledge: Disease Process*

INTERVENTIONS	RATIONALES
Assess knowledge of disorder, signs and symptoms for infant or child as appropriate, replacement therapy.	Provides information needed to develop plan of instruction to ensure compliance with medical regimen.
Teach parents and child about cause of thyroid deficiency and need for prompt treatment in infants and for gradual increases in thyroxine in children to achieve euthyroidism.	Provides thyroid replacement over 4 to 8 weeks in the child without causing hyperthyroidism.
Teach parents and child about thyroid replacement including administering daily for life without missing doses, crushing and mixing with food, giving at breakfast time.	Ensures compliance with correct administration of thyroid replacement via oral route.

INTERVENTIONS	RATIONALES
Teach parents and child to report nervousness, irritability, tachycardia, diarrhea.	Indicates an excess of thyroid hormone and need for and adjustment in dosage.
Reassure parents and child that improvement will be gradual as hormone levels are achieved and sleep, elimination, appetite, growth, and activity levels will improve.	Promotes comfort and reduces anxiety caused by physical and mental changes brought about by the disorder, maintains realistic expectations from the treatment.

NIC: *Teaching: Disease Process*

Evaluation

(Date/time of evaluation of goal)

(Has goal been met? Not met? Partially met?)

(What did clients say about the cause and treatment of hypothyroidism?)

(Revisions to care plan? D/C care plan? Continue care plan?)

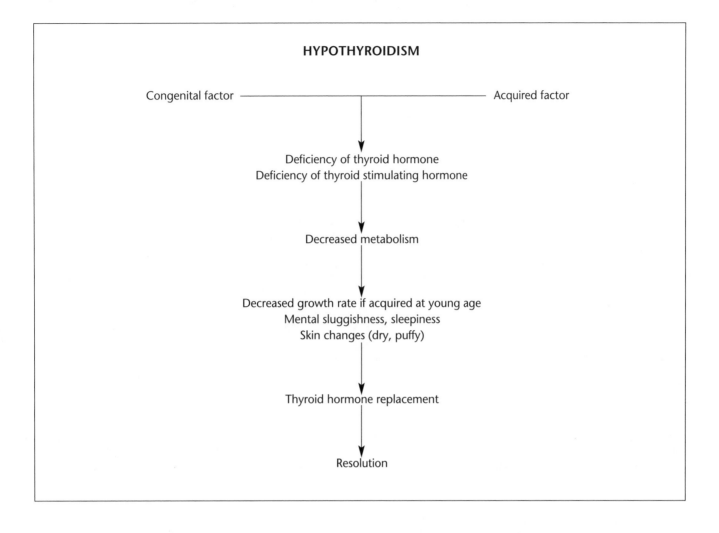

HYPOTHYROIDISM

Congenital factor ———————————— Acquired factor

Deficiency of thyroid hormone
Deficiency of thyroid stimulating hormone

Decreased metabolism

Decreased growth rate if acquired at young age
Mental sluggishness, sleepiness
Skin changes (dry, puffy)

Thyroid hormone replacement

Resolution

UNIT 10

INTEGUMENTARY SYSTEM

CHAPTER 10.0

INTEGUMENTARY SYSTEM: BASIC CARE PLAN

The integumentary system includes the skin and associated structures or appendages, which are hair, nails, and sensory skin receptors. Skin acts as a barrier to retain body fluids and electrolytes, a regulator of body heat, and a receptor of sensory stimuli (tactile, pain, heat and cold). It is made up of three layers including the epidermis (outer layer), the dermis (thicker layer directly under the epidermis), and the subcutaneous (fat and connective tissue under the dermis). Its appearance reflects the general health of an infant or child. Changes in the skin that alter appearance are a source of psychological stress and embarrassment to children. Common integumentary conditions of childhood are infections, lesions, wounds, and dermatitis disorders.

INTEGUMENTARY GROWTH AND DEVELOPMENT

Integumentary component structure and function:

- Skin is 1 mm thick at birth and increases to twice this thickness by maturity.
- Perspiration is present in the child over 1 month of age.
- Lanugo disappears by 3 months of age.
- Hair is soft and fine in texture in the young child and takes on adult characteristics with growth.
- Nails are soft in infant and young child and become hardened with growth and development.
- Pubic and axillary hair appear between 8 to 12 years of age, with axillary hair occurring 6 months later than pubic hair and facial hair in males occurring 6 months later than pubic hair; texture becomes coarse and curly with growth and development.

NURSING DIAGNOSES

RISK FOR IMPAIRED SKIN INTEGRITY

Related to: (Specify: external mechanical factors of shearing, pressure, restraint forces; external factor of radiation; external factor of immobilization; external factors of excretions, secretions, humidity, infection.)

Defining Characteristics: (Specify: redness; edema; irritation of skin, perianal area, buttocks; excoriation or maceration of skin; enforced bed rest; induration or fissure in skin; scratching; rash; scales; crusting disruption of skin surface; destruction of skin layers with or without necrosis; open wound with drainage; pressure from cast, splint, brace, or other appliance/device; prolonged placement in one position.)

Related to: (Specify: internal factors of altered nutrition, circulation, sensation, skin turgor, metabolic rate, pigmentation and internal factors of medications, skeletal prominence, immunosuppression, developmental status, communicable disease.)

Defining Characteristics: (Specify: thin, fragile skin; temperature elevation; dryness; flakiness; pruritus; pallor; cyanosis; redness; jaundice; allergic response to food, medication; dermatitis; rash; muscle tissue wasting; weakness; decreased muscle strength; edema; disruption of skin surface; eruptions [papule, macule, vesicle]; loss of tactile perception in extremities.)

Goal: Client's skin will remain intact by (date and time to evaluate).

Outcome Criteria

✔ (Specify outcome criteria based on potential problems, e.g., no redness, edema, healed lesion.)

NOC: *Risk Control*

INTERVENTIONS	RATIONALES
Assess skin and mucous membranes for color changes, warmth, dryness, firmness, swelling or edema, lesions or breaks, and infection or inflammation of the oral cavity, nose, eyes, ears, and scalp.	Provides information about potential for disruption of skin integrity in any part of the body to ensure identification and intervention before impairment becomes too severe or extensive.
Assess mobility status, ability to move in bed, use of restraints and length of time restraint used, enforced bed rest as part of medical regimen, presence of any immobilization device.	Reveals ability for movement, external factors that produce pressure leading to skin breakdown as circulation of oxygen and nutrients is reduced.
Assess for any skin rashes, dermatitis, pruritis, and scratching.	Reveals skin conditions that lead to impairment.
Assess for open wounds and type of drainage (serosanguineous or purulent), peristomal skin, diarrhea and effect on perianal area, diaper rash from prolonged exposure to ammonia from urine decomposition.	Reveals presence of secretions and excretions that lead to skin impairment especially in infants and young children who have thinner, more sensitive skin.
(Assess skin under cast edges, tightness of cast, color and sensation in toes or fingers, redness and fit discomfort under any immobilization or assistive [prosthetic] device.)	Reveals skin impairment causes and neurocirculatory effects of cast, splint, brace application.
Assess nutritional and hydration status including dehydration or fluid imbalances and obesity or emaciation with muscle wasting and weakness.	Reveals information regarding ability to maintain healthy skin and mucous membranes with proper nutrition and circulation to tissues and the preservation of muscle mass and strength needed to pad bony prominences and allow movement and position change.
(Assess effect of radiation therapy, presence and extent of burns, chemotherapy on skin, mucous membranes, and areas of vulnerability.)	Provides rationale for preventive measures to treat risk for burns, stomatitis, impairment, and infection caused by immunosuppression.
Assess skin cleanliness and examine bony prominences for changes, condition of hair and nails, use of cleansing products, and skin response; include assessment of effect of contact allergens that cause skin changes.	Provides information about removal of dirt, irritants, bacteria, sweat, urine, feces to promote skin integrity and offers an assessment opportunity.

INTERVENTIONS	RATIONALES
Provide bathing in bed, tub, or shower (specify); use warm water and mild soap and rinse well, with a soft towel pat dry and (avoid rubbing) including all folds, crevices, and creases.	Promotes health and cleanliness of skin, reduces accumulation of body secretions and excretions, and reduces bacteria in skin folds where bacterial growth is enhanced.
Provide careful cleansing of eyes with either warm, sterile water or saline and soft cloth from inner to outer aspect of eye; nasal mucosa with warm water and application of a protective lubricant; oral mucosa with a peroxide solution mouthwash.	Promotes intact mucous membranes from irritation and breakdown caused by pressure or inflammation from tubes or by suctioning, chemotherapy, or NPO status; rapidly dividing epithelial tissue of oral and nasal mucosa leads to breakdown when receiving chemotherapeutic agents.
Provide hair shampooing, nail trimming as ordered; cut nails straight across with round-tipped scissors; dry hair well, rubbing gently with soft towel.	Promotes cleanliness and prevents skin irritation or breaking caused by scratching with long nails.
Apply emollients, lotions to skin, bony prominences with gentle massage using fingers and/or hands as ordered.	Protects and softens skin and promotes circulation to vulnerable parts.
(Apply skin adhesive barrier to peristomal area including tracheostomy, urinary or bowel diversion, and over bony prominences if immobilized or too weak or ill to move in bed.)	Protects skin that is exposed to secretions and excretion or pressure.
Provide position change q 1 to 2h as indicated with prone, supine, side or elevated position utilized; if child is able, encourage to change positions on own.	Prevents prolonged pressure on any one area leading to skin and tissue breakdown.
Maintain body alignment and encourage to maintain correct posture when sitting, lying, and walking.	Promotes even pressure on body parts.
Pad bony prominences and susceptible parts with sheepskin, foam rubber, pillows, alternating pads and mattress, special apparatus such as Stryker frame.	Protects vulnerable parts from pressure and redistribution weight and improves circulation.
Maintain tight, wrinkle-free linens and bed free of crumbs, sharp toys, and dampness from urine or feces.	Prevents irritation and excoriation of skin.

(continues)

(continued)

INTERVENTIONS	RATIONALES
(Correct tight dressings by loosening tape, correct dry and sticking dressings with saline solution before removing, secure tubing away from skin contact, correct fit of any prosthesis or immobilization device, petal edges of cast with soft adhesive material.)	Reduces external sources of pressure that decrease circulation or irritate skin.
Apply topical skin medications (ointments, solutions) as ordered (specify); bathe or soak area or extremity.	Promotes healing and prevents infection (action).
Provide bath with oatmeal or other emollients, mitts on hands, temporary soft restraints as needed.	Soothes pruritis and prevents scratching.
Provide nutritional diet that is high in protein and calories and includes vitamins A and C.	Promotes tissue healing with synthesis of protein to meet metabolic needs and formation of collagen and connective tissue by vitamins A and C.
(If wound present, provide dressing change, irrigations, debridement, wet or dry dressing, Op-site as ordered specific to wound.)	Promotes healing and prevents infection and further skin breakdown.
Teach parents to remove environmental irritants, chemical agents, and allergens that have an outward effect on the child's skin (fabrics, soaps, lotions, toys, dust, pollens, plants, animals, others).	Prevents or controls skin rashes or eruptions caused by contact with offending substances.
Teach parents and child about bathing and personal hygiene measures regarding toileting, mouth and teeth care, nail and hair care, and to avoid wearing tight-fitting clothing.	Promotes cleanliness and removes infectious agents from the skin.
Teach parents and child about nutritional diet and fluids to provide or replenish needed intake if skin disruption is present.	Promotes healing of any skin wound or breakdown.

INTERVENTIONS	RATIONALES
(Instruct parents in dressing change using sterile technique, allow for return demonstration.)	Promotes wound cleanliness and healing.
(Inform parents to maintain mobility of child, avoid allowing child to remain in same position over 1 hour.)	Promotes circulation to skin and tissues.
Teach parents to report any changes in skin color, irritation, pain or absence of sensations, breaks in skin.	Allows for adjustment of device prosthesis or appliance.
Teach parents to report any redness, swelling, pain, purulent drainage from skin or mucous membrane, lesions or open wounds.	Provides early interventions if skin infection present.
Instruct in application of lotions or ointments (antiseptic, antibiotic, or palliative) to skin and irritated areas as ordered (specify).	Protects skin and promotes comfort.
Advise child to avoid scratching or picking at skin or squeezing eruptions.	Prevents further damage to skin and risk for infection.
Teach parents about safety to prevent burn injuries (specify).	Provides information for protective measures.
Teach parents on first aid measures for skin insults (e.g., burns, insect bites) (specify).	Provides information for early intervention.

NIC: *Teaching: Disease Process*

Evaluation

(Date/time of evaluation of goal)

(Has goal been met? Not met? Partially met?)

(Provide data related to the outcome criteria for the specific client.)

(Revisions to care plan? D/C care plan? Continue care plan?)

CHAPTER 10.1

BURNS

Burns are injuries to the skin and underlying tissues caused by flames, electricity, contact with hot articles or water, or radiation therapy. Burns affect children of all ages. They are classified according to severity, source, and extent of surface involved. Most burn injuries occur in children under 5 years of age. Severe burns affect all systems with local responses that include edema, circulatory stasis, and fluid loss. Systemic responses include circulation alteration, anemia, fluid loss, metabolic alteration, acidosis, and stress response. Burns that involve over 10% of body surface require hospitalization with management of ventilation, fluid and electrolyte imbalance, pain control, nutrition, wound care, infection prevention, skin grafting, and rehabilitation.

MEDICAL CARE

Analgesics: for pain relief.

Antimicrobials: applied topically as ointment to affected areas.

Vitamins/Minerals: to facilitate growth and replace depleted stores.

Complete Blood Count (CBC): reveals decreased RBC, Hgb, HCT.

Electrolyte Panel: reveals decreases because of loss from burned areas.

Proteins: reveals decreases with protein breakdown and losses.

Blood Urea Nitrogen/Creatinine: reveals increases as tissue is destroyed and in presence of oliguria.

Wound Culture: reveals and identifies infectious organism if present and sensitivity to anti-infective treatment.

COMMON NURSING DIAGNOSES

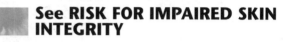 See RISK FOR IMPAIRED SKIN INTEGRITY

Related to: Burn.

Defining Characteristics: (Specify: disruption of skin surface or layers, destruction of skin layers, edema, altered circulation, altered nutritional state, altered metabolic state.)

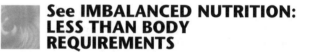 See IMBALANCED NUTRITION: LESS THAN BODY REQUIREMENTS

Related to: (Specify: inability to ingest, metabolize nutrients.)

Defining Characteristics: (Specify: catabolism, protein and fat wasting, anorexia, diarrhea, weight loss.)

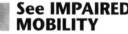 See IMPAIRED PHYSICAL MOBILITY

Related to: (Specify: pain and discomfort, musculoskeletal impairment.)

Defining Characteristics: (Specify: limited range of motion, impaired joint flexibility, scar formation, reluctance to attempt movement.)

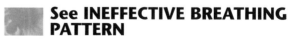 See INEFFECTIVE BREATHING PATTERN

Related to: Musculoskeletal impairment.

Defining Characteristics: (Specify: trauma/edema of airway, oral or nasal membranes, restlessness, tachypnea, dyspnea.)

See RISK FOR DEFICIENT FLUID VOLUME

Related to: Excessive losses.

Defining Characteristics: (Specify: loss of protective skin, blood loss from stress ulcer, electrolyte imbalance, reduced cardiac output with reduced plasma and blood volume.)

See DELAYED GROWTH AND DEVELOPMENT

Related to: Effects of long-term disability.

Defining Characteristics: (Specify: altered physical growth, inability to perform self-care or self-control activities appropriate for age.)

ADDITIONAL NURSING DIAGNOSES

 ## PAIN

Related to: Burn injury.

Defining Characteristics: (Specify: communication [verbal or nonverbal] of pain descriptors depending on severity and type of burn, moaning, crying, restlessness, guarding of injured area.)

Goal: Client will experience decreased pain by (date and time to evaluate).

Outcome Criteria

✔ Pain is rated as less than (specify level and pain scale used).

NOC: *Pain Level*

INTERVENTIONS	RATIONALES
Assess pain in burned area for severity and degree of burn (specify frequency).	Provides information about pain that varies in severity with extent and depth of burn, cause of burn injury (chemical, thermal).
Administer analgesic as ordered (specify) depending on severity of pain and status of other systems; administer before procedures and care are performed; anticipate need before pain becomes severe.	Relieves and controls pain response caused by injury to superficial nerve endings (action of drug).

INTERVENTIONS	RATIONALES
Provide relaxation, diversionary activities (specify).	Provides nonpharmacologic relief of pain.
Place in position of comfort, change q 2h, and handle injured parts gently.	Promotes comfort and prevents additional pain caused by rough handling or pressure on injured body parts.
Avoid touching painful parts, use bed cradle over injured, painful parts.	Prevents contact with linens of hard surfaces that cause pain.
Apply ointment to healing skin that is itchy and flaking, as ordered (specify).	Provides relief from discomfort of itching with use of an antihistamine cream.
Teach parents about methods to relieve pain including quiet play, reading to child, television, music, games, soft toys, other activities to interest to child.	Provides information about interventions that may distract child from any discomfort experienced.
Instruct parents and child to protect injured areas from contact with pain including stimuli.	Prevents further injury and pain.

NIC: *Pain Management*

Evaluation

(Date/time of evaluation of goal)

(Has goal been met? Not met? Partially met?)

(What is pain rating? Specify scale used)

(Revisions to care plan? D/C care plan? Continue care plan?)

RISK FOR INFECTION

Related to: Inadequate primary defenses.

Defining Characteristics: (Specify: broken skin, traumatized tissue, new skin graft, fever, purulent drainage from open wound or under eschar, positive wound culture.)

Goal: Client will not experience infection by (date and time to evaluate).

Outcome Criteria

✔ Temperature remains <101° F.

✔ Wound is without redness, edema, odor, or purulent drainage.

NOC: *Risk Detection*

INTERVENTIONS	RATIONALES
Assess healing wounds for changes in color, odor and drainage. Assess VS and temperature elevation.	Provides information indicating infection of wound or skin graft area.
Administer antibiotics, as ordered (specify).	(Action of drug.)
Perform protective isolation as appropriate including mask, gown, gloves; perform hand-washing before giving any care; discourage visits from those who are suffering from an infection or who are ill.	Protects child from exposure to infectious organisms.
Apply antimicrobial wet dressings to wound or antimicrobial ointment as ordered when performing a dressing change.	Destroys infectious agents and protects wound from infection.
Use sterile technique to perform all dressing changes and wound care.	Protects wound from pathogens and reduces risk of infection.
Instruct parents in handwashing technique and importance of procedure in caring for child.	Provides method of controlling exposure to infectious agents.
Instruct parents in healing process and expected changes in skin during healing; how to assess wound and graft for signs of infection that should be reported.	Provides information about process of healing and changes to note that should be reported.
Instruct parents to avoid any contact with family, friends, visitors that are ill with an infection.	Prevents transmission of infectious agents to the child.
Instruct parents in administration of antimicrobial therapy via PO or topical application.	Promotes compliance with medication regimen to prevent or treat infection.

NIC: *Surveillance*

Evaluation

(Date/time of evaluation of goal)

(Has goal been met? Not met? Partially met?)

(What is temperature? Describe wound. Is there any redness, edema, odor, or purulent drainage?)

(Revisions to care plan? D/C care plan? Continue care plan?)

DISTURBED BODY IMAGE

Related to: Biophysical and psychosocial factors.

Defining Characteristics: (Specify: verbal and nonverbal responses to change in body appearance [scarring, deformity], loss of control, dependence, negative feelings about body, multiple stressors and change in daily living limitations and social relationships.)

Goal: Child will experience improved body image by (date and time to evaluate).

Outcome Criteria

✔ Child expresses feelings about how they look.

✔ Child identifies at least 1 positive thing about self.

NOC: *Body Image*

INTERVENTIONS	RATIONALES
Assess child for feelings about multiple restrictions in lifestyle, change in appearance, difficulty in school and social situations, inability to keep up with peers and participate in activities.	Provides information about status of self-concept and body image that require special attention.
Encourage expression of feelings and concerns and support communications with parents, teachers, and peers.	Provides opportunity to vent feelings and reduce negative feelings about changes in appearance.
Avoid negative comments and stress positive aspect of activities and accomplishments.	Enhances body image and confidence.
Note withdrawal behavior and signs of depression.	Reveals responses to body image changes and possible poor adjustment to changes.
Show support and acceptance of changes in appearance of child; provide privacy as needed.	Promotes trust and demonstrates respect for child.
Allow as much control and decision making by child as possible.	Promotes independence and gives child some control over the situation.
Allow and encourage parental and peer visits when possible.	Promotes social acceptance by peers and support by parents.
Inform parents of importance of maintaining support for child regardless of their needs.	Encourages acceptance of the child with special needs, long-term rehabilitation needs, life-long activity restrictions.

(continues)

(continued)

INTERVENTIONS	RATIONALES
Inform parents and child of impact of the disease on body systems and risk of scarring, physical disability; correct any misinformation and inform of ways to cope with body changes.	Provides correct information to assist in dealing with negative feelings about body.
Instruct parents of need for flexibility in care of child and need to integrate care and routines into family activities; to allow child to participate in peer activities.	Promotes well-being of child and sense of belonging and control of life events by participating in normal activities for age and enhancing developmental task achievement.
Inform parents and child about how to deal with peer and school perceptions of appearance and how to tell others about change in appearance.	Prevents stigmatization of child by those who are not apprised of the child's disease; attitude of others will affect child's body image.
Inform of clothing, wigs, scarves, makeup that may assist in preserving body image.	Provides suggestions for aids that will camouflage scarring or disfigurement.

INTERVENTIONS	RATIONALES
Suggest psychological counseling or child life worker and inform of functions performed by these professionals.	Assists to improve self-esteem and to learn coping and problem solving skills.

NIC: *Self-Esteem Enhancement*

Evaluation

(Date/time of evaluation of goal)

(Has goal been met? Not met? Partially met?)

(What feelings did child verbalize about how he or she looks? What positive thing about self did child identify? Use quotes.)

(Revisions to care plan? D/C care plan? Continue care plan?)

BURNS

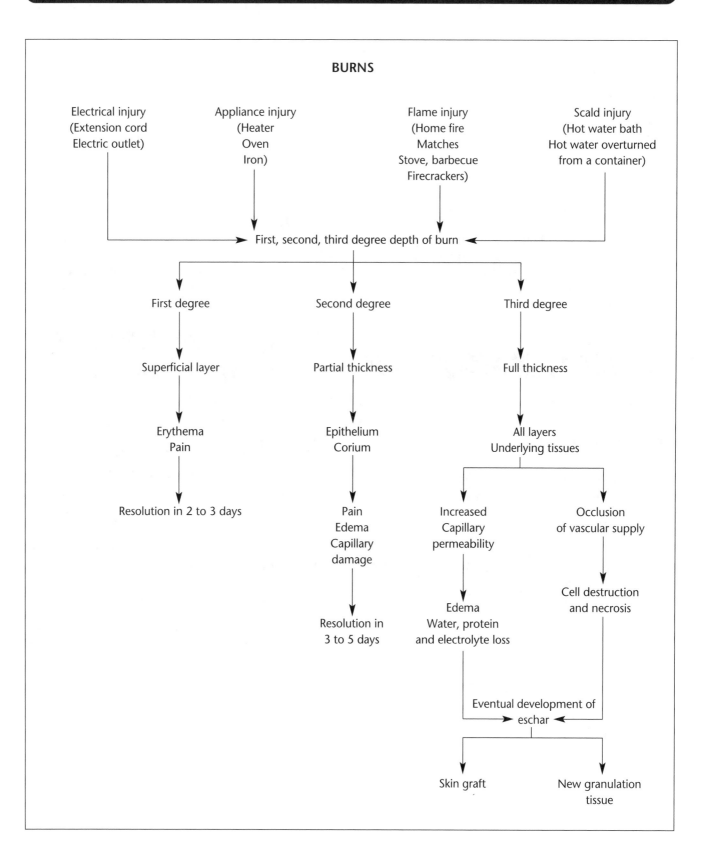

CHAPTER 10.2

CELLULITIS

Cellulitis is an infection of the skin and underlying subcutaneous tissue affecting the lymph nodes within the area of inflammation. It may follow an upper respiratory infection and become systemic in its symptomology. The most common areas affected are the face, periorbital area, and extremities. Treatment includes antibiotic therapy.

MEDICAL CARE

Antipyretics/Analgesics: to reduce fever and/or control pain.

Antibiotics: based on culture identification of organism and sensitivity to drugs.

Wound Aspirate/Blood Culture: reveals and identifies infectious agent if present and sensitivity to specific antimicrobial treatment.

COMMON NURSING DIAGNOSES

See HYPERTHERMIA

Related to: Illness (infection).

Defining Characteristics: Increase in body temperature above normal range, flushed skin that is warm to touch, increased pulse and respiration rate.

See RISK FOR DEFICIENT FLUID VOLUME

Related to: (Specify: altered intake; excessive losses through normal routes.)

Defining Characteristics: (Specify: temperature elevation, diaphoresis, insensible losses, dry, hot skin and mucous membranes.)

See RISK FOR IMPAIRED SKIN INTEGRITY

Related to: Infection of skin layers.

Defining Characteristics: (Specify: redness, swelling, induration, warmth, pain at affected areas, destruction of skin layers.)

ADDITIONAL NURSING DIAGNOSES

DEFICIENT KNOWLEDGE

Related to: Lack of information about condition.

Defining Characteristics: (Specify: request for information about cause and treatment of the condition, measures to prevent spread of the infection.)

Goal: Clients will obtain information about cellulitis by (date and time to evaluate).

Outcome Criteria

✔ Clients verbalize understanding about the cause and treatment of cellulitis.

NOC: *Knowledge: Disease Process*

INTERVENTIONS	RATIONALES
Assess knowledge of treatment of an infection, possible complications, extent of infection, and risk of spread.	Provides information needed to plan teaching that will assist parents in caring for child with an infection involving skin layers.
Inform parents of cause of the infection and manifestations to note including pain, redness, swelling, warmth of a localized infection and to report increasing temperature, enlarged lymph nodes in the region, and a red streak along the lymph pathway in a systemic infection.	Provides information indicating cellulitis and spreading of infection systemically.

INTERVENTIONS	RATIONALES
Administer antibiotics as ordered (specify), teaching parents about administration with dose, time, frequency, side effects, and instruct to take until entire prescription is ingested.	Provides treatment to destroy causative agent by inhibiting cell wall synthesis; route is dependent upon site and severity of the infection.
Inform parents that culture is done to determine treatment.	Provides identification of microorganism and sensitivity to specific antibiotics.
Instruct parents to apply warm compresses or soaks to affected area or limb.	Promotes vasodilation and circulation to the area to promote healing.
Instruct parents in dressing change using sterile technique if an incision and drainage has been done at infection site, and instruct in proper disposal of soiled dressing.	Promotes wound cleanliness and prevents introduction of additional pathogens.
Instruct parents and child in handwashing technique and	Prevents transmission of infectious agents.

INTERVENTIONS	RATIONALES
instruct them to perform this before and after giving care to the child.	
Inform parents to immobilize limb and maintain bed rest for the child.	Promotes healing and reduces pain caused by movement if an extremity is involved.

NIC: *Teaching: Disease Process*

Evaluation

(Date/time of evaluation of goal)

(Has goal been met? Not met? Partially met?)

(Did clients verbalize understanding about cause and treatment for cellulitis? Use quotes.)

(Revisions to care plan? D/C care plan? Continue care plan?)

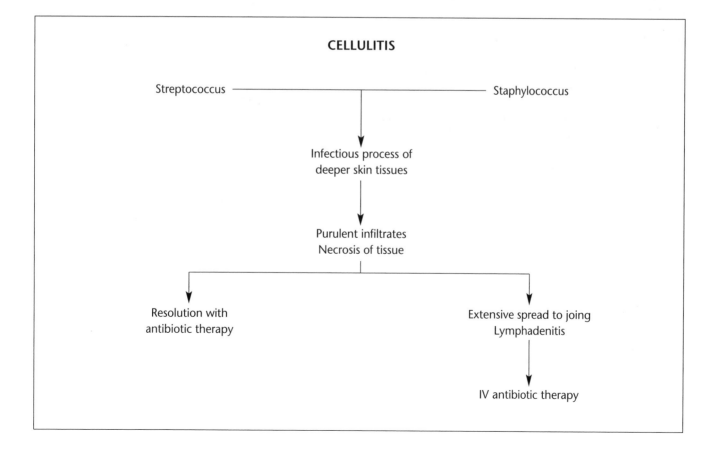

CHAPTER 10.3

DERMATITIS

Dermatitis is an inflammatory condition of the superficial layer of the skin. It may be caused by contact with an allergen, urine, or feces, and it may cause irritation characterized by erythema, papules, or vesicles. Treatment includes actions to prevent infection and skin breakdown.

MEDICAL CARE

Anti-inflammatories: hydrocortisone in cream, lotion, ointment forms to apply topically to suppress inflammatory process and modify immune response to hypersensitivities.

Antihistamines: to relieve allergic response and promote rest.

Antipruritics: applied topically as compresses, lotion, or for bathing to allay itching.

Skin Protectors: applied topically to protect skin against contact with irritants.

COMMON NURSING DIAGNOSES

See RISK FOR IMPAIRED SKIN INTEGRITY

Related to: (Specify: excretions and secretions, contact with allergens or irritants.)

Defining Characteristics: (Specify: rash, erythema, papule, vesicle, lesions, disruptions of skin surface, itching.)

ADDITIONAL NURSING DIAGNOSES

DEFICIENT KNOWLEDGE

Related to: Lack of information about disorder.

Defining Characteristics: (Specify: request for information about cause and treatments of dermatitis and measures to prevent recurrence.)

Goal: Clients will obtain information about dermatitis by (date and time to evaluate).

Outcome Criteria

✔ Clients verbalize understanding of cause and treatment for dermatitis (specify for individual child).

NOC: *Knowledge: Disease Process*

INTERVENTIONS	RATIONALES
Assess type and extent of dermatitis including site and offending irritant, presence of redness, papules, vesicles, breaks in skin, excoriation, itching.	Provides information about rash resulting from contact that may be chemical or physical and most commonly is caused by ammonia from diaper, plant, animal, cloth, soap, or sun exposure.
Inform of potential factors causing eruptions/dermatitis and how to avoid contact with offending agents (specify: e.g., clothing covering all part of body, to wash after contact with substance, to use hypoallergic soaps, proper use of skin applications, and proper changing and laundering of diapers).	Provides information to assist in avoiding contact with substances that cause dermatitis.
(Teach about application of ointment or lotion as ordered to treat diaper rash, to cleanse and dry area well during diaper change, to expose irritated area to the air; laundering diapers by soaking, using mild soap, double rinsing, and drying well in clothes dryer or in sun.)	Promotes healing of skin irritation caused by ammonia in diapers.
Teach parents about palliative treatments (specify: such as application of warm, wet compresses and lotion or paste to the affected areas, and baths; discourage child from scratching the areas.)	Promotes comfort and healing, allays pruritis, and prevents infection if skin is broken down.

INTERVENTIONS	RATIONALES
Instruct parents in administration of antibiotics, anti-inflammatories, antihistamines as ordered.	Reduces allergic reactions and prevents complications associated with dermatitis.
Inform parents to avoid dressing child in tight clothing, to wash new clothing before wearing, to rinse clothing well during laundering.	Promotes comfort and prevents risk of contact with substance that may cause rash.
Inform parents to use sun protection with a minimum sun protection factor of 15 such as PABA.	Protects skin from sunburn by blocking or absorbing ultraviolet rays.
Suggest toys, games, television, and activities preferred by child; maintain short, smooth nails.	Provides diversion to prevent scratching.

NIC: *Teaching: Disease Process*

Evaluation

(Date/time of evaluation of goal)

(Has goal been met? Not met? Partially met?)

(Did clients verbalize understanding about cause and treatment for dermatitis? Use quotes.)

(Revisions to care plan? D/C care plan? Continue care plan?)

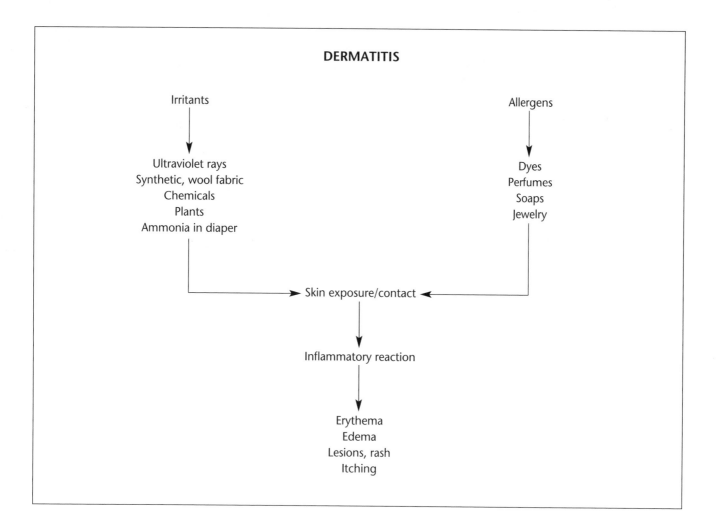

DERMATITIS

Irritants

Allergens

Ultraviolet rays
Synthetic, wool fabric
Chemicals
Plants
Ammonia in diaper

Dyes
Perfumes
Soaps
Jewelry

Skin exposure/contact

Inflammatory reaction

Erythema
Edema
Lesions, rash
Itching

BIBLIOGRAPHY

Alfaro-LaFevre, R. (2004). *Critical thinking in nursing: A practical approach* (3rd ed.). Philadelphia: W.B. Saunders Co.

American Academy of Pediatrics. (2000). Pickering, L. (Ed.). *2000 Red book: Report of the committee on infectious diseases* (25th ed.). Elk Grove, IL: Author.

Ball, J. W., & Binder, R. C. (2002). *Pediatric nursing: Caring for children* (3rd ed.). Upper Saddle River, NJ: Prentice Hall.

Barnum, B.S. (1999). *Teaching nursing in the era of managed care.* New York: Springer Publishing.

Behrman, R. E., Kleigman, R. M., Jenson, H. B. (2004). *Nelson's textbook of pediatrics* (17th ed.). Philadelphia: W.B. Saunders.

Betz, C., Snowden, L. A., & Betz, L. (2004). *Mosby's pediatric nursing reference* (5th ed.). St. Louis: Mosby.

Brazelton, T. B. (1984). *Neonatal behavioral assessment scale* (2nd ed.). London: Heinemann.

Burns, C., Barber, N., Brady, M., & Dunn, A. (2000). *Pediatric primary care: A handbook for nurse practitioners.* Philadelphia: W.B. Saunders.

Carpenito, L. J. (2004). *Handbook of nursing diagnosis* (10th ed.). Philadelphia: Lippincott Williams & Wilkins.

Carpenito, L. J. (2004). *Nursing diagnosis: Application to clinical practice* (10th ed.). Philadelphia: Lippincott Williams & Wilkins.

Daly, K. A., Selvius, R. E., & Lindgren, M. S. (1997). Knowledge and attitudes about otitis media risk: Implications for prevention. *Pediatrics, 100*(6), 931–936.

DeLaune, S.C., & Ladner, P.K. (2002). *Fundamentals of nursing: Standards and practice* (2nd ed.). Clifton Park, NY: Thomson Delmar Learning.

Dochterman, J. M., & Bulechek, G.M. (2004). *Nursing Interventions Classificaton (NIC)* (4th ed.). St. Louis: Mosby, Inc.

Fischbach, F. T. (2004). *A manual of laboratory and diagnostic tests* (7th ed.). Philadelphia: Lippincott Williams & Wilkins.

Fleming, D. F. (1999). Challenging traditional insulin injection practices. *American Journal of Nursing, 99*(2), 72–74.

Foley, G. V., Fochtman, D., & Mooney, K. H. (1997). *Nursing care of the child with cancer* (3rd ed.). Philadelphia: W.B. Saunders.

Gardner, P. (2003). *Nursing process in action.* Clifton Park, NY: Thomson Delmar Learning.

Harkreader, H. (2004). *Fundamentals of nursing: Caring and clinical judgment* (2nd ed.). Philadelphia: W.B. Saunders Co.

Hazinski, M. F. (1999). *Manual of pediatric critical care.* St. Louis: Mosby.

Jackson, P. L., & Vessey, J. A. (2000). *Primary care of the child with a chronic condition* (3rd ed.). St. Louis: Mosby.

Kaditis, A. G., & Wald, E. R. (1999). Viral group: Current diagnosis and treatment. *Contemporary Pediatrics, 16*(2), 139–153.

Kee, J. L. (2001). *Laboratory and diagnostic tests with nursing implications* (6th ed.). Norwalk, CT: Appleton & Lange.

Kelly-Heidenthal, P. (2003). *Nursing leadership and management.* Clifton Park, NY: Thomson Delmar Learning.

Kozier, B., Erb, G., Blais, K., & Wilkinson, J. (2004). *Fundamentals of nursing: Concepts process and practice* (7th ed.). Upper Saddle River, NJ: Pearson Education.

McCance, K. L., & Huether, S. E. (2002). *Pathophysiology: The biologic basis for disease in adults and children* (4th ed.). St. Louis: Mosby.

Meyers, T. A., Eichhorn, D. J., Guzzetta, C. E., Clark, A. P., Klein, J. D., Taliaferro, E., & Calvin, A. (2000). Family presence during invasive procedures and resuscitation. *American Journal of Nursing, 100*(2), 32–42.

Moorhead, S., Johnson, M., & Maas, M. (2004). *Nursing outcomes classifications (NOC)* (3rd ed.). St. Louis: Mosby, Inc.

Nettina, S. (2001). *The Lippincott manual of nursing practice* (7th ed.). Philadelphia: Lippincott Williams & Wilkins.

North American Nursing Diagnosis Association. (2003). *Nursing diagnoses: Definitions & classification 2003–2004.* Philadelphia: Author.

Olds, S. B., London, M. L., & Ladewig, P. A. (2000). *Maternal-newborn nursing: A family and community-based approach* (6th ed.). Upper Saddle River, NJ: Prentice Hall.

Pasero, C. (1999). Pain control: Epidural analgesia in children. *American Journal of Nursing, (99)*5, 20.

Pizzo, P. A., & Poplack, D. G. (2001). *Principle and practice of pediatric oncology* (4th ed., pp. 1343–1355). Philadelphia: Lippincott Williams & Wilkins.

Porth, C. M. (2002). *Pathophysiology. Concepts of altered health states* (6th ed.). Philadelphia: Lippincott Williams & Wilkins.

Rudolph, C. D., Hostetter, M. K., Siegel, N. J., & Lister, G. E. (2002). *Rudolph's pediatrics* (21st ed.). Stamford, CT: Appleton & Lange.

Smeltzer, S., & Bare, B. (2004). *Brunner and Suddarth's textbook of medical-surgical nursing* (10th ed.). Philadelphia: Lippincott Williams & Wilkins.

Ulrich, S., & Canale, W. (2001). *Nursing care planning guides: For adults in acute, extended and home care settings* (5th ed.). Philadelphia: W. B. Saunders Co.

Whaley, L. F., & Wong, D. L. (1999). *Nursing care of infants and children* (6th ed.). St. Louis: Mosby Year Book.

White, L. (2003). *Documentation and the Nursing Process.* Clifton Park, NY: Thomson Delmar Learning.

Wilkinson, J. M. (2000). *Nursing diagnosis handbook* (7th ed.). Upper Saddle River, NJ: Prentice Hall.

Wilson, B. A., Shannon, M. T., & Stand, C. L. (2000). *Nurse's drug guide 2000.* Stamford, CT: Appleton & Lange.

Wolfe, J., Grier, H. E., Klar, N., Levin, S. B., Ellenbogen, J. M., Salem-Schaltz, S., Emanuel, E. J., & Weeks, J. C. (2000). Symptoms and suffering at the end of life in children with cancer. *New England Journal of Medicine, 342*(5), 326–333.

Wong, D. L., Hockenberry-Easton, M., Wilson, D., Winkelstein, M., & Schwartz, P. (2001). *Wong's Essentials of Pediatric Nursing* (6th ed.). St. Louis: Mosby.

Yoos, H. L., & McMullen, A. (1999). Symptom perception and evaluation in childhood asthma. *Nursing Research, 48*(1), 2–8.

APPENDIX A

NANDA NURSING DIAGNOSES

Activity Intolerance
Acute Confusion
Acute Pain
Adult Failure To Thrive
Anticipatory Grieving
Anxiety
Autonomic Dysreflexia

Bathing/Hygiene Self-Care Deficit
Bowel Incontinence

Caregiver Role Strain
Chronic Confusion
Chronic Low Self-Esteem
Chronic Pain
Chronic Sorrow
Compromised Family Coping
Constipation

Death Anxiety
Decisional Conflict (specify)
Decreased Cardiac Output
Decreased Intracranial Adaptive Capacity
Defensive Coping
Deficient Diversional Activity
Deficient Fluid Volume
Deficient Knowledge (specify)
Delayed Growth And Development
Delayed Surgical Recovery
Diarrhea
Disabled Family Coping
Disorganized Infant Behavior
Disturbed Body Image
Disturbed Energy Field
Disturbed Personal Identity
Disturbed Sensory Perception (specify: visual, auditory,
    kinesthetic, gustatory, tactile, olfactory)
Disturbed Sleep Pattern
Disturbed Thought Processes
Dressing/Grooming Self-Care Deficit
Dysfunctional Family Processes: Alcoholism
Dysfunctional Grieving
Dysfunctional Ventilatory Weaning Response

Effective Breast-Feeding
Effective Therapeutic Regimen Management
Excess Fluid Volume

Fatigue
Fear
Feeding Self-Care Deficit
Functional Urinary Incontinence

Health-Seeking Behaviors (specify)
Hopelessness
Hyperthermia
Hypothermia

Imbalanced Nutrition: Less Than Body Requirements
Imbalanced Nutrition: More Than Body Requirements
Impaired Adjustment
Impaired Bed Mobility
Impaired Dentition
Impaired Environmental Interpretation Syndrome
Impaired Gas Exchange
Impaired Home Maintenance
Impaired Memory
Impaired Oral Mucous Membrane
Impaired Parenting
Impaired Physical Mobility
Impaired Skin Integrity
Impaired Social Interaction
Impaired Spontaneous Ventilation
Impaired Swallowing
Impaired Tissue Integrity
Impaired Transfer Ability
Impaired Urinary Elimination
Impaired Verbal Communication
Impaired Walking
Impaired Wheelchair Mobility
Ineffective Airway Clearance
Ineffective Breast-Feeding
Ineffective Breathing Pattern
Ineffective Community Coping
Ineffective Community Therapeutic Regimen
    Management
Ineffective Coping

Ineffective Denial
Ineffective Family Therapeutic Regimen Management
Ineffective Health Maintenance
Ineffective Infant Feeding Pattern
Ineffective Protection
Ineffective Role Performance
Ineffective Sexuality Patterns
Ineffective Therapeutic Regimen Management
Ineffective Thermoregulation
Ineffective Tissue Perfusion (specify type: renal, cerebral, cardiopulmonary, gastrointestinal, peripheral)
Interrupted Breast-Feeding
Interrupted Family Processes

Latex Allergy Response

Nausea
Noncompliance (specify)

Parental Role Conflict
Perceived Constipation
Post-Trauma Syndrome
Powerlessness

Rape-Trauma Syndrome
Rape-Trauma Syndrome: Compound Reaction
Rape-Trauma Syndrome: Silent Reaction
Readiness for Enhanced Communicaton
Readiness for Enhanced Community Coping
Readiness for Enhanced Coping
Readiness for Enhanced Family Coping
Readiness for Enhanced Family Processes
Readiness for Enhanced Fluid Balance
Readiness for Enhanced Knowledge (specify)
Readiness for Enhanced Nutrition
Readiness for Enhanced Organized Infant Behavior
Readiness for Enhanced Parenting
Readiness for Enhanced Self-Concept
Readiness for Enhanced Sleep
Readiness for Enhanced Spiritual Well-Being
Readiness for Enhanced Therapeutic Regimen Management
Readiness for Enhanced Urinary Elimination
Reflex Urinary Incontinence
Relocation Stress Syndrome
Risk for Activity Intolerance
Risk for Aspiration
Risk for Autonomic Dysreflexia
Risk for Caregiver Role Strain
Risk for Constipation

Risk for Deficient Fluid Volume
Risk for Delayed Development
Risk for Disorganized Infant Behavior
Risk for Disproportionate Growth
Risk for Disuse Syndrome
Risk for Falls
Risk for Imbalanced Body Temperature
Risk for Imbalanced Fluid Volume
Risk for Imbalanced Nutrition: More Than Body Requirements
Risk for Impaired Parent/Infant/Child Attachment
Risk for Impaired Parenting
Risk for Impaired Skin Integrity
Risk for Infection
Risk for Injury
Risk for Latex Allergy Response
Risk for Loneliness
Risk for Other-Directed Violence
Risk for Perioperative-Positioning Injury
Risk for Peripheral Neurovascular Dysfunction
Risk for Poisoning
Risk for Post-Trauma Syndrome
Risk for Powerlessness
Risk for Relocation Stress Syndrome
Risk for Self-Directed Violence
Risk for Self-Mutilation
Risk for Situational Low Self-Esteem
Risk for Spiritual Distress
Risk for Sudden Infant Death Syndrome
Risk for Suffocation
Risk for Suicide
Risk for Trauma
Risk for Urge Urinary Incontinence

Self-Mutilation
Sexual Dysfunction
Situational Low Self-Esteem
Sleep Deprivation
Social Isolation
Spiritual Distress
Stress Urinary Incontinence

Toileting Self-Care Deficit
Total Urinary Incontinence

Unilateral Neglect
Urinary Retention
Urge Urinary Incontenance

Wandering

APPENDIX B

NURSING OUTCOMES CLASSIFICATIONS (NOC)

Abuse Cessation
Abuse Protection
Abuse Recovery Status
Abuse Recovery: Emotional
Abuse Recovery: Financial
Abuse Recovery: Physical
Abuse Recovery: Sexual
Abusive Behavior Self-Restraint
Acceptance: Health Status
Activity Tolerance
Adaptation to Physical Disability
Adherence Behavior
Aggression Self-Control
Allergic Response: Localized
Allergic Response: Systemic
Ambulation
Ambulation: Wheelchair
Anxiety Level
Anxiety Self-Control
Appetite
Aspiration Prevention
Asthma Self-Management

Balance
Blood Coagulation
Blood-Glucose Level
Blood Loss Severity
Blood Transfusion Reaction
Body Image
Body Mechanics Performance
Body Positioning: Self-Initiated
Bone Healing
Bowel Continence
Bowel Elimination
Breastfeeding Establishment: Infant
Breastfeeding Establishment: Maternal
Breastfeeding: Maintenance
Breastfeeding: Weaning

Cardiac Disease Self-Management
Cardiac Pump Effectiveness
Caregiver Adaptation to Patient Institutionalization

Caregiver Emotional Health
Caregiver Home Care Readiness
Caregiver Lifestyle Disruption
Caregiver-Patient Relationship
Caregiver Performance: Direct Care
Caregiver Performance: Indirect Care
Caregiver Physical Health
Caregiver Stressors
Caregiver Well-Being
Caregiving Endurance Potential
Child Adaptation to Hospitalization
Child Development: 1 Month
Child Development: 2 Months
Child Development: 4 Months
Child Development: 6 Months
Child Development: 12 Months
Child Development: 2 Years
Child Development: 3 Years
Child Development: 4 Years
Child Development: Middle Childhood
Child Development: Adolescence
Circulation Status
Client Satisfaction: Access to Care Resources
Client Satisfaction: Caring
Client Satisfaction: Communication
Client Satisfaction: Continuity of Care
Client Satisfaction: Cultural Needs Fulfillment
Client Satisfaction: Functional Assistance
Client Satisfaction: Physical Care
Client Satisfaction: Physical Environment
Client Satisfaction: Protection of Rights
Client Satisfaction: Psychological Care
Client Satisfaction: Safety
Client Satisfaction: Symptom Control
Client Satisfaction: Teaching
Client Satisfaction: Technical Aspects of Care
Cognition
Cognitive Orientation
Comfort Level
Comfortable Death
Communication
Communication: Expressive

Communication: Receptive
Community Competence
Community Disaster Readiness
Community Health Status
Community Health Status: Immunity
Community Risk Control: Chronic Disease
Community Risk Control: Communicable Disease
Community Risk Control: Lead Exposure
Community Risk Control: Violence
Community Violence Level
Compliance Behavior
Concentration
Coordinated Movement
Coping

Decision Making
Depression Level
Depression Self-Control
Diabetes Self-Management
Dignified Life Closure
Discharge Readiness: Independent Living
Discharge Readiness: Supported Living
Distorted Thought Self-Control

Electrolyte and Acid/Base Balance
Endurance
Energy Conservation

Fall Prevention Behavior
Falls Occurrence
Family Coping
Family Functioning
Family Health Status
Family Integrity
Family Normalization
Family Participation in Professional Care
Family Physical Environment
Family Resiliency
Family Social Climate
Family Support During Treatment
Fear Level
Fear Level: Child
Fear Self-Control
Fetal Status: Antepartum
Fetal Status: Intrapartum
Fluid Balance
Fluid Overload Severity

Grief Resolution
Growth

Health Beliefs
Health Beliefs: Perceived Ability to Perform
Health Beliefs: Perceived Control
Health Beliefs: Perceived Resources
Health Beliefs: Perceived Threat
Health Orientation

Health-Promoting Behavior
Health-Seeking Behavior
Hearing Compensation Behavior
Hemodialysis Access
Hope
Hydration
Hyperactivity Level

Identity
Immobility Consequences: Physiological
Immobility Consequences: Psycho-Cognitive
Immune Hypersensitivity Response
Immune Status
Immunization Behavior
Impulse Self-Control
Infection Severity
Infection Severity: Newborn
Information Processing

Joint Movement: Ankle
Joint Movement: Elbow
Joint Movement: Fingers
Joint Movement: Hip
Joint Movement: Knee
Joint Movement: Neck
Joint Movement: Passive
Joint Movement: Shoulder
Joint Movement: Spine
Joint Movement: Wrist

Kidney Function
Knowledge: Body Mechanics
Knowledge: Breastfeeding
Knowledge: Cardiac Disease Management
Knowledge: Child Physical Safety
Knowledge: Conception Prevention
Knowledge: Diabetes Management
Knowledge: Diet
Knowledge: Disease Process
Knowledge: Energy Conservation
Knowledge: Fall Prevention
Knowledge: Fertility Promotion
Knowledge: Health Behavior
Knowledge: Health Promotion
Knowledge: Health Resources
Knowledge: Illness Care
Knowledge: Infant Care
Knowledge: Infection Control
Knowledge: Labor and Delivery
Knowledge: Medication
Knowledge: Ostomy Care
Knowledge: Parenting
Knowledge: Personal Safety
Knowledge: Postpartum Maternal Health
Knowledge: Preconception Maternal Health
Knowledge: Pregnancy
Knowledge: Prescribed Activity

Knowledge: Sexual Functioning
Knowledge: Substance Abuse Control
Knowledge: Treatment Procedure(s)
Knowledge: Treatment Regimen

Leisure Participation
Loneliness Severity

Maternal Status: Antepartum
Maternal Status: Intrapartum
Maternal Status: Postpartum
Mechanical Ventilation Response: Adult
Mechanical Ventilation Weaning Response: Adult
Medication Response
Memory
Mobility
Mood Equilibrium
Motivation

Nausea & Vomiting Control
Nausea & Vomiting: Disruptive Effects
Nausea & Vomiting Severity
Neglect Cessation
Neglect Recovery
Neurological Status
Neurological Status: Autonomic
Neurological Status: Central Motor Control
Neurological Status: Consciousness
Neurological Status: Cranial Sensory/Motor Function
Neurological Status: Spinal Sensory/Motor Function
Newborn Adaptation
Nutritional Status
Nutritional Status: Biochemical Measures
Nutritional Status: Energy
Nutritional Status: Food and Fluid Intake
Nutritional Status: Nutrient Intake

Oral Health
Ostomy Self-Care

Pain: Adverse Psychological Response
Pain Control
Pain: Disruptive Effects
Pain Level
Parent-Infant Attachment
Parenting: Adolescent Physical Safety
Parenting: Early/Middle Childhood Physical Safety
Parenting: Infant/Toddler Physical Safety
Parenting Performance
Parenting: Psychosocial Safety
Participation in Health Care Decisions
Personal Autonomy
Personal Health Status
Personal Safety Behavior
Personal Well-Being
Physical Aging
Physical Fitness

Physical Injury Severity
Physical Maturation: Female
Physical Maturation: Male
Play Participation
Post Procedure Recovery Status
Prenatal Health Behavior
Preterm Infant Organization
Psychomotor Energy
Psychosocial Adjustment: Life Change

Quality of Life

Respiratory Status: Airway Patency
Respiratory Status: Gas Exchange
Respiratory Status: Ventilation
Rest
Risk Control
Risk Control: Alcohol Use
Risk Control: Cancer
Risk Control: Cardiovascular Health
Risk Control: Drug Use
Risk Control: Hearing Impairment
Risk Control: Sexually Transmitted Diseases (STDs)
Risk Control: Tobacco Use
Risk Control: Unintended Pregnancy
Risk Control: Visual Impairment
Risk Detection
Role Performance

Safe Home Environment
Seizure Control
Self-Care Status
Self-Care: Activities of Daily Living (ADL)
Self-Care: Bathing
Self-Care: Dressing
Self-Care: Eating
Self-Care: Hygiene
Self-Care: Instrumental Activities of Daily Living (IADL)
Self-Care: Nonparenteral Medication
Self-Care: Oral Hygiene
Self-Care: Parenteral Medication
Self-Care: Toileting
Self-Direction of Care
Self-Esteem
Self-Mutilation Restraint
Sensory Function Status
Sensory Function: Cutaneous
Sensory Function: Hearing
Sensory Function: Proprioception
Sensory Function: Taste and Smell
Sensory Function: Vision
Sexual Functioning
Sexual Identity
Skeletal Function
Sleep
Social Interaction Skills
Social Involvement

Social Support
Spiritual Health
Stress Level
Student Health Status
Substance Addiction Consequences
Suffering Severity
Suicide Self-Restraint
Swallowing Status
Swallowing Status: Esophageal Phase
Swallowing Status: Oral Phrase
Swallowing Status: Pharyngeal Phase
Symptom Control
Symptom Severity
Symptom Severity: Perimenopause
Symptom Severity: Premenstrual Syndrome (PMS)
Systemic Toxin Clearance: Dialysis

Thermoregulation
Thermoregulation: Neonate
Tissue Integrity: Skin and Mucous Membranes

Tissue Perfusion: Abdominal Organs
Tissue Perfusion: Cardiac
Tissue Perfusion: Cerebral
Tissue Perfusion: Peripheral
Tissue Perfusion: Pulmonary
Transfer Performance
Treatment Behavior: Illness or Injury

Urinary Continence
Urinary Elimination

Vision Compensation Behavior
Vital Signs

Weight: Body Mass
Weight Control
Will to Live
Wound Healing: Primary Intention
Wound Healing: Primary Intention

APPENDIX C

NURSING INTERVENTIONS CLASSIFICATIONS (NIC)

Abuse Protection Support
Abuse Protection Support: Child
Abuse Protection Support: Domestic Partner
Abuse Protection Support: Elder
Abuse Protection Support: Religious
Acid-Base Management
Acid-Base Management: Metabolic Acidosis
Acid-Base Management: Metabolic Alkalosis
Acid-Base Management: Respiratory Acidosis
Acid-Base Management: Respiratory Alkalosis
Acid-Base Monitoring
Active Listening
Activity Therapy
Acupressure
Admission Care
Airway Insertion And Stabilization
Airway Management
Airway Suctioning
Allergy Management
Amnioinfusion
Amputation Care
Analgesic Administration
Analgesic Administration: Intraspinal
Anaphylaxis Management
Anesthesia Administration
Anger Control Assistance
Animal-Assisted Therapy
Anticipatory Guidance
Anxiety Reduction
Area Restriction
Aromatherapy
Art Therapy
Artificial Airway Management
Aspiration Precautions
Assertiveness Training
Asthma Management
Attachment Promotion
Autogenic Training
Autotransfusion

Bathing
Bed Rest Care
Bedside Laboratory Testing
Behavior Management

Behavior Management: Overactivity/Inattention
Behavior Management: Self-Harm
Behavior Management: Sexual
Behavior Modification
Behavior Modification: Social Skills
Bibliotherapy
Biofeedback
Bioterrorism Preparedness
Birthing
Bladder Irrigation
Bleeding Precautions
Bleeding Reduction
Bleeding Reduction: Antepartum Uterus
Bleeding Reduction: Gastrointestinal
Bleeding Reduction: Nasal
Bleeding Reduction: Postpartum Uterus
Bleeding Reduction: Wound
Blood Products Administration
Body Image Enhancement
Body Mechanics Promotion
Bottle Feeding
Bowel Incontinence Care
Bowel Incontinence Care: Encopresis
Bowel Irrigation
Bowel Management
Bowel Training
Breast Examination
Breastfeeding Assistance

Calming Technique
Capillary Blood Sample
Cardiac Care
Cardiac Care: Acute
Cardiac Care: Rehabilitative
Cardiac Precautions
Caregiver Support
Care Management
Cast Care: Maintenance
Cast Care, Wet
Cerebral Edema Management
Cerebral Perfusion Promotion
Cesarean Section Care
Chemical Restraint
Chemotherapy Management

Chest Physiotherapy
Childbirth Preparation
Circulatory Care: Arterial Insufficiency
Circulatory Care: Mechanical Assist Device
Circulatory Care: Venous Insufficiency
Circulatory Precautions
Circumcision Care
Code Management
Cognitive Restructuring
Cognitive Stimulation
Communicable Disease Management
Communication Enhancement: Hearing Deficit
Communication Enhancement: Speech Deficit
Communication Enhancement: Visual Deficit
Community Disaster Preparedness
Community Health Development
Complex Relationship Building
Conflict Mediation
Constipation/Impaction Management
Consultation
Contact Lens Care
Controlled Substance Checking
Coping Enhancement
Cost Containment
Cough Enhancement
Counseling
Crisis Intervention
Critical Path Development
Culture Brokerage
Cutaneous Stimulation

Decision-Making Support
Delegation
Delirium Management
Delusion Management
Dementia Management
Dementia Management: Bathing
Deposition/Testimony
Developmental Care
Developmental Enhancement: Adolescent
Developmental Enhancement: Child
Dialysis Access Maintenance
Diarrhea Management
Diet Staging
Discharge Planning
Distraction
Documentation
Dressing
Dying Care
Dysreflexia Management
Dysrhythmia Management

Ear Care
Eating Disorders Management
Electroconvulsive Therapy (ECT) Management
Electrolyte Management
Electrolyte Management: Hypercalcemia

Electrolyte Management: Hyperkalemia
Electrolyte Management: Hypermagnesemia
Electrolyte Management: Hypernatremia
Electrolyte Management: Hyperphosphatemia
Electrolyte Management: Hypocalcemia
Electrolyte Management: Hypokalemia
Electrolyte Management: Hypomagnesemia
Electrolyte Management: Hyponatremia
Electrolyte Management: Hypophosphatemia
Electrolyte Monitoring
Electronic Fetal Monitoring: Antepartum
Electronic Fetal Monitoring: Intrapartum
Elopement Precautions
Embolus Care: Peripheral
Embolus Care: Pulmonary
Embolus Precautions
Emergency Care
Emergency Cart Checking
Emotional Support
Endotracheal Extubation
Energy Management
Enteral Tube Feeding
Environmental Management
Environmental Management: Attachment Process
Environmental Management: Comfort
Environmental Management: Community
Environmental Management: Home Preparation
Environmental Management: Safety
Environmental Management: Violence Prevention
Environmental Management: Worker Safety
Environmental Risk Protection
Examination Assistance
Exercise Promotion
Exercise Promotion: Strength Training
Exercise Promotion: Stretching
Exercise Therapy: Ambulation
Exercise Therapy: Balance
Exercise Therapy: Joint Mobility
Exercise Therapy: Muscle Control
Eye Care

Fall Prevention
Family Integrity Promotion
Family Integrity Promotion: Childbearing Family
Family Involvement Promotion
Family Mobilization
Family Planning: Contraception
Family Planning: Infertility
Family Planning: Unplanned Pregnancy
Family Presence Facilitation
Family Process Maintenance
Family Support
Family Therapy
Feeding
Fertility Preservation
Fever Treatment
Financial Resource Assistance

Fire-Setting Precautions
First Aid
Fiscal Resource Management
Flatulence Reduction
Fluid/Electrolyte Management
Fluid Management
Fluid Monitoring
Fluid Resuscitation
Foot Care
Forgiveness Facilitation

Gastrointestinal Intubation
Genetic Counseling
Grief Work Facilitation
Grief Work Facilitation: Perinatal Death
Guilt Work Facilitation

Hair Care
Hallucination Management
Health Care Information Exchange
Health Education
Health Policy Monitoring
Health Screening
Health System Guidance
Heat/Cold Application
Heat Exposure Treatment
Hemodialysis Therapy
Hemodynamic Regulation
Hemofiltration Therapy
Hemorrhage Control
High-Risk Pregnancy Care
Home Maintenance Assistance
Hope Instillation
Hormone Replacement Therapy
Humor
Hyperglycemia Management
Hypervolemia Management
Hypnosis
Hypoglycemia Management
Hypothermia Treatment
Hypovolemia Management

Immunization/Vaccination Administration
Impulse Control Training
Incident Reporting
Incision Site Care
Infant Care
Infection Control
Infection Control: Intraoperative
Infection Protection
Insurance Authorization
Intracranial Pressure (ICP) Monitoring
Intrapartal Care
Intrapartal Care: High-Risk Delivery
Intravenous (IV) Insertion
Intravenous (IV) Therapy
Invasive Hemodynamic Monitoring

Kangaroo Care

Labor Induction
Labor Suppression
Laboratory Data Interpretation
Lactation Counseling
Lactation Suppression
Laser Precautions
Latex Precautions
Learning Facilitation
Learning Readiness Enhancement
Leech Therapy
Limit Setting
Lower Extremity Monitoring

Malignant Hyperthermia Precautions
Mechanical Ventilation
Mechanical Ventilatory Weaning
Medication Administration
Medication Administration: Ear
Medication Administration: Enteral
Medication Administration: Eye
Medication Administration: Inhalation
Medication Administration: Interpleural
Medication Administration: Intradermal
Medication Administration: Intramuscular (IM)
Medication Administration: Intraosseous
Medication Administration: Intraspinal
Medication Administration: Intravenous (IV)
Medication Administration: Nasal
Medication Administration: Oral
Medication Administration: Rectal
Medication Administration: Skin
Medication Administration: Subcutaneous
Medication Administration: Vaginal
Medication Administration: Ventricular Reservoir
Medication Management
Medication Prescribing
Meditation Facilitation
Memory Training
Milieu Therapy
Mood Management
Multidisciplinary Care Conference
Music Therapy
Mutual Goal Setting

Nail Care
Nausea Management
Neurologic Monitoring
Newborn Care
Newborn Monitoring
Nonnutritive Sucking
Normalization Promotion
Nutrition Management
Nutrition Therapy
Nutritional Counseling
Nutritional Monitoring

Oral Health Maintenance
Oral Health Promotion
Oral Health Restoration
Order Transcription
Organ Procurement
Ostomy Care
Oxygen Therapy

Pain Management
Parent Education: Adolescent
Parent Education: Childrearing Family
Parent Education: Infant
Parenting Promotion
Pass Facilitation
Patient Contracting
Patient Controlled Analgesia (PCA) Assistance
Patient Rights Protection
Peer Review
Pelvic Muscle Exercise
Perineal Care
Peripheral Sensation Management
Peripherally Inserted Central (PIC) Catheter Care
Peritoneal Dialysis Therapy
Pessary Management
Phlebotomy: Arterial Blood Sample
Phlebotomy: Blood Unit Acquisition
Phlebotomy: Cannulated Vessel
Phlebotomy: Venous Blood Sample
Phototherapy: Mood/Sleep Regulation
Phototherapy: Neonate
Physical Restraint
Physician Support
Pneumatic Tourniquet Precautions
Positioning
Positioning: Intraoperative
Positioning: Neurologic
Positioning: Wheelchair
Postanesthesia Care
Postmortem Care
Postpartal Care
Preceptor: Employee
Preceptor: Student
Preconception Counseling
Pregnancy Termination Care
Premenstrual Syndrome (PMS) Management
Prenatal Care
Preoperative Coordination
Preparatory Sensory Information
Presence
Pressure Management
Pressure Ulcer Care
Pressure Ulcer Prevention
Product Evaluation
Program Development
Progressive Muscle Relaxation
Prompted Voiding

Prosthesis Care
Pruritus Management

Quality Monitoring

Radiation Therapy Management
Rape-Trauma Treatment
Reality Orientation
Recreation Therapy
Rectal Prolapse Management
Referral
Religious Addiction Prevention
Religious Ritual Enhancement
Relocation Stress Reduction
Reminiscence Therapy
Reproductive Technology Management
Research Data Collection
Resiliency Promotion
Respiratory Monitoring
Respite Care
Resuscitation
Resuscitation: Fetus
Resuscitation: Neonate
Risk Identification
Risk Identification: Childbearing Family
Risk Identification: Genetic
Role Enhancement

Seclusion
Security Enhancement
Sedation Management
Seizure Management
Seizure Precautions
Self-Awareness Enhancement
Self-Care Assistance
Self-Care Assistance: Bathing/Hygiene
Self-Care Assistance: Dressing/Grooming
Self-Care Assistance: Feeding
Self-Care Assistance: IADL
Self-Care Assistance: Toileting
Self-Care Assistance: Transfer
Self-Esteem Enhancement
Self-Hypnosis Facilitation
Self-Modification Assistance
Self-Responsibility Facilitation
Sexual Counseling
Shift Report
Shock Management
Shock Management: Cardiac
Shock Management: Vasogenic
Shock Management: Volume
Shock Prevention
Sibling Support
Simple Guided Imagery
Simple Massage
Simple Relaxation Therapy

Skin Care: Donor Site
Skin Care: Graft Site
Skin Care: Topical Treatments
Skin Surveillance
Sleep Enhancement
Smoking Cessation Assistance
Socialization Enhancement
Specimen Management
Spiritual Growth Facilitation
Spiritual Support
Splinting
Sports-Injury Prevention: Youth
Staff Development
Staff Supervision
Subarachnoid Hemorrhage Precautions
Substance Use Prevention
Substance Use Treatment
Substance Use Treatment: Alcohol Withdrawal
Substance Use Treatment: Drug Withdrawal
Substance Use Treatment: Overdose
Suicide Prevention
Supply Management
Support Group
Support System Enhancement
Surgical Assistance
Surgical Precautions
Surgical Preparation
Surveillance
Surveillance: Community
Surveillance: Late Pregnancy
Surveillance: Remote Electronic
Surveillance: Safety
Sustenance Support
Suturing
Swallowing Therapy

Teaching: Disease Process
Teaching: Foot Care
Teaching: Group
Teaching: Individual
Teaching: Infant Nutrition
Teaching: Infant Safety
Teaching: Infant Stimulation
Teaching: Preoperative
Teaching: Prescribed Activity/Exercise
Teaching: Prescribed Diet
Teaching: Prescribed Medication
Teaching: Procedure/Treatment
Teaching: Psychomotor Skill
Teaching: Safe Sex
Teaching: Sexuality
Teaching: Toddler Nutrition
Teaching: Toddler Safety

Teaching: Toilet Training
Technology Management
Telephone Consultation
Telephone Follow-Up
Temperature Regulation
Temperature Regulation: Intraoperative
Temporary Pacemaker Management
Therapeutic Play
Therapeutic Touch
Therapy Group
Total Parenteral Nutrition (TPN) Administration
Touch
Traction/Immobilization Care
Transcutaneous Electrical Nerve Stimulation (TENS)
Transport
Trauma Therapy: Child
Triage: Disaster
Triage: Emergency Center
Triage: Telephone
Truth Telling
Tube Care
Tube Care: Chest
Tube Care: Gastrointestinal
Tube Care: Umbilical Line
Tube Care: Urinary
Tube Care: Ventriculostomy/Lumbar Drain

Ultrasonography: Limited Obstetric
Unilateral Neglect Management
Urinary Bladder Training
Urinary Catheterization
Urinary Catheterization: Intermittent
Urinary Elimination Management
Urinary Habit Training
Urinary Incontinence Care
Urinary Incontinence Care: Enuresis
Urinary Retention Care

Values Clarification
Vehicle Safety Promotion
Venous Access Device (VAD) Maintenance
Ventilation Assistance
Visitation Facilitation
Vital Signs Monitoring
Vomiting Management

Weight Gain Assistance
Weight Management
Weight Reduction Assistance
Wound Care
Wound Care: Closed Drainage
Wound Irrigation

APPENDIX D

ABBREVIATIONS

↑: increase
↓: decrease
→: leads to
>: greater than
<: less than
°: degree
AAP: American Academy of Pediatrics
ABO: refers to the blood types A, B, or O
ABG: arterial blood gas
ADHD: attention deficit hyperactivity disorder
AFDC: Aid to Families with Dependent Children
AIDS: acquired immunodeficiency syndrome
ALT: alanine aminotransferase (also SGPT)
APTT: activated partial thromboplastin time
ARDS: adult respiratory distress syndrome
AROM: artificial rupture of membranes
ASD: atrial septal defect
AST: aspartate aminotransferase (also SGOT)
BBT: basal body temperature
BM: bowel movement
BP: blood pressure
BRP: bathroom privileges
BUN: blood urea nitrogen
C: centigrade
cal: calories
CBC: complete blood count
cc: cubic centimeters
CD & I: clean, dry, and intact
CHF: congestive heart failure
Cl⁻: chloride
CNS: central nervous system
c/o: complains of
CO: cardiac output
CO_2: carbon dioxide

CPAP: continuous positive airway pressure
CPT: chest physiotherapy
CRP: C-reactive protein
CSF: cerebral spinal fluid
CT: computerized axial tomography
CVP: central venous pressure
CVA: cerebral vascular accident
DAT: diet as tolerated
D/C: discharge
DCFS: Department of Children and Family Services
DIC: disseminating intravascular coagulation
dL: deciliter
DNA: deoxyribonucleic acid
dsg: dressing
DtaP: diptheria, tetanus, activated pertussis
DTR: deep tendon reflexes
EBL: estimated blood loss
ECMO: extracorporeal membrane oxygenation
ECT: electroconvulsive therapy
EEG: electroencephalogram
e.g.: for example
ELISA: enzyme-linked immunosorbent assay
F: Fahrenheit
FFP: fresh frozen plasma
FiO_2: fraction of inspired oxygen
FVE: fluid volume excess
FVD: fluid volume deficit
GBS: group B streptococcus
GC: gonorrhea
GFR: glomerular filtration rate
GI: gastrointestinal
gm: gram
GTT: glucose tolerance test
GU: genitourinary

H$^+$: hydrogen ion

Hct: hematocrit

Hgb: hemoglobin

Hib: *Haemophilus influenzae*, type b

HIE: hypoxic-ischemic encephalopathy

HIV: human immunodeficiency virus

H$_2$O: water

HOB: head of bed

hr: hour

HR: heart rate

Ht: height

HTN: hypertension

hx: history

I&O: intake & output

ICP: intracranial pressure

ID: identification

IDDM: insulin-dependent diabetes mellitus

Ig: immune globulin

IM: intramuscular

IMV: intermittent mechanical ventilation

IPPB: intermittent positive pressure breathing

IPV: inactivated poliovirus vaccine

IV: intravenous

IVP: intravenous push

K$^+$: potassium

KVO: keep vein open

kcal: kilo calories

kg: kilogram

L: liter

LOC: level of consciousness

LR: lactated Ringer's

MAE: moves all extremities

mEq: milliequivalent

mg: milligram

mL: milliliter

mm Hg: millimeters of mercury

MRI: magnetic resonance imaging

Mg^{2+}: magnesium

MMR: measles, mumps, rubella vaccine

Na$^+$: sodium

NIC: nursing interventions classification

NPO: nothing by mouth

NTD: neural tube defect

N&V: nausea and vomiting

O$_2$: oxygen

OG: orogastric

OTC: over-the-counter

OR: operating room

oz: ounce

P: pulse

PaCO$_2$: arterial carbon dioxide pressure

PaO$_2$: arterial oxygen pressure

PCA: patient controlled analgesia

PEEP: positive end expiratory pressure

PO: by mouth

PO$_2$: partial pressure of oxygen

PO$_4$$^{3-}$: phosphorus

PPV: positive pressure ventilation

prn: as needed

PT: prothrombin time

PTT: partial thromboplastin time

PVC: premature ventricular contraction

PVR: pulmonary vascular resistance

q: every

R: respirations

RBC: red blood cell

REEDA: redness, edema, echymosis, approximation

RN: registered nurse

SaO$_2$: oxygen saturation

SC: subcutaneous

SGOT: serum glutamic-oxaloacetic transaminase (AST)

SGPT: serum glutamic-pyruvic transaminase (ALT)

sp. gr.: specific gravity

SR: side rails

s/s: signs and symptoms

STD: sexually transmitted disease

SVR: systemic vascular resistance

T: temperature

TCDB: turn, cough, and deep breathe

TCM: transcutaneous monitoring

TcPaO$_2$: transcutaneous partial pressure of oxygen

TcPaCO$_2$: transcutaneous partial pressure of carbon dioxide

Td: tetanus toxid vaccine

TEF: tracheoesophageal fistula

TGV: transposition of the great vessels

TPN: total parenteral nutrition

TPR: temperature, pulse, respirations

TSH: thyroid stimulating hormone

UA: urinalysis

URI: upper respiratory infection

UTI: urinary tract infection

VP: ventriculoperitoneal

VS: vital signs

VSD: ventricular septal defect

WBC: white blood cell

WIC: women, infants, and children program

WNL: within normal limits

Wt: weight

w/o: without

ZDT: zidovudine

INDEX

Note: **Bold** type indicates main entries which are nursing diagnoses.

Acquired immunodeficiency syndrome. *See* HIV/AIDS

Activity intolerance
 anemia, 335–336
 asthma, 79
 chronic renal failure, 187
 congenital heart disease, 40–41
 congestive heart failure, 47
 cystic fibrosis, 96–97
 glomerulonephritis, 193
 hepatitis, 163

Adjustment, impaired
 inflammatory bowel disease, 172–173

Airway clearance, ineffective
 asthma, 77–78
 cleft lip/palate, 150
 croup, 107
 cystic fibrosis, 95
 dying child, 23–24
 epiglottitis, 103
 gastroesophageal reflux disease, 158
 Guillain-Barré syndrome, 292
 HIV/AIDS, 328
 respiratory system: basic care plan, 67–69
 tonsillitis, 119
 tracheostomy, 123

Allergic rhinitis, 132–134
 medical care, 132
 nursing diagnoses
  ineffective breathing pattern, 132
  risk for infection, 132–133
 schematic, 134

Anemia, 333–339
 medical care, 333–334
  diagnostic evaluation for aplastic anemia, 334
  diagnostic evaluation for iron deficiency anemia, 333
  diagnostic evaluation for sickle cell anemia, 333
  treatment for aplastic anemia, 334
  treatment for iron deficiency anemia, 333

 treatment for sickle cell anemia, 334
 nursing diagnoses
  activity intolerance, 335–336
  deficient knowledge, 337–338
  imbalanced nutrition, 334
  ineffective tissue perfusion, 334
  pain, 335
  risk for deficient fluid volume, 334
  risk for impaired skin integrity, 334–335
  risk for infection, 336–337
  risk for injury, 337
 schematic, 339

Anxiety
 appendicitis, 147–148
 asthma, 78–79
 brain tumor, 289–290
 bronchiolitis, 85–86
 child abuse, 19
 cleft lip/palate, 150–151
 congestive heart failure, 46–47
 croup, 108
 cryptorchidism, 210–211
 cystic fibrosis, 98–99
 dying child, 26–27
 epiglottitis, 104
 gastroesophageal reflux disease, 160–161
 Guillain-Barré syndrome, 294–295
 HIV/AIDS, 328–329
 hospitalized child, 12–14
 hypospadias/epispadias, 197–198
 inflammatory bowel disease, 171–172
 Kawasaki disease, 58–59
 meningitis, 298
 osteogenic sarcoma, 252
 osteomyelitis, 257
 pyloric stenosis, 179–180
 Reye's syndrome 308–309
 tonsillitis, 119
 tracheostomy, 123–124
 vesicoureteral reflux, 218–219
 Wilm's tumor, 224–225

NOTES

License Agreement for Delmar Learning, a division of Thomson Learning, Inc.

Educational Software/Data

You the customer, and Delmar Learning, a division of Thomson Learning, Inc. incur certain benefits, rights, and obligations to each other when you open this package and use the software/data it contains. BE SURE YOU READ THE LICENSE AGREEMENT CAREFULLY, SINCE BY USING THE SOFTWARE/DATA YOU INDICATE YOU HAVE READ, UNDERSTOOD, AND ACCEPTED THE TERMS OF THIS AGREEMENT.

Your rights:

1. You enjoy a non-exclusive license to use the software/data on a single microcomputer in consideration for payment of the required license fee, (which may be included in the purchase price of an accompanying print component), or receipt of this software/data, and your acceptance of the terms and conditions of this agreement.

2. You acknowledge that you do not own the aforesaid software/data. You also acknowledge that the software/data is furnished "as is," and contains copyrighted and/or proprietary and confidential information of Delmar Learning, a division of Thomson Learning, Inc. or its licensors.

There are limitations on your rights:

1. You may not copy or print the software/data for any reason whatsoever, except to install it on a hard drive on a single microcomputer and to make one archival copy, unless copying or printing is expressly permitted in writing or statements recorded on the diskette(s).

2. You may not revise, translate, convert, disassemble or otherwise reverse engineer the software/data except that you may add to or rearrange any data recorded on the media as part of the normal use of thesoftware/data.

3. You may not sell, license, lease, rent, loan or otherwise distribute or network the software/data except that you may give the software/data to a student or an instructor for use at school or, temporarily at home.

Should you fail to abide by the Copyright Law of the United States as it applies to this software/data your license to use it will become invalid. You agree to erase or otherwise destroy the software/data immediately after receiving note of termination of this agreement for violation of its provisions from Delmar Learning.

Delmar Learning, a division of Thomson Learning, Inc. gives you a LIMITED WARRANTY covering the enclosed software/data. The LIMITED WARRANTY follows this License.

This license is the entire agreement between you and Delmar Learning, a division of Thomson Learning, Inc. interpreted and enforced under New York law.

LIMITED WARRANTY

Delmar Learning, a division of Thomson Learning, Inc. warrants to the original licensee/purchaser of this copy of microcomputer software/data and the media on which it is recorded that the media will be free from defects in material and workmanship for ninety (90) days from the date of original purchase. All implied warranties are limited in duration to this ninety (90) day period. THEREAFTER, ANY IMPLIED WARRANTIES, INCLUDING IMPLIED WARRANTIES OF MERCHANTABILITY AND FITNESS FOR A PARTICULAR PURPOSE, ARE EXCLUDED. THIS WARRANTY IS IN LIEU OF ALL OTHER WARRANTIES, WHETHER ORAL OR WRITTEN, EXPRESS OR IMPLIED.

If you believe the media is defective please return it during the ninety (90) day period to the address shown below. Defective media will be replaced without charge provided that it has not been subjected to misuse or damage.

This warranty does not extend to the software or information recorded on the media. The software and information are provided "AS IS." Any statements made about the utility of the software or information are not to be considered as express or implied warranties.

Limitation of liability: Our liability to you for any losses shall be limited to direct damages, and shall not exceed the amount you paid for the software. In no event will we be liable to you for any indirect, special, incidental, or consequential damages (including loss of profits) even if we have been advised of the possibility of such damages.

Some states do not allow the exclusion or limitation of incidental or consequential damages, or limitations on the duration of implied warranties, so the above limitation or exclusion may not apply to you. This warranty gives you specific legal rights, and you may also have other rights which vary from state to state. Address all correspondence to: Delmar Learning, a division of Thomson Learning, Inc., 5 Maxwell Drive, P.O. Box 8007, Clifton Park, NY 12065-8007. Attention: Technology Department.

SYSTEM REQUIREMENTS

The CD-ROM version will be developed to run on client systems with the following minimum configuration:

- Operating System: Microsoft Windows 98 SE, Windows 2000, Windows XP
- Processor: Pentium PC 120 MHz or higher
- RAM: 64 MB of RAM or better
- Free Drive Space: 25 MB free disk space
- CD-ROM Drive—necessary for installation only
- Internet Connection Speed: 56K or better in order to view web links provided in program but is not required.
- Screen Resolution: 800 × 600 pixels or better
- Color Depth: 16-bit color (thousands of colors) or 24-bit color (millions of colors)
- Sound card: N/A

SET UP INSTRUCTIONS

To install the program, simply run the "X:\setup.exe", where X is the drive letter of you CD-ROM drive. Follow the on screen prompts to complete the installation. You may also:

1. Double click My Computer
2. Double click the Control Panel icon
3. Double click Add/Remove Programs
4. Click the Install button and follow the on screen prompts from there.